KV-636-131

Family guide
to
common
ailments

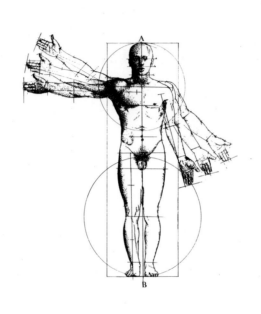

Family guide to common ailments

Medical Advisor
Dr. Joan Gomez M.B.B.S., M.R.C.Psych., D.B.M.

Additional Contributions
Dr. Nicola McClure M.B.B.S.M.R.C.S., L.R.C.P.
and Nigel Perryman

HAMLYN

London New York Sydney Toronto

Published by
The Hamlyn Publishing Group Limited
London New York Sydney Toronto
Astronaut House, Feltham, Middlesex,
England

Copyright © 1981 Quarto Limited
All rights reserved. No part of this
publication may be reproduced, stored in
a retrieval system, or transmitted, in any
form or by any means, electronic,
mechanical, photocopying, recording or
otherwise, without the permission of the
Hamlyn Publishing Group Limited and
the copyright holder.

ISBN 0 600 33210 1
Typeset by Tradespools Limited
Printed in Hong Kong by
Lee Fung Asco Ltd.

This book was designed and
produced by
Quarto Publishing Limited, 32 Kingly
Court, London W1.

Medical Advisor Dr. Joan Gomez
M.B.B.S., M.R.C.Psych., D.B.M.
Glossary of Symptoms and Medical
Terms, You and Your Health, You and
Your Doctor Dr. Nicola McClure
M.B.B.S.M.R.C.S., L.R.C.P.
and Nigel Perryman

Editorial Director: Jeremy Harwood
Art Director: Robert Morley
Editor and Caption Writer: James Roberts
Art Editor: Clive Hayball
Visualization and Artwork: Quill
(Nigel Osborne, Jim Marks, Paul Cooper,
David Weeks, Tony Lodge, Paul Roland,
Paul Eustace, Nicola Beger)

The publishers also wish to thank:
Marion Appleton, Robert Ashby,
Turissa Bregy, Nick Clark, Moira Clinch,
Chris Forsey, Victoria Funk, Roger
Daniels, Des Lynch, Ivan Lapper, David
Mallet, Jerry Llewellyn Smith, Tessa
Stone, The Paul Press, Reuker UK, John
Watney Photography, Science Photo
Library London, Tom West and
Associates, The Women's National
Cancer Control Campaign, The Royal
National Throat, Nose and Ear Hospital,
The Maudsley Hospital (Guttman
Maclay Collection), St. Mary's Hospital
Medical School, St. George's Hospital,
Tooting, St. James' Hospital, Tooting.

Contents

You and Your Doctor

NEARLY ALL OF US, no matter how healthy, have to see a doctor at some time in our lives. It may just be a matter of routine, such as a *vaccination*, *developmental check* or common illness of childhood. Later in life there may be a medical check-up for insurance purposes, a blood test before getting married or the special care needed during pregnancy.

Some people will go and see the doctor with a specific pain or discomfort, while others just feel generally unwell. Many patients have a nagging and ill-defined worry which they want to talk through with a doctor and often advice and support are needed more than a course of drugs. Whatever it is that makes you decide to consult a doctor, a good relationship with trust and understanding on both sides can be crucial to the successful treatment of your problem. To achieve this it is important to understand how the doctor finds out what is wrong with you and how he or she decides what to do.

The consultation

Often the time that you can spend with your doctor is limited, and it is important to make the best possible use of the few minutes that you have. This can be done by reducing the chances of misunderstanding and trying to eliminate any hesitation or personal reticence that you may feel.

Once you have made up your mind to tell the doctor your problem it is important to know how to describe it in the most accurate way, so that you avoid any confusion or misunderstanding. *Pain*, for example, is difficult to put into words. Generally the doctor needs to know how severe it is, whether it is constant or intermittent, how long you have had it, and, of course, where it is. The location of the pain is in itself a problem, because many people have a very inaccurate idea of where the various organs of the body really are. The illustrations will help you to understand this, and show you how the various body systems discussed earlier in the book really fit together. However, it is important that you do not run away with the idea that a pain that you think is in one particular organ means that that organ is diseased, because pain can be *referred* from one part of the body to another part that is completely healthy. So self-diagnosis can be misleading – and often dangerous.

The doctor also needs to know the general nature of the pain – whether it is sharp or dull, stabbing or throbbing. Do not hesitate to describe it in detail. Many people describe *angina* as a constricting pain in the chest; a feeling that someone is actually sitting on their chest. This may sound silly to you – but in fact it is not so at all. Such a description means something

quite specific to a doctor; it is characteristic of angina. It is much better to try and describe a pain in this way than to use medical words, which often mean one thing to you and something quite different to a doctor – as you will see from the *Glossary of Medical Terms and Symptoms. Indigestion*, for example, is a broad term that to a doctor covers a number of specific symptoms, yet the word means something different to nearly every patient.

Diagnosis

When the doctor feels that he has a good idea of the pain or problem that is worrying you he will try and pin down its cause. (It may take some time to reach this stage, because a surprisingly high proportion of people go to the doctor with a minor complaint and refuse at first to admit to their real worry.) The doctor has to

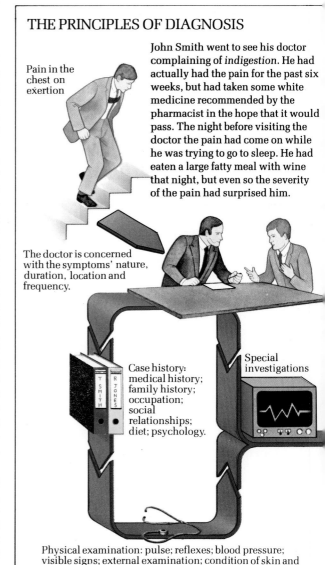

THE PRINCIPLES OF DIAGNOSIS

John Smith went to see his doctor complaining of *indigestion*. He had actually had the pain for the past six weeks, but had taken some white medicine recommended by the pharmacist in the hope that it would pass. The night before visiting the doctor the pain had come on while he was trying to go to sleep. He had eaten a large fatty meal with wine that night, but even so the severity of the pain had surprised him.

Pain in the chest on exertion

The doctor is concerned with the symptoms' nature, duration, location and frequency.

Case history: medical history; family history; occupation; social relationships; diet; psychology.

Special investigations

Physical examination: pulse; reflexes; blood pressure; visible signs; external examination; condition of skin and muscles; temperature; vaginal or rectal examination.

relate your symptoms to a whole host of other factors before he works out what, if anything, is wrong with you, because there is rarely any one symptom that indicates one specific disease. Some of the questions that the doctor will ask you may well seem irrelevant. They are not, and it is essential that you answer them truthfully and in full. To leave something out because you think that it is unimportant can be very dangerous.

There are two main parts to the doctor's investigation – the case history and the physical examination. Every doctor has his own methods, and you should never feel that you have not been properly treated if he misses out some of the steps. If you have been consulting the same family doctor for some years, many of the questions will be unnecessary because he will have the information in your records.

The case history is divided into a number of parts. Your original symptom will already have been discussed in detail, but in addition the doctor will want to know all about your personal medical history, including all the illnesses you have had since childhood. If you are female, he will want to know about your periods and the form of *contraception*, if any, that you use. The history of your medical treatment is important – what drugs you have been prescribed in the recent past, whether you are still taking any, whether you are taking any patent remedies and whether you have ever had surgery. Again, you must never leave out anything because you think that it is unimportant, or because you assume that the doctor already knows the answer. He will ask about your family's medical history, because some diseases are to an extent *hereditary*. Next the

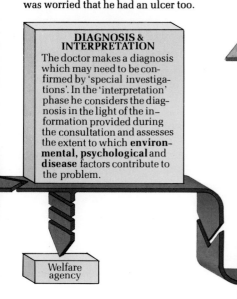
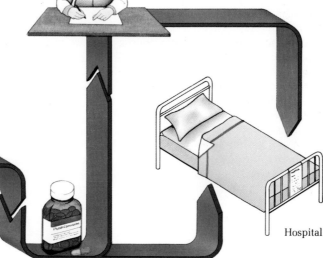

On close questioning this 'indigestion' turned out to have been a tight feeling in the chest, usually on exertion.

Mr Smith was a 46-year-old businessman whose work involved travelling and entertaining. His job seemed to put him under a certain amount of pressure, and a few years earlier he had been treated for high blood pressure. His father had died at the age of 65 from a heart attack, but more recently his brother had had a *duodenal ulcer*. As he had read that ulcers were associated with his kind of life-style, Mr Smith was worried that he had an ulcer too.

On examination he seemed slightly overweight and his *blood pressure* was a little lower than usual. The doctor was able to hear some *crackles*, or *crepitations*, in his chest, indicating fluid in the lungs, and he seemed a little short of breath.

The doctor thought that John Smith's indigestion sounded much more like *angina* and that he might even have had a slight heart attack

the night before – certainly the case history and physical examination pointed that way. The only way to be sure was to make further tests.

An *E.C.G.* was run, and Mr Smith's blood was analysed to see if any of the *enzymes* that are found when heart muscle is damaged were present. Both tests showed that Mr Smith had had a small localized *myocardial infarction*, or heart attack. He was admitted straight away to the coronary care unit of the local hospital.

Ten days later John Smith was back in the doctor's office, looking much better; the pain had gone.

Consultant

DIAGNOSIS & INTERPRETATION
The doctor makes a diagnosis which may need to be confirmed by 'special investigations'. In the 'interpretation' phase he considers the diagnosis in the light of the information provided during the consultation and assesses the extent to which **environmental, psychological** and **disease** factors contribute to the problem.

Welfare agency

Family doctor's treatment

Hospital

doctor will try to build up a complete picture of your life-style. He needs to know your job history and the exact nature of your present occupation; your relationships at work and at home; your diet and your past and present use of alcohol and tobacco. He will probably ask a whole host of seemingly irrelevant questions, but any one of them might just give him the vital clue that he needs.

The second part of the investigation is the physical examination. Part of it has been going on during your talk. The doctor will have noted your weight, build, coloration and mental state, as well as any *facies* – the classic look of a disease, for example the typically coarse facial features of thyroid deficiency. The rest of the examination will probably concentrate on the body system that appears to be the problem, but could cover the whole body. The doctor will check the various body reflexes and pulses and listen to and feel the different organs of the chest and abdomen. He will take your blood pressure and examine your eyes, ears and mouth with specialized instruments, and look at the general condition, color, temperature and tone of your skin and muscles. In some cases the doctor will want to examine your urine and stools, and a *rectal* or *vaginal* examination may be needed.

Interpretation

By now the doctor has a whole mass of facts about you and your problem, and he has to interpret them. He must decide how much of the problem can be explained by your environment, how much by your mental attitude and *psychology*, and how much by a disease process.

The doctor cannot do very much about problems caused by your environment except refer you to a welfare agency – a doctor cannot prescribe better housing. If the problem seems to have a psychological basis he will either give you *counselling* himself, and possibly a course of drugs, or refer you to a specialist *psychiatrist*. More usually the doctor will recognize a disease that does not require hospitalization and start treatment himself.

Sometimes the doctor will not know what the exact problem is. He may say: "This looks like a minor virus infection. I'm sure that it isn't serious, but if it isn't better in a few days contact me". This is quite reasonable, especially as there is really no effective treatment for minor conditions like influenza or the common cold. Occasionally the doctor will think that he has identified the problem but need some confirmation of his opinion. Then you will be asked to take some further tests – which are often called *special investigations*.

Special Investigations

You should not think that because the doctor has asked for some further tests that you are seriously ill. Several relatively minor conditions – for example *anaemia* – can only be diagnosed with certainty after a blood test. In America many of these tests can be done in the family practitioner's office, and in Britain more and more surgeries and health centers now have the capability of carrying out special investigations. The tests can range from a simple blood sample and analysis to the use of a sophisticated *E.C.G.* machine or an *X-ray* or *ultrasound* scan. The vast majority of these tests are quite painless, and whenever there is a chance of discomfort a *local anaesthetic* will be given. After analysis the results of the various special investigations that your doctor has ordered can be examined, along with the case history and physical examination, enabling the doctor to make a firm diagnosis and decide on a course of treatment. Alternatively he or she may decide to refer you to a specialist in the particular disorder.

Treatment

When the doctor has decided what lies at the root of your problem he will work out a course of treatment. Unless you ask, he may not explain what is wrong with you, how the illness will progress and what the treatment he prescribes will do to help. This is because many people actually prefer not to know the detail and implications of what is wrong with them.

It may be more convenient not to know what is happening to your body, but it is not particularly sensible – after all, you always ask the mechanic what is wrong with your car, and your body is rather more important. At the same time you should accept the treatment that the doctor suggests and try to avoid preconceptions about the sort of treatment you should have.

When you understand the treatment that the doctor has prescribed you must follow it exactly. If you have been given a course of drugs to take, complete the course – whether or not you feel better before the course is finished. If you are told to lose weight, to take more exercise, to give up smoking or to cut down on alcohol, do what the doctor tells you – there will have been a good reason for the advice.

Ultimately the responsibility for your health is in your own hands. But if you do have to visit your doctor the trust and understanding that leads to a good doctor-patient relationship should help you to get the best from the wealth of knowledge, ability and experience that makes up modern medicine.

Guide to ailments

Respiratory/Introduction

Respiration is the process by which the body takes in the oxygen it needs and expels the carbon dioxide produced as a result of reactions within the body.

The central feature of the respiratory system, the lungs, are like sponges encased in bags, which expand and relax at varying rates, depending on the body's requirements. Inhalation is the result of action by the diaphragm and the intercostal muscles. Exhalation is usually a more passive process.

Linking the lungs to the nose and mouth are the pharynx, larynx and trachea (windpipe). This divides into the two bronchi, the right and left, which sub-divide into smaller bronchi in the lobes of the lungs. These smaller bronchi sub-divide again into bronchioles and these in turn terminate in the alveolar ducts which lead into the alveolar sacs.

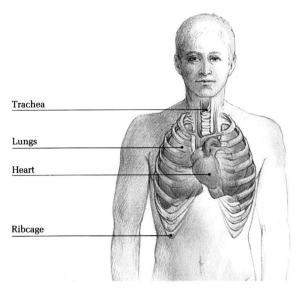

Trachea

Lungs

Heart

Ribcage

Normal air: 21% oxygen, 79% nitrogen

Exhaled air: 16.5% oxygen, 80% nitrogen, 3.5% carbon dioxide

Air is inhaled

Oxygen begins to be absorbed by the blood

Carbon dioxide replaces used oxygen

Nitrogen

Oxygen

Carbon dioxide

Location of the Lungs
The ribs radiate from the spine at the back to the sternum at the front, and form a protective cage for the heart and lungs. The heart separates the two lungs, and they are attached to it and to the trachea. Apart from this they lie free. The top of each lung reaches to the collar bone, the base to the diaphragm.

Breathing rates.
An adult person's lungs hold about 3 liters of air at rest, increasing this to 3.5 liters with each inhalation at rest but up to as much as 6 liters during deep breathing. At a resting rate of 15 inhalations a minute, 7.5 liters of air are inhaled. Of this about 5.5 liters reach the alveoli. On exertion the total volume breathed in can be increased 15 fold, and the oxygen absorbed 30 fold.

How You Breathe
Respiration provides the metabolism of the body with its vital supply of oxygen. The lungs are central to this process as it is here, through the alveoli, that oxygen is exchanged for carbon dioxide. The diagram above shows the constituents of the air which enters the body and which leaves it. The amount of nitrogen remains constant but the amount and proportion of oxygen is less when the air is exhaled. The proportion of carbon dioxide is correspondingly increased. Originally negligible (0.03%) it now occupies 3.5% of the total volume.

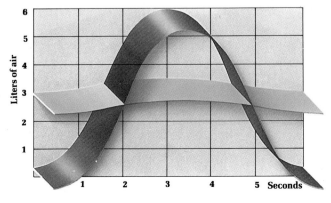

Liters of air

6
5
4
3
2
1

1   2   3   4   5   Seconds

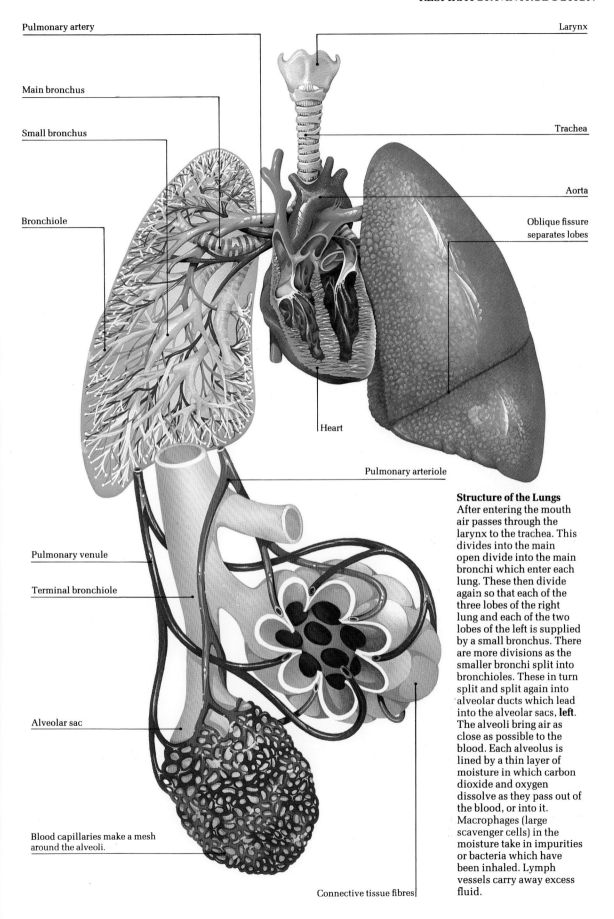

Pulmonary artery

Larynx

Main bronchus

Small bronchus

Trachea

Bronchiole

Aorta

Oblique fissure
separates lobes

Heart

Pulmonary arteriole

Pulmonary venule

Terminal bronchiole

Alveolar sac

Blood capillaries make a mesh
around the alveoli.

Connective tissue fibres

Structure of the Lungs
After entering the mouth
air passes through the
larynx to the trachea. This
divides into the main
open divide into the main
bronchi which enter each
lung. These then divide
again so that each of the
three lobes of the right
lung and each of the two
lobes of the left is supplied
by a small bronchus. There
are more divisions as the
smaller bronchi split into
bronchioles. These in turn
split and split again into
alveolar ducts which lead
into the alveolar sacs, **left**.
The alveoli bring air as
close as possible to the
blood. Each alveolus is
lined by a thin layer of
moisture in which carbon
dioxide and oxygen
dissolve as they pass out of
the blood, or into it.
Macrophages (large
scavenger cells) in the
moisture take in impurities
or bacteria which have
been inhaled. Lymph
vessels carry away excess
fluid.

The main work of the lungs is carried out in the tiny alveoli which spread throughout their volume. The size and number of these alveoli gives them a huge combined surface area — thirty times greater, in fact, than the total surface area of the skin. The body receives all of its oxygen by a process of absorption through their linings, so the greater their surface area, the greater the quantity of oxygen that can be absorbed over a given period.

The respiratory system is also responsible for the voice. The volume of sound depends on the flow of expired air through the tight vocal cords. Pitch depends on the exact tightness of the cords and their length, which changes with age. Resonance depends on chest shape. Vowels are made by the mouth, whilst changing the position of the palate, lips and tongue will produce consonants.

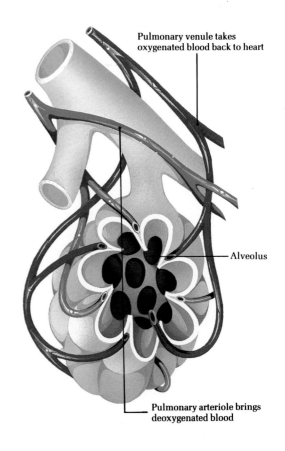

Pulmonary venule takes oxygenated blood back to heart

Alveolus

Pulmonary arteriole brings deoxygenated blood

The Principles of Gas Exchange

The pulmonary arteriole brings carbon dioxide dissolved in blood to the capillaries around the alveolus. One cell at a time, the blood is allowed into the capillary. Through differences in pressure, the dissolved carbon dioxide passes through the capillary wall, through the adjoining alveolar wall, and into the thin film of moisture that lines the alveolus. Oxygen from inhaled air takes a reverse path, dissolving in the moisture lining the alveolus and passing through alveolar and capillary walls. It combines with the haemoglobin in the blood to form oxyhaemoglobin, and pulmonary venules take the oxygenated blood back to the heart.

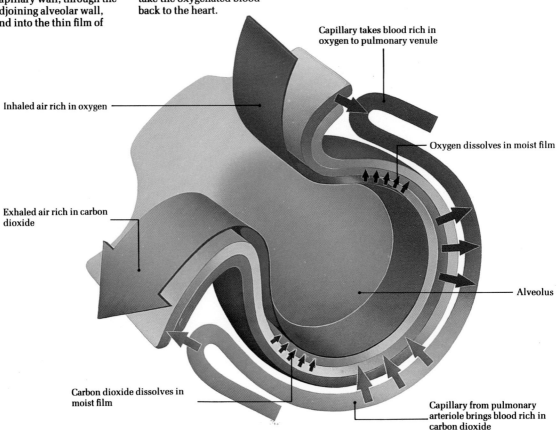

Capillary takes blood rich in oxygen to pulmonary venule

Inhaled air rich in oxygen

Oxygen dissolves in moist film

Exhaled air rich in carbon dioxide

Alveolus

Carbon dioxide dissolves in moist film

Capillary from pulmonary arteriole brings blood rich in carbon dioxide

The Role of the Muscles in Breathing
The muscles most active in breathing are those of the diaphragm. The intercostal muscles, which run in a double layer between each rib, are also important. In inspiration (inhaling) the diaphragm gets flatter and the rib cage more voluminous. In this way the elastic lungs are allowed to expand. Expiration (exhaling) takes place through the lungs' relaxation.

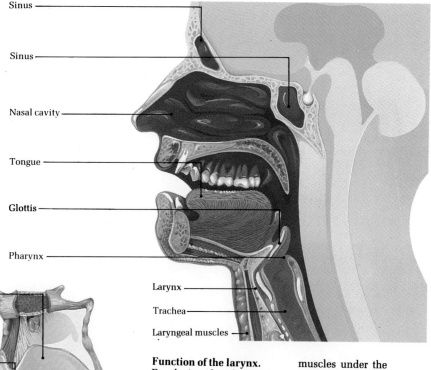

Rest

Inspiration

Expiration

Trachea

Lungs

Location of the larynx.
The larynx, often called the 'Adam's Apple', separates the passage which carries air from the passage which carries food and water. At the top it reaches the root of the tongue, opening into the pharynx to form part of the pharynx wall. The lower part continues into the trachea.

Sinus

Sinus

Nasal cavity

Tongue

Glottis

Pharynx

Larynx

Trachea

Laryngeal muscles

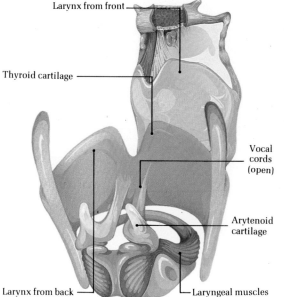

Larynx from front

Thyroid cartilage

Vocal cords (open)

Arytenoid cartilage

Larynx from back

Laryngeal muscles

Function of the larynx.
By closing the glottis, the larynx prevents food and water from entering the windpipe. By housing the vocal cords, and moving them with muscles under the control of the speech center in the brain, it produces voice. When the laryngeal muscles draw the vocal cords towards each other, they vibrate through the resulting movement of air and make sounds. The sound is louder if the air is faster. It is higher if the cords are tighter – an effect brought about by the laryngeal muscles pulling the small cartilages like the arytenoid at the back of the larynx.

13

Pneumonia

Pneumonia is a disease of the lungs, in which whole segments of the organ, including the working tissue, become inflamed. Either one or both lungs can be affected; in the latter case, the disease is defined as bi-lateral pneumonia.

What happens is quite simple to understand. Normally, the lung consists of a spongy mass of air-filled sacs. In pneumonia, the affected parts of the lungs become solid and therefore are unable to perform their job of taking in oxygen and disposing of waste gases. Luckily, it is uncommon for pneumonia to affect the whole lung – the lower segments are the ones most frequently affected. This is because the organs are divided into about ten separate sections, each with its own blood supply and bronchial tube system. Infection does not spread easily from one section to another.

Anyone can develop pneumonia. Victims can range from a new-born baby to an 80-year-old invalid spending most of his or her time in bed. The commonest way of developing the disease is from a spread of infection down the bronchial tubes when you are already suffering from BRONCHITIS. Those at greatest risk are the elderly, smokers, the under-nourished, those with other illnesses such as diabetes, and those rendered immobile.

Among young and middle-aged adults, excessive drinkers are particularly susceptible to the disease. It is the greatest health risk in delirium tremens (see ALCOHOLISM), the alcoholic state in which the victim frequently hallucinates and suffers from nightmares even when awake. Sufferers from DIABETES mellitus and the overweight are also prone to contracting pneumonia.

Pneumonia can also have physical causes –

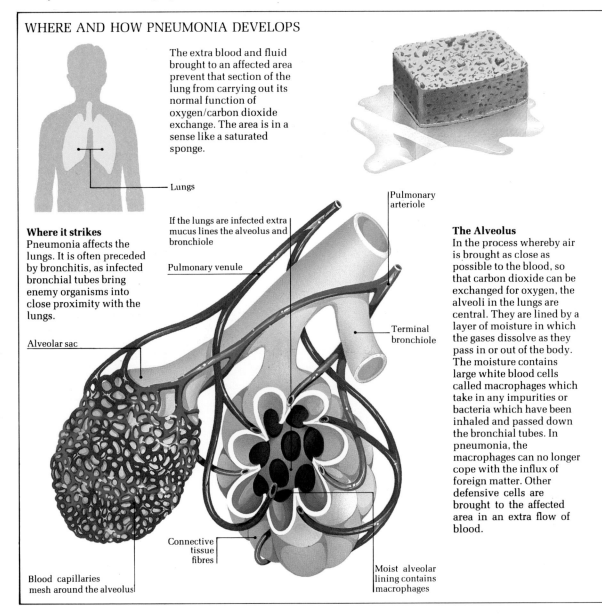

WHERE AND HOW PNEUMONIA DEVELOPS

The extra blood and fluid brought to an affected area prevent that section of the lung from carrying out its normal function of oxygen/carbon dioxide exchange. The area is in a sense like a saturated sponge.

Lungs

Where it strikes
Pneumonia affects the lungs. It is often preceded by bronchitis, as infected bronchial tubes bring enemy organisms into close proximity with the lungs.

Alveolar sac

If the lungs are infected extra mucus lines the alveolus and bronchiole

Pulmonary venule

Pulmonary arteriole

Terminal bronchiole

Connective tissue fibres

Blood capillaries mesh around the alveolus

Moist alveolar lining contains macrophages

The Alveolus
In the process whereby air is brought as close as possible to the blood, so that carbon dioxide can be exchanged for oxygen, the alveoli in the lungs are central. They are lined by a layer of moisture in which the gases dissolve as they pass in or out of the body. The moisture contains large white blood cells called macrophages which take in any impurities or bacteria which have been inhaled and passed down the bronchial tubes. In pneumonia, the macrophages can no longer cope with the influx of foreign matter. Other defensive cells are brought to the affected area in an extra flow of blood.

if, for instance, something like a peanut is swallowed 'the wrong way' into the respiratory system and so blocks off a section of lung. Inhaling vomit, or other material from the mouth, when unconscious through, say, drunkenness or a head injury can lead to the disease, while inhaling irritant gases, petrol or kerosene fumes, or getting drops of the laxative, liquid paraffin, into the lungs may also cause pneumonia to develop.

Physical symptoms

Pneumonia is almost always the result of an invasion of the lung tissues by bacteria, viruses, or, occasionally, fungi. Infection spreads down the bronchial tubes into the lungs, where the germs settle in the tissues of the air sacs and surrounding cells. The lungs react to the attack by becoming inflamed. The affected part swells

as extra blood flows to the scene, carrying antibodies to help combat the infection, and fluid is poured out to dilute and wash away the irritating substances.

When the lung tissue is full of fluid, the effect is somewhat similar to drowning. With less usable tissue to breathe with, you have to inhale and exhale more rapidly in order to satisfy your body's requirements of oxygen. The rate may increase from sixteen breaths a minute to between thirty and sixty, while the little muscles by your nostrils may expand to make a forlorn attempt to widen the air entry at your nose.

If the infection spreads through to the surface of the affected segments, the outside covering of the lungs – the pleura – may become inflamed. This is pleurisy, the commonest complication of pneumonia.

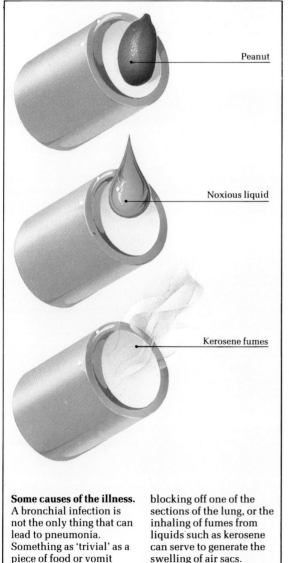

Peanut

Noxious liquid

Kerosene fumes

Some causes of the illness. A bronchial infection is not the only thing that can lead to pneumonia. Something as 'trivial' as a piece of food or vomit blocking off one of the sections of the lung, or the inhaling of fumes from liquids such as kerosene can serve to generate the swelling of air sacs.

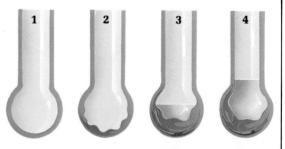

How the lungs are disabled.
1. An infection reaches the alveolar sac.
2. Phagocyte-carrying blood flows to the sac to destroy the infection and swells the lining.

3. Extra fluid comes out of the lining to wash the infection away.
4. Because of this influx, there is no room for the proper function of gas exchange.

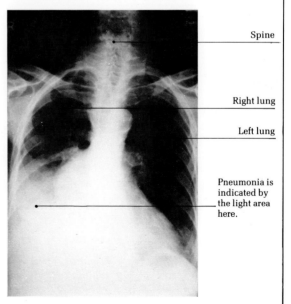

Spine

Right lung

Left lung

Pneumonia is indicated by the light area here.

The X-ray photograph above revealed that pneumonia had set in at the base of the right lung.

The onset of pneumonia can be sudden. You may feel ill very suddenly; perhaps the first indication of the disease is an attack of shaking, in which, although you have a high fever, you feel deadly cold. Your body temperature may be as high as 38.9° to 40.6°C (102° to 105°F). Your skin will be hot and moist, but pale, and you may develop herpes blisters – painful sores – on your lip. You will start off with a dry painful cough, which will become less painful when you start to cough up sputum from the lungs. This will be either green, yellow, or blood-stained rusty in colour.

As the effort of breathing at more than three times your usual rate is exhausting, you will feel generally tired. If you develop pleurisy, each breath may produce a specific pain in one part of your chest. This is uncomfortable, but not dangerous.

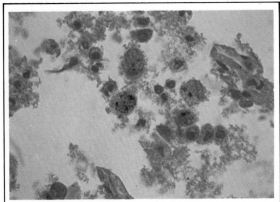

In the photograph above, magnified 600 times, pneumonia bacilli show as black spots.

PRESCRIPTION

Diagnosis
The doctor checks your breathing rate, takes your temperature (this is normally raised), and examines your chest. Tapping the chest produces a duller-pitched note over the infected, solid areas and is a clear indication of the disease. Blood and other bacteriological tests – particularly of the phlegm produced when you cough – confirm the existence of infection and indicate which particular organism is the cause of it. A chest x-ray may be necessary.

Treatment
Bed rest is essential. Keep yourself propped up on pillows. If you have a fever, tepid sponging will not only make you more comfortable, but also reduce fluid and salt loss through sweating. Your fluid intake should be around six pints a day; fruit squash is the most suitable fluid to drink. Oxygen may be given if breathing becomes acutely strained. Specific medicines are prescribed to relieve any cough, deal with the infection and cope with any organisms that may strike during the period of lowered resistance. Antibiotics, penicillin in particular, are the usual treatment. If necessary, injections are normally given over the first few days of the illness. The acute stage of the disease lasts, as a rule, for a week to ten days. During recovery, a high-protein diet is important, while a further period of convalescence is sometimes necessary.

Diagnosis and treatment

Your doctor will count your breathing rate, take your temperature and examine your chest. If you have pneumonia, he or she will hear abnormalities in your breath sounds and a local creaking sound if you have developed pleurisy. If there are areas which have become solid, a different pitch will be detected when the various parts of the chest are tapped. This is just like tapping a half-filled bottle; the note is duller over the part full of fluid than the air-filled part.

A blood test should also be taken. This will show the signs of infection, including the increase in the 'soldier' cells—polymorphonuclear leukocytes—the body produces to fight against the disease. It will also show how much oxygen and carbon dioxide there is in your blood as an indication of how efficiently your lungs are coping. A chest x-ray may be necessary to confirm the diagnosis. This will show up any area of solid lung, while the effects of treatment can be monitored by taking further films.

A sample of the phlegm you cough up will be sent to a laboratory to find out which organisms are present and which medicines are likely to deal with them most effectively. However, this need not delay treatment. Your doctor may prescribe medication immediately, modifying it in the light of the results of the tests.

It is essential to stay in bed, propped up on several pillows. If your temperature is very high, tepid sponging will make you more comfortable. It will also help to prevent you losing too much fluid and salt in your sweat. You need to drink about six pints of fruit squash, or other fluid, each day and to take extra salt. In the acute, early stages of the disease, solid food is not important; later you will have to make up for lack of appetite with a nourishing high-protein diet. You may be given oxygen temporarily.

You may be given medicine to relieve the pain caused by your cough, but the most important part of the treatment is chemotherapy – that is, prescribing drugs to help to kill the enemy organism. Of these drugs, penicillin is still the best; before the introduction of penicillin, one in four victims of pneumonia used to die but now the fatality rate is one in twenty, depending on the degree of fitness of the victim. Depending on the nature of the infecting organism, you may need to have injections for the first few days of your illness.

Further rest is necessary and you will remain more susceptible to attacks of pneumonia in the future. Deep-breathing exercises as a regular routine are beneficial.

Influenza

Influenza is commonly a short-lived, feverish illness, caused by any one of several types of virus, usually categorized as A, B and C and sub-divided into individual strains. Influenza sufferers feel ill, have aches and pains in many of their muscles and have the symptoms of a cold, headache, sore throat and sometimes chest infection.

Influenza is an extremely common disease. There are no barriers of age, sex or country affecting it. Its seriousness varies enormously, according to the strain of virus causing it; babies, the old and those with heart or chest diseases are those least able to cope with the infection.

Physical symptoms

The most important influenza viruses are types A and B; type C usually causes only a very mild illness. The infection is carried in the breath, or, more accurately, in the virus-laden moisture expelled during coughs and sneezes. The illness is at its most infectious during its first two days, though it is possible for someone to pass on the disease without knowing they have it.

When the virus reaches your nose, it settles in the lining, where it kills the cells on the surface. From there, it may spread downwards to involve the trachea (windpipe) and the bronchial tubes. The throat is often inflamed and extremely uncomfortable. If the lung tissue is involved, PNEUMONIA may develop. The influenza virus may invade the air sacs, the essential working area of the lungs; alternatively, it may so lower the general resistance to infection that another organism, staphylococcus, can gain a foothold and produce staphylococcal pneumonia.

THE NORMAL COURSE OF INFLUENZA

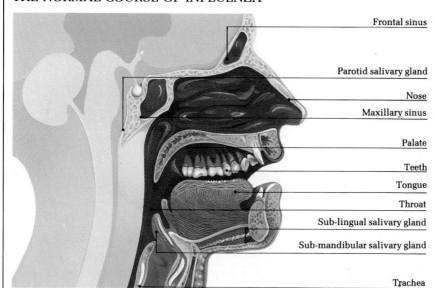

Frontal sinus

Parotid salivary gland

Nose

Maxillary sinus

Palate

Teeth

Tongue

Throat

Sub-lingual salivary gland

Sub-mandibular salivary gland

Trachea

Where influenza strikes
Influenza strikes the nose, throat and possibly the trachea and bronchial tubes. The influenza virus lands in your nose and starts to kill the cells on the surface. As it works its way towards your windpipe and bronchial tubes it will make your throat sore and inflamed. You may start shivering or aching in your limbs. The effort required to deal with everyday tasks suddenly seems much greater. To retire to bed will be a great relief.

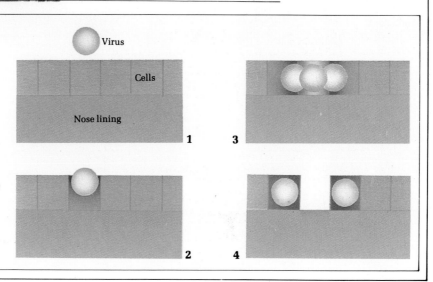

How the virus grows
When an influenza virus reaches the cells that line the nasal passages (1) it can start to kill them (2). As it is gaining this foothold its presence will not really be noticeable, but once established it reproduces itself by replication (3) and simultaneously destroys the cells in the surrounding tissue (4). The actions of the body's defences at this point are probably the first noticeable signs of 'flu.

Virus

Cells

Nose lining

1

3

2

4

It takes two or three days after the initial infection for the full range of symptoms to appear. In the interim, the virus has established itself in the body and is now reproducing itself at the expense of your tissues. Quite suddenly, you will feel shivery and ill. You may have a headache, while your temperature is raised, perhaps to 39° C (102° F). Your limbs ache.

The next day, you develop a dry cough but cannot produce any phlegm to relieve it. You may have a sore throat, sore eyes and a blocked nose. After a few days of this, in the ordinary course of the illness, your temperature returns to normal and the symptoms subside. You are left feeling weak and will get tired easily for a few weeks. Your spirits may be low.

Diagnosis and treatment
Normally, there is no need for special medical treatment. If you develop chest symptoms, you will be prescribed antibiotics, while, if it is an isolated occurrence, laboratory examination of the material from a throat swab will reveal the virus if it is present.

Go to bed immediately – this is just as much a protection for others as it is helpful to you. Drink plenty of fluids, especially fruit juices, and take soluble aspirin as a gargle which you swallow for the sore throat and muscle pain. Do not expect, or demand, too much of yourself for the next few weeks.

Research on protection from, and treatment of, influenza is extremely active. At the moment, vaccination gives approximately sixty per cent protection against influenza for about twelve months, provided it is carried out before an epidemic occurs. However, each new epidemic demands a new injection.

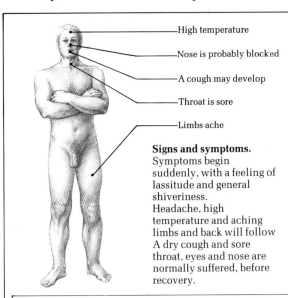

High temperature

Nose is probably blocked

A cough may develop

Throat is sore

Limbs ache

Signs and symptoms.
Symptoms begin suddenly, with a feeling of lassitude and general shiveriness. Headache, high temperature and aching limbs and back will follow A dry cough and sore throat, eyes and nose are normally suffered, before recovery.

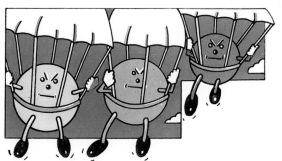

How you get influenza.
There are three major sorts of virus, two more serious than the third. They are typically caught by breathing in the air that an infected person has breathed out. An infected person may not realize that he is carrying the virus, although he is most likely to transmit it during its first two days.

PRESCRIPTION

Diagnosis
The account of your symptoms, along with a temperature measurement, is normally sufficient indication of influenza. Your doctor will be aware of any epidemic.

Treatment
Treatment by special medicines such as antibiotics is normally unnecessary in influenza. These are only needed if the infection spreads to the chest. If you go to bed, you will feel more comfortable and probably help to speed up your recovery. You will also be more likely to keep the virus to yourself. It is important to take plenty of liquids, and the weakness and aching which seem to permeate your body should be relieved to some extent by aspirin.

An attack by a particular sort of influenza virus gives a patient immunity to that strain. An injected vaccine will have a similar effect. But each new epidemic of influenza is caused by a new strain, so complete immunity cannot be given by injections.

Your symptoms will abate after a few days, but do not be surprised if you feel weak for rather longer.

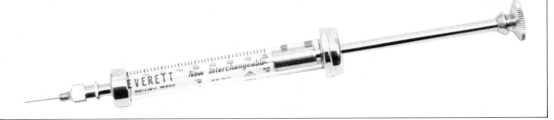

Chronic Bronchitis

Bronchitis is inflammation of the mucous linings of the main tubes leading from the windpipe to the lungs. There are two forms – acute and chronic. The former is less serious than the latter, though it should be treated promptly; chronic bronchitis, however, can be a killer disease. It means that you have had a phlegm-laden winter cough for two years without a break and are gradually becoming less and less resistant to all respiratory infections and more breathless on effort.

Physical symptoms
Chronic bronchitis is intimately bound up with the way the lungs work and how the body reacts to deal with any threat to their efficient working. This is particularly important where the airways are concerned – the nose and mouth, windpipe, the left and right bronchial tubes and their smaller and smaller branches – the bronchioles – which lead into the tiny air sacs of the lungs. Since it is vital that the main passages are kept clear, they have a lining that is extremely sensitive to any foreign element inside them. If, for instance, a crumb goes down 'the wrong way', you cough, choke and splutter violently. Similarly, if you have a small accumulation of mucus and bacterial debris in your bronchial tubes, you have to cough it up.

If, however, the lining itself is swollen because of irritation from germs, smoke or dust, this also makes you cough, although there is nothing produced to show for it. When you cough, the pressure inside the delicate air sacs increases; if you continue coughing for months and years, they lose their elasticity and their walls break. This condition is called emphy-

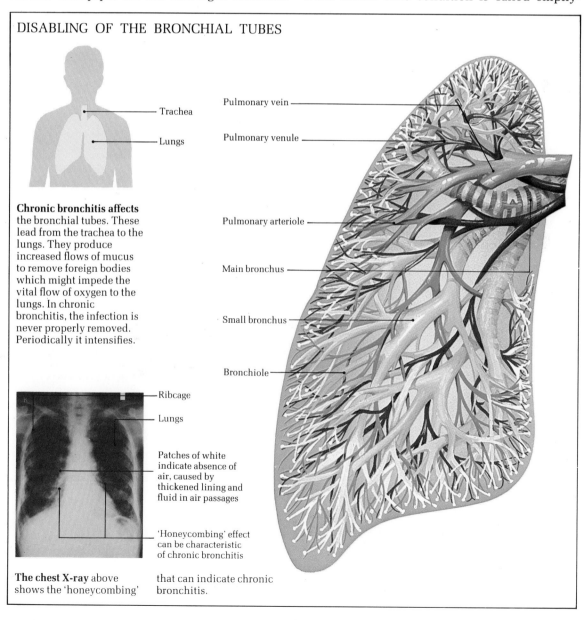

DISABLING OF THE BRONCHIAL TUBES

Trachea

Lungs

Chronic bronchitis affects the bronchial tubes. These lead from the trachea to the lungs. They produce increased flows of mucus to remove foreign bodies which might impede the vital flow of oxygen to the lungs. In chronic bronchitis, the infection is never properly removed. Periodically it intensifies.

Pulmonary vein

Pulmonary venule

Pulmonary arteriole

Main bronchus

Small bronchus

Bronchiole

Ribcage

Lungs

Patches of white indicate absence of air, caused by thickened lining and fluid in air passages

'Honeycombing' effect can be characteristic of chronic bronchitis

The chest X-ray above shows the 'honeycombing' that can indicate chronic bronchitis.

sema and is usual in long-standing chronic bronchitis.

Another major problem comes with the cleaning of the airways. Normally, these are kept slightly moist by a sticky fluid called mucus; microscopic hairs inside the bronchial tubes – the cilia – continually waft this upwards, cleaning away germs and any tiny particles of soot and dust which are inhaled. Tobacco smoke in particular – alcohol has the same effect to some extent – not only paralyses the cilia but also the guard cells – macrophages – which are the body's first line of defence against invading germs and viruses.

This has particular relevance to bronchitis. When an infection settles in your bronchial tubes, they try to get rid of it by producing more mucus to wash it away. In chronic bronchitis, however, the infection is subdued, but not

beaten; every now and then, perhaps when you are tired or cold, the germs get the upper hand. The result is a severe attack, with fever, pus and perhaps blood in your phlegm. The bronchial lining becomes more and more damaged with each attack until, eventually, the cilia are destroyed and there is constant over-production of mucus. This builds up overnight and in the morning you may feel wheezy, only recovering through a hot drink and a hawking cough. The irritating effect of a cigarette on your tubes may help you to clear the air passages – but, while this seems to help at the time, the long-term effect is disastrous. In bronchitis, each cigarette is a small nail in your coffin.

Having started out with a winter cough and attacks of wheezing, you will now be coughing throughout the year. Over the years, as emphysema develops, you become more and more short of breath, while your lips take on a bluish tinge, as you are less able to take in the oxygen you need. Your chest is always partly expanded and you may reach a stage when you use your neck muscles to help you breathe and cope with your breathlessness.

Diagnosis and treatment

Your doctor will want to x-ray your chest, mainly to ensure that you have not contracted lung cancer, tuberculosis or pneumonia. He will probably have your sputum, or phlegm, examined for germs, including tuberculosis, and for cancer cells. This will also help him to choose the right medicine to deal with any bacteria that may be present. A blood test is likely to show that you have more red blood cells than normal; this is an attempt by your body to compensate for poor oxygen exchange by producing more oxygen-transporting cells. An electrocardiogram will tell him or her how your heart is standing up to the strain, while the efficiency of your breathing will be monitored at regular intervals.

You must give up smoking completely, avoid sleeping tablets and keep your alcohol intake low. In cold weather, sleep with your windows shut, but keep the room door open to provide adequate ventilation. Move to a clean-air district if you can. If your breathing is impeded by a layer of fat, reduce your weight. On the other hand, it is important to eat plenty of protein and vitamins.

Your doctor will help by prescribing antibiotics and physiotherapy whenever you have an acute attack. Broncho-dilator tablets or aerosol sprays can help by opening up your tubes and making breathing easier; it is vital, however, to follow the doctor's instructions exactly, as these can be dangerous if used to excess.

PRESCRIPTION

Diagnosis
A chest X-ray, and analysis of your phlegm will be the main diagnostic tool, but your doctor will want to check on your heart, to see how it is standing up to the increased strain.

Treatment
Smoking is especially dangerous once chronic bronchitis has set in, so smokers must give up the habit altogether. If it is at all possible, it is also best to live away from highly polluted areas. An excess of body fat will put extra strain on the heart and lungs. Antibiotics will help to fight infection, and you will also be given tablets or sprays which make breathing easier. Take careful note of all the instructions on medicaments such as these. Below: a vitallometer helps to determine how seriously the lungs are affected by chronic bronchitis. In measuring the speed of air exhalation, it monitors two sorts of change, obstructive and restrictive. Obstructive changes characterize bronchitis: the volume of air in the lungs is not much diminished, but it takes longer than normal to expel it. If the lung capacity is reduced too (a 'restrictive' change) emphysema is indicated. Obstructive changes make the oxygen/carbon dioxide exchange less efficient, and faster breathing is an attempt to make up for this. This obviously has repercussions on the heart.

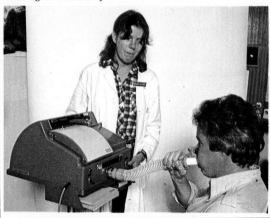

Bronchial Asthma

Bronchial asthma is a respiratory disorder. In it, the airways in the lungs – the bronchial tubes – periodically become unduly narrowed, producing attacks of breathlessness and wheezing. There are two main types – extrinsic asthma and intrinsic asthma. The first, so-called because it is brought on by external agents, is a largely allergic disease that starts in childhood. Intrinsic asthma, also called late-onset asthma, starts in adult life, often at middle age. It is the result of infection of the upper or lower respiratory tract. Examples of such infections include SINUSITIS.

Asthma affects both sexes, all races and all social classes. In extrinsic asthma, it is likely that other members of a family will also have allergic diseases. In intrinsic asthma, it is common for other members of a family to be asthma sufferers.

Physical symptoms

Three reactions take place in the body to produce an asthmatic attack. Firstly, the muscle in the wall of the bronchial tubes tightens. The body also reacts through the swelling of the lining of the bronchial tubes and the production of extra mucus.

A permanently runny nose, or chest troubles in general – especially wheezing bronchitis – are common in asthmatics and their families. Presumably, this is the weak chink in their bodily armor. Very occasionally, a condition known as *status asthmaticus* develops – an asthma attack which is prolonged for hours because the smaller airways have become plugged with sticky mucus. It is more normal, however, for asthma attacks to last acutely only for an hour or so, although a degree of wheeziness and shortness of breath may continue for

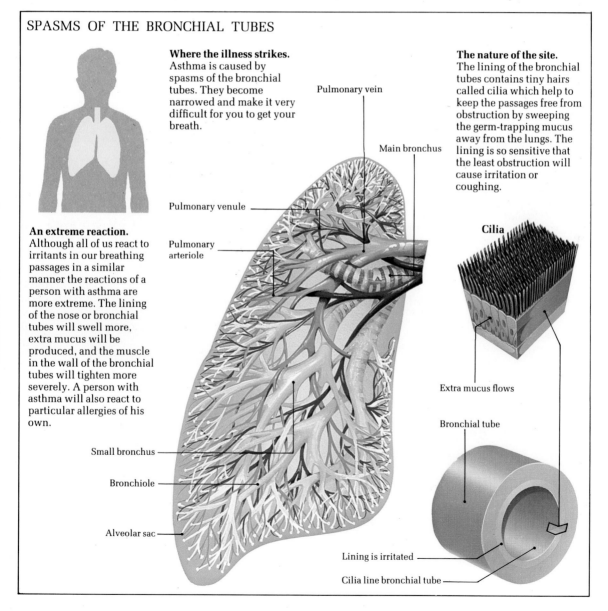

SPASMS OF THE BRONCHIAL TUBES

Where the illness strikes.
Asthma is caused by spasms of the bronchial tubes. They become narrowed and make it very difficult for you to get your breath.

The nature of the site.
The lining of the bronchial tubes contains tiny hairs called cilia which help to keep the passages free from obstruction by sweeping the germ-trapping mucus away from the lungs. The lining is so sensitive that the least obstruction will cause irritation or coughing.

An extreme reaction.
Although all of us react to irritants in our breathing passages in a similar manner the reactions of a person with asthma are more extreme. The lining of the nose or bronchial tubes will swell more, extra mucus will be produced, and the muscle in the wall of the bronchial tubes will tighten more severely. A person with asthma will also react to particular allergies of his own.

Pulmonary vein

Main bronchus

Pulmonary venule

Pulmonary arteriole

Cilia

Extra mucus flows

Bronchial tube

Small bronchus

Bronchiole

Alveolar sac

Lining is irritated

Cilia line bronchial tube

over a week.

Asthmatic attacks often start suddenly, with difficulty in breathing and a feeling of tightness inside your chest, like a drawstring strangling the exit from your lungs. You cannot exhale easily through the narrowed airways; the more anxious you become about this disability, the worse the muscle spasm. You want to draw in another breath desperately, but you know you must first get rid of the stale air already in your lungs. Your chest is slightly over-expanded. You may wheeze as you breathe out – the hardest task – and have a dry cough which produces only small amounts of sticky mucus.

Occasionally, with much painful coughing, you bring up a stringy plug of mucus, so shaped because it had exactly fitted into a small tube. This plug is known as a cast and it is beneficial, though unpleasant, to expel it.

Your breathing rate may not be fast – it is too difficult to speed it up – but your pulse will be racing, mainly because of your anxiety.

Many asthmatics breathe normally between attacks. However, in long-standing asthma, emphysema (see CHRONIC BRONCHITIS) may develop. This will give some degree of permanent breathlessness.

Diagnosis and treatment
Seventy per cent of children grow out of their asthma in adolescence; for the others, excellent treatment is now available. Testing your breathing with an instrument called a spirometer at different times of the day and before and after giving you a bronchial dilator medicine will help in assessing whether your symptoms are due to asthma and what tends to bring on the attacks. Your doctor will take blood

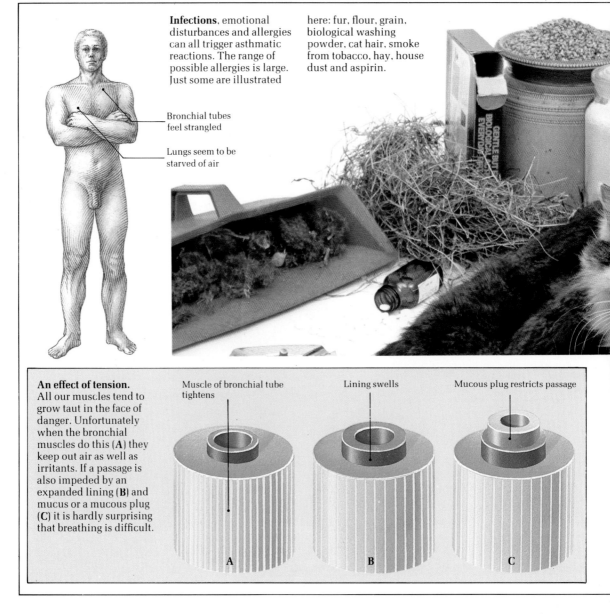

Infections, emotional disturbances and allergies can all trigger asthmatic reactions. The range of possible allergies is large. Just some are illustrated here: fur, flour, grain, biological washing powder, cat hair, smoke from tobacco, hay, house dust and aspirin.

Bronchial tubes feel strangled

Lungs seem to be starved of air

An effect of tension. All our muscles tend to grow taut in the face of danger. Unfortunately when the bronchial muscles do this (**A**) they keep out air as well as irritants. If a passage is also impeded by an expanded lining (**B**) and mucus or a mucous plug (**C**) it is hardly surprising that breathing is difficult.

Muscle of bronchial tube tightens

Lining swells

Mucous plug restricts passage

A

B

C

samples to assess the degree of infection and to look for an excess of eosinophil cells. These occur in both types of asthma. Examination of your sputum – the material you cough up – may also show eosinophil cells and casts of the smaller airways. A chest x-ray will be taken to check for pneumonia and other lung disorders. In uncomplicated asthma, the film is usually normal, though the diaphragm may be rather low if the lung is over-inflated.

Hyper-sensitivity tests may be performed. Tiny drops of various extracts, such as house dust and pollen, are dotted along your arms and the skin scratched with a needle. After ten minutes, red wheals may appear, according to your sensitivity. Sometimes a minute injection is made into the skin if the results are in doubt.

The obvious action to take is to avoid all possible causes of sensitivity and infection.

Unfortunately, hypo-sensitization by injections of increasing amounts of the materials to which you are especially sensitive only helps a few asthmatics, but there are other remedies that can be effective. Using an inhaler is a useful preventative, as it stops the cycle of events within your body that leads to spasm of the bronchial muscles in reaction to an irritant. Broncho-dilators, which actively relax your bronchial muscles, may be taken by mouth or used as an aerosol inhaler. They are useful before, during and after an attack. In severe asthma, which is resistant to other forms of treatment, steroid medication is of the utmost value. In some cases, this may have to be continued between attacks. The undesirable side-effects of steroids tend to be avoided if they are inhaled directly into the bronchial tubes, but they are best avoided in pregnancy.

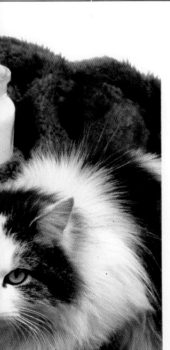

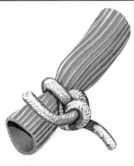

How it feels
At the onset of an attack you may feel that access to the lungs is being cut off by a tightening grip around the tubes that feed them. This is the effect of the spasm of the bronchial tube muscles. If you are prone to anxiety, the spasm may be intensified.

Although the body's
reactions are so powerful, the irritant may appear to resist all of them.

PRESCRIPTION

Diagnosis
Your doctor will carry out tests that determine what brings on attacks, what, if any, degree of infection is present, and that establish the presence or otherwise of the cells associated with bronchial asthma. He or she will also want to eliminate other lung disorders by appropriate tests.

Treatment
Many forms of drug treatment imitate the action of adrenaline in the body— that is, they widen or 'dilate' the bronchial tubes. It is important when using any drug of this nature not to exceed the stated dose. If they do not work at the given limit, they will not work above it, and may cause considerable harm.

It is important to have plenty to drink before an attack becomes too severe, so that dryness in the throat will not make the mucus less moist, and more difficult to shift.

It is sometimes necessary to learn from a physiotherapist how to cough more effectively.

If an allergic reaction is behind an attack, steroid drugs might suppress the reaction. A patient can be desensitized to a particular allergen by a course of an appropriate drug. Below: the use of bronchial dilators is an important method of relieving an attack, but it is necessary always to follow the doctor's and manufacturer's instructions carefully.

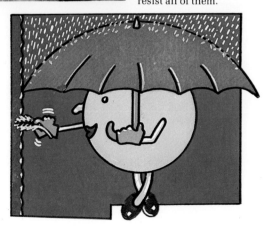

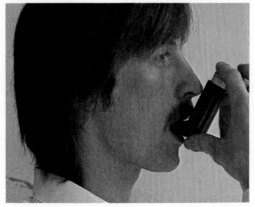

Laryngitis

Laryngitis occurs when the mucous membrane of the voice box (larynx), including the vocal chords, becomes inflamed. It may be acute – that is, a short, sharp infection, usually developing in the course of a cold – or chronic, in which your voice is never clear and gradually changes to a lower pitch.

Attacks of acute laryngitis can be precipitated by shouting, singing or speech-making, particularly if you are not trained in voice reproduction. It is particularly likely if you are subject to a blocked nose, SINUSITIS, or if your work is sedentary in a stuffy atmosphere. Several attacks of this kind may well lead to the development of the chronic condition.

Physical symptoms

The inflammation which is the chief cause of laryngitis may spread downwards from the nose and throat when you have a common cold, sore throat, influenza, or such infections as measles. The inflamed larynx will look red and swollen, while the vocal cords, which normally have a bright, pearly lustre, are dull and pink. In chronic laryngitis, there are signs of prolonged irritation – from tobacco smoke, for instance – and of over-production of sticky mucus, as in alcohol abuse. Small swellings on the vocal cords—known as singers' nodes—occur in either sex, usually in young adults. They are the result of damage from using the voice during an attack of acute laryngitis.

You may be slightly feverish in acute laryngitis, but, otherwise, the symptoms are much the same whether the condition is acute or chronic. You will probably have a dry, tickling discomfort in the neck, together with a dry cough that produces little sputum. The main

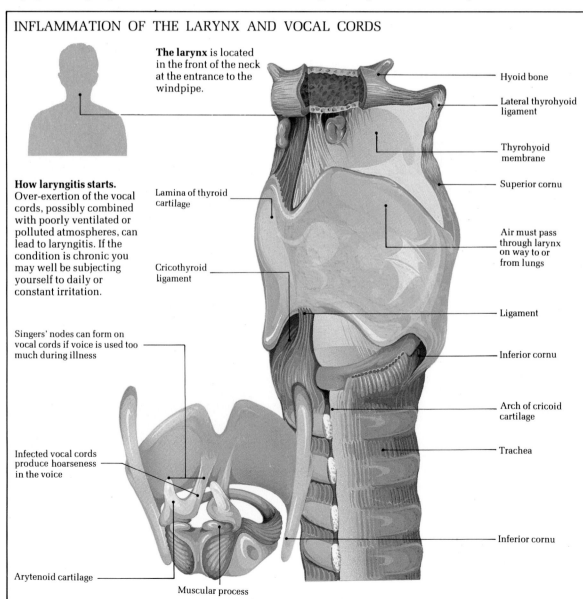

INFLAMMATION OF THE LARYNX AND VOCAL CORDS

The larynx is located in the front of the neck at the entrance to the windpipe.

Hyoid bone

Lateral thyrohyoid ligament

Thyrohyoid membrane

Superior cornu

How laryngitis starts. Over-exertion of the vocal cords, possibly combined with poorly ventilated or polluted atmospheres, can lead to laryngitis. If the condition is chronic you may well be subjecting yourself to daily or constant irritation.

Lamina of thyroid cartilage

Air must pass through larynx on way to or from lungs

Cricothyroid ligament

Ligament

Singers' nodes can form on vocal cords if voice is used too much during illness

Inferior cornu

Arch of cricoid cartilage

Infected vocal cords produce hoarseness in the voice

Trachea

Inferior cornu

Arytenoid cartilage

Muscular process

problem is hoarseness. On waking, talking will be uncomfortable and your voice will sound hoarse. The feeling will increase as you use your voice until it nearly vanishes.

Diagnosis and treatment

Proper treatment of laryngitis is vital, particularly if the victim is a child. If a child's small, undeveloped larynx becomes swollen, he or she may have difficulty in breathing. The air must pass through the larynx to reach or leave the lungs.

It is normal procedure to pass a swab over the tissues as far back as the doctor can reach for bacteriological examination to establish what infecting organisms may be involved. Antibiotics will be given if there is no marked improvement after two days or so; otherwise no special tests are required, unless the hoarseness persists for six weeks or more. In that case, the doctor will examine your larynx with a mirror at the back of your throat, or, if that does not give a good enough view, with a laryngoscope to check whether there is a polyp, or any other kind of tumor, present. Your thyroid gland will also be tested, since lack of thyroid hormone causes hoarseness or enlarged thyroid.

Rest in a warm, well-ventilated room and do not even try to speak. Steam inhalations every four hours are helpful. Honey and lemon juice, or another linctus, may help you not to cough.

In chronic laryngitis, the vital part of the treatment is to locate the underlying cause of the condition. It can be cigarettes, drink, dust or poor ventilation – take a long, hard look at your way of life. The trouble may be infective, so check that your nose, throat, sinuses or teeth do not need attention.

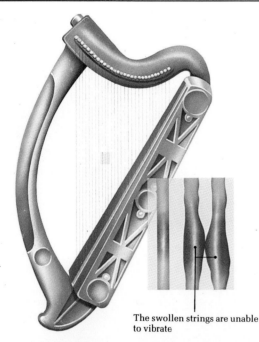

The swollen strings are unable to vibrate

How your voice is affected. The vocal cords produce sound through vibration, in a manner comparable to that of the strings of a musical instrument. If the cords become swollen and inflamed their sound-producing capacities will be severely diminished.

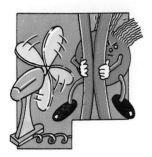

The hoarseness which characterizes the illness becomes more acute the more you try to use your voice. You may find that your ability to speak disappears altogether as the air is drawn in vain past your vocal cords.

PRESCRIPTION

Diagnosis
If you describe the symptoms of sore throat, dry cough and hoarseness to your doctor, this, along with a straightforward throat examination, should be enough for a diagnosis of laryngitis. If the symptoms persist, an examination with a laryngoscope will be necessary.

Treatment
An attack of laryngitis rarely lasts more than a few days. Keep warm and stay indoors, as one of the main irritants of laryngitis is cold air. Normally, inhaled air is warmed as it passes through the nasal passages. If the nose is blocked, this obviously cannot happen. The coldness and dryness of the throat can be partly relieved by the warmed moisture of inhaled steam. This remedy may also help to clear the nasal passages. It is advisable to put as little strain on the vocal cords as possible, so keep your efforts at speaking down to the absolute minimum. Treatments which may ease the discomfort without actually curing the disease include traditional cough mixtures, honey and lemon drinks and additions to the steam inhalation such as menthol.

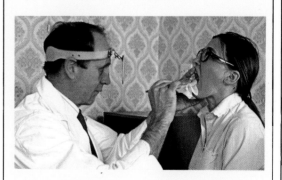

The laryngologist is looking for an absence of lustre on the vocal cords. He will also check for other diseases that give similar symptoms.

Lung Cancer

Lung cancer (bronchial carcinoma) is a malignant tumor which develops anywhere within the branches of the bronchial tree. It is the leading cause of death from cancer in Western society, particularly among men, though proportionately fewer deaths occur from it in Australia and the USA than in England. Over ninety per cent of cases result from smoking; the likeliest candidates for the disease smoke twenty-five or more cigarettes a day for many years, preferring high tar, strong tobacco varieties without filter tips to filtered ones, a pipe, or cigars. Typical male sufferers are aged between forty-five and sixty-five, who are heavy cigarette smokers.

Physical symptoms

Lung cancer is usually asymptomatic – that is, without symptoms – in its early stages. After many years of irritation, the cells lining the breathing tubes may start multiplying faster than is necessary for normal replacement purposes of wear and tear. The usual type of growth, accounting for fifty-six per cent of lung cancer cases, comes from the squamous cells, usually in the larger bronchial tubes. The cancer grows very slowly. Much more rapid to develop is the oat-cell type, which also appears in the larger tubes. Another type – not related to smoking and affecting the sexes equally – develops in the mucus glands, which lubricate and clean the bronchial tubes. These cancers are usually found near the outer edges of the lung.

The disease progresses in two ways. A growth may finally block the affected tube, leading to the likelihood of infection developing in the part of the lung that has been

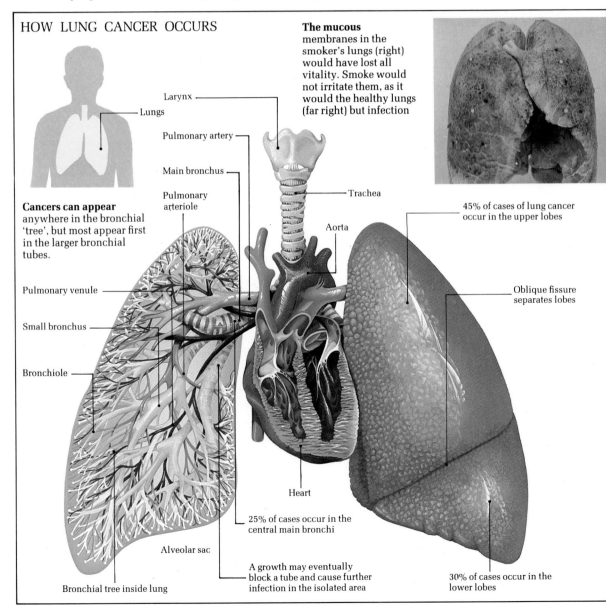

HOW LUNG CANCER OCCURS

The mucous membranes in the smoker's lungs (right) would have lost all vitality. Smoke would not irritate them, as it would the healthy lungs (far right) but infection

Larynx

Lungs

Pulmonary artery

Main bronchus

Pulmonary arteriole

Trachea

Aorta

Cancers can appear anywhere in the bronchial 'tree', but most appear first in the larger bronchial tubes.

Pulmonary venule

Small bronchus

Bronchiole

45% of cases of lung cancer occur in the upper lobes

Oblique fissure separates lobes

Heart

25% of cases occur in the central main bronchi

Alveolar sac

A growth may eventually block a tube and cause further infection in the isolated area

30% of cases occur in the lower lobes

Bronchial tree inside lung

isolated. Additionally, malignant cells may get carried in the lymphatic vessels to the glands in the chest, or in the blood stream to other parts of the body, especially the liver.

Diagnosis and treatment

One of the chief forms of diagnosis is through chest x-ray, which will detect the presence of lung cancer in the absence of all physical symptoms. If you are a man of forty-five or more – and a smoker – symptoms which should arouse your suspicions are a persistent cough – particularly if there is blood in the phlegm – breathlessness and chest pain. The last may be more noticeable after drinking. You may notice that you are losing weight or feeling unaccountably depressed. You may have an unexpected bout of pneumonia or pleurisy.

If you have the slightest suspicion of lung cancer, ask your doctor to send you for a chest x-ray. Some lung cancers can be cured and the sooner treatment is started the better. Surgical removal of the tumor produces good results where it is applicable. In some cases, however – particularly with oat-cell cancer – radical radiotherapy is the most effective treatment. This is also useful in stopping pain, if this is troublesome. Chemotherapy, the use of drugs which selectively kill cancer cells if injected into the blood stream, may be used alone or in conjunction with radiotherapy.

The best course of action is to lessen the risk of contracting the disease at all. If you are in the risk area – you smoke heavily but have not so far developed a cancer – give the habit up immediately. After six weeks of discomfort, every day is a step further away from the risk of contracting the disease.

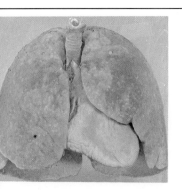

would easily set in, and breathing difficulties would strain the heart.

Cell division
Over a given period A-B healthy cells will reproduce at a rate in accordance with the needs of the body (top). Cancerous cells reproduce at a vastly increased rate (bottom).

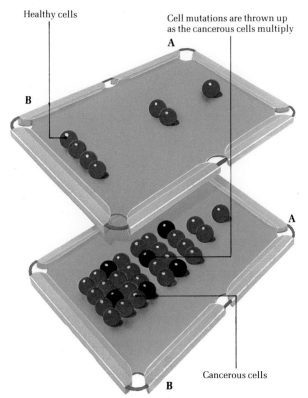

Healthy cells

Cell mutations are thrown up as the cancerous cells multiply

A

B

A

B

Cancerous cells

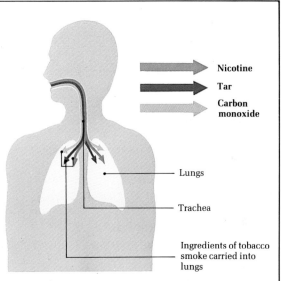

Nicotine

Tar

Carbon monoxide

Lungs

Trachea

Ingredients of tobacco smoke carried into lungs

The contents of tobacco smoke
The three main poisonous ingredients of tobacco smoke are: tar, carbon monoxide and nicotine. Tar irritates and disables the air passages and massively increases the chances of getting lung cancer. Poor lungs put extra strain on the heart. Carbon monoxide may contribute to defective eyesight. Nicotine overactivates the heart, suppresses appetite and restricts blood vessels.

PRESCRIPTION

Diagnosis
A chest X-ray will detect the presence of lung cancer before symptoms show.

Treatment
Up to one half of the cases of lung cancer found by routine chest X-ray can be operated on, so it is a good idea to have check-ups with reasonable regularity. When symptoms first start to appear, it may be too late for treatment. The most effective form of treatment is removal of the tumor. Radiotherapy may also be necessary. Drugs are used, too, to kill the cancer cells.

Sinusitis

Sinusitis is an inflammation of the mucous membranes that line the sinuses, the four air-containing cavities within the bones of the face. It can be either acute or chronic. The first form consists of short, sharp attacks, which can be brought about by the spread of germs into the sinuses as a result, say, of heavy nose-blowing during another respiratory infection. Chronic sinusitis usually only develops if you have some condition that tends to block one or more of the drainage holes to the nose.

Physical symptoms

When you have a cold, the inflammation usually spreads into your sinuses in passing. If, however, you are generally run down, or if a particularly virulent organism is attacking you, one or more of your sinuses may become acutely inflamed. The swelling of the lining that results impairs the outflow of infected mucus, as the cilia – microscopic hairs along the cells which normally sweep the mucus out – find it impossible to shift it along (see CHRONIC BRONCHITIS). If an outlet is completely blocked, pus collects in the sinus, causing a throbbing pain and a general feeling of illness.

In acute sinusitis, the infection is generally quick to clear up, given the proper treatment. In chronic sinusitis, however, the infection does not subside. The lining of the affected sinus becomes permanently thickened and sticky material may remain inside it.

The classic symptoms of acute sinusitis are headache and a heavy, aching feeling in the face, which becomes worse when you bend down – to fasten your shoe, for instance. Your nose also runs. If a sinus becomes blocked, the pain intensifies and your nose will not dis-

INFLAMMATION IN THE SINUSES

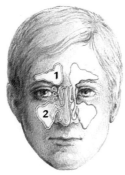

Front view
1 Frontal sinuses
2 Maxillary sinuses

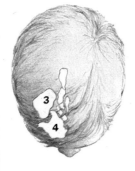

Top view
3 Sphenoidal sinuses
4 Ethmoidal sinuses

Location of sinus cavities.
The paranasal sinuses – hollow cavities located in the bones at the front of the skull – are the seat of sinusitis. Their only known functions are to act as resonators for the voice, and to reduce the weight of

the skull.
The lining of the sinus is continuous with the lining of the nose. So inflammation through a cold may spread to the sinuses, swell the lining, and block the flow of infected mucus.

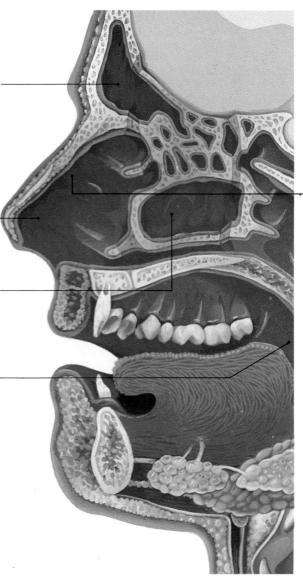

Frontal sinus – symptom of infection here is pain around the eye and possibly a swollen lid

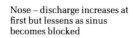

Nose – discharge increases at first but lessens as sinus becomes blocked

Maxillary sinus – symptom of infection here is toothache

Throat-infected mucus can drain down throat, especially at night, to cause further infection.

charge as freely as it does in the preliminary stages of the disease. If blockage occurs in a maxillary sinus – that is, in the upper jaw – your teeth may ache and you may mistakenly blame one of them for the pain. If you press the bone over an acutely infected sinus, it is unpleasantly painful.

In chronic sinusitis, there is little tenderness. It is therefore possible to tolerate a nose that is often blocked, or runny, and a mild, dull feeling in your face. Colds in the head are worse than normal and last longer. Frequent attacks of sore throat, laryngitis or bronchitis may occur.

Diagnosis and treatment

Your doctor will look up your nose to examine the exits from the sinuses and will palpate your face for tenderness. Trans-illumination – shin-ing a torch inside your mouth with the lips shut or against the bone just below your eyebrows – should produce a glow, which will be obscured if there is inflammation. An x-ray will show up thickened lining and pus.

If you have acute sinusitis, stay indoors resting, though you will feel better upright than lying down. Use nasal drops or a spray every four hours to make the mucous membranes shrink. Follow this up fifteen minutes later with a steam inhalation. This will help the sinuses to drain. Pain killers, such as soluble aspirin will help; if the condition is severe, your doctor will prescribe a suitable antibiotic. If a sinus remains blocked after a week's treatment, it is sometimes necessary for the doctor to puncture the sinus and wash it out.

In chronic sinusitis, the best and most sensible form of treatment is surgical.

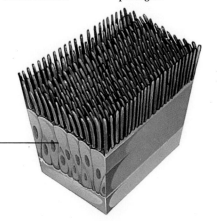

Enlarged section of the sinus wall, showing the cilia. Cilia are microscopic hairs which become clogged with mucus in sinusitis, so that they can no longer clear the passages.

PRESCRIPTION

Diagnosis
Your doctor will be able to see the exits from your sinuses by looking up your nose. He or she may check for inflammation by shining a torch against the areas most likely to be affected, and may arrange for an X-ray.

Treatment
It is important to treat sinusitis properly because some of its side-effects or complications can be dangerous. Treatment is normally through antibiotics, which destroy most infections quite efficiently. Nose drops shrink the mucous membrane, and so give quick relief, but it is best not to make a habit of using them. Their usefulness diminishes with frequency and they may make things worse in the end. Your doctor may decide that your sinuses should be rinsed.

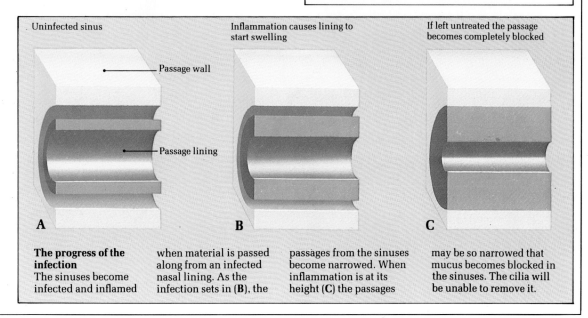

Uninfected sinus

Inflammation causes lining to start swelling

If left untreated the passage becomes completely blocked

Passage wall

Passage lining

A   B   C

The progress of the infection
The sinuses become infected and inflamed when material is passed along from an infected nasal lining. As the infection sets in (**B**), the passages from the sinuses become narrowed. When inflammation is at its height (**C**) the passages may be so narrowed that mucus becomes blocked in the sinuses. The cilia will be unable to remove it.

Hayfever

Hay fever, sometimes called pollenosis, is a form of allergy. In it, the mucous membrane lining the nose is sensitive to one or more kinds of pollen and, as a result, swells and becomes inflamed. It is an extremely common complaint; it is estimated, for instance, to affect between five and ten per cent of the population of the USA (the only country for which there are official figures).

Physical symptoms

Doctors define hay fever as a typical allergen-antibody reaction. What basically happens is that, if your genes carry the requisite allergic tendency, your body will develop a substance called reaginic-antibody or I.g.E. In hay fever, this antibody is to be found in the lining of the nose and bronchial tubes, eyes and skin. When an antigen – in this case, a pollen – comes into contact with I.g.E. antibody, a reaction takes place on the surface of the cell and various substances, including histamine, are released. As a result, the surrounding tissue swells full of fluid and there is a watery discharge, with an outpouring of mucus on the surface. In other words, the body reacts as though a powerful infection has arrived, rather than harmless grains of pollen.

Grass pollen is a very common antigen, but all pollens can cause the disease. When the pollen season arrives, you will sneeze almost constantly. Usually, your nose runs like a tap, though it may remain congested and blocked. Your eyes will be sore, red and watery, because pollen grains have got on to the conjunctiva, the transparent 'skin' over the eyes. ASTHMA, or at least mild wheezing, may appear when the pollen season is at its peak. Urticaria – itchy

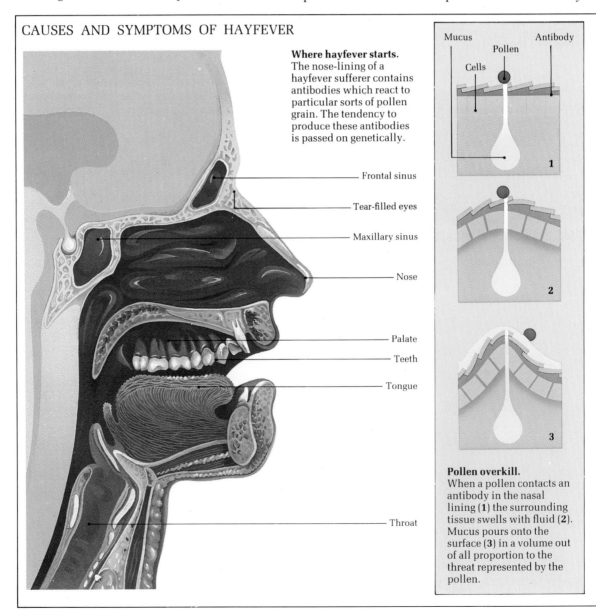

CAUSES AND SYMPTOMS OF HAYFEVER

Where hayfever starts.
The nose-lining of a hayfever sufferer contains antibodies which react to particular sorts of pollen grain. The tendency to produce these antibodies is passed on genetically.

Mucus — Pollen — Antibody — Cells

Frontal sinus
Tear-filled eyes
Maxillary sinus
Nose
Palate
Teeth
Tongue
Throat

1

2

3

Pollen overkill.
When a pollen contacts an antibody in the nasal lining (**1**) the surrounding tissue swells with fluid (**2**). Mucus pours onto the surface (**3**) in a volume out of all proportion to the threat represented by the pollen.

wheals – may crop out on the skin where you have been in contact with grass. Itching inside your ears, on the roof of your mouth and in your throat may be a constant source of irritation. You may well feel generally ill and you can even develop a mild fever.

Diagnosis and treatment

Sensitivity testing is essential for effective treatment. This should be carried out well in advance, as systematic desensitization must be started at least four months before the pollen season begins. You will be tested on one, or both, arms with a range of pollen extracts and probably some other common allergens, such as house dust mite, fungi and horse hair. The most effective method is to make a series of pricks, each of which contains about a millionth of a millimetre of allergenic extracts,

into the skin itself. If a weal develops in a few minutes, you are sensitive to the extract.

Following this, a vaccine, made to suit your sensitivity reactions, is injected in increasing strengths every week until the course is completed. Usually, this must be repeated annually for three years.

Even so, you should avoid potential risk areas. Never walk through long grass or ragweed, keep your bedroom and car windows closed and avoid country holidays in the pollen season. Antihistamine drugs damp down the symptoms, but will make you sleepy, especially with alcohol, and you should not drive while taking them. Decongestant sprays containing ephedrine will make your nose more comfortable, while cortico-steroid eye drops will help your eye symptoms. Anti-asthmatic drugs may also be helpful.

Symptoms.
When your particular pollen or allergen is in the air you will sneeze repeatedly and, while your nose may simply become congested, it will probably run profusely. An irritating itching in the roof of the mouth and throat and sore, runny eyes are also likely.

There is normally a significant amount of pollen in the air only for the two summer months. During these months there will be between 0 and 400 grains per cubic meter of air. At 50 grains per cubic meter, anyone who is going to have an attack will have started sneezing.

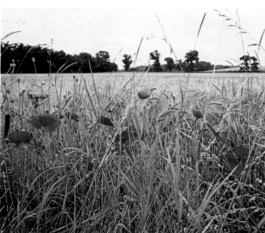

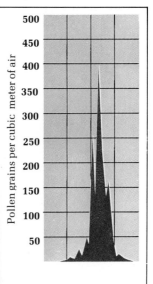

PRESCRIPTION

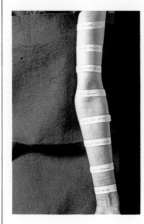

Diagnosis
Your doctor will attempt to find which allergen is bringing on the symptoms.

Treatment
Histamine is one of the substances released when the body reacts to an allergen to which it is sensitive. The symptoms of sneezing and heavy discharge of mucus are triggered by it. Drugs which combat the production of histamine—antihistamines—are

consequently used to combat hayfever symptoms They are reasonably effective, but tend to make the patient sleepy. Some people undergo courses of injections. These must be preceded by tests (see left) which isolate the particular sensitivity of an individual. The patient on the left has shown a marked reaction to rat scurf and a less marked one to rat serum. He has only reacted to grass pollen slightly, if at all. Once the allergen has

been determined a suitable vaccine is then injected in a course lasting several weeks, normally preceding the onset of the hayfever 'season'. The success rate of this method is between 70 and 80 per cent.

Digestive/Introduction

Food gives us energy and the basic materials that the body needs for growth or to replace tissue. The digestive system breaks down food into the simpler forms that can be used for these purposes. The substances responsible for the breakdown are called enzymes. Each one of these – starting with ptyalin in the saliva – promotes one sort of chemical change. The small intestine is the site of most of the digestion. The blood takes many nutrients from here to the liver, to be stored and released when needed. Carbohydrates in food are ultimately burned for energy. Proteins are mainly used in the building of body tissue, but can also be used for fuel. Fats pass into the circulation for use or storage all over the body. Most vitamins cannot be synthesized by the body; others cannot be stored. All these must be ingested in the diet.

The first stage.
Apart from chewing and swallowing, the mouth produces a starch-reducing enzyme, ptyalin, which is released in the saliva. It also modifies the temperature of food.

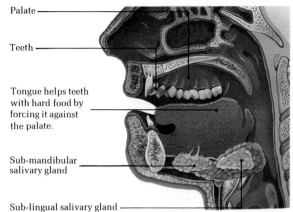

Palate
Teeth
Tongue helps teeth with hard food by forcing it against the palate.
Sub-mandibular salivary gland
Sub-lingual salivary gland

What the system has to do.
Food consists of proteins, fats, carbohydrates, water, salts and vitamins. It is the function of the digestive system to reduce food to a form which can be absorbed by the blood stream, and used by the cells of the body.

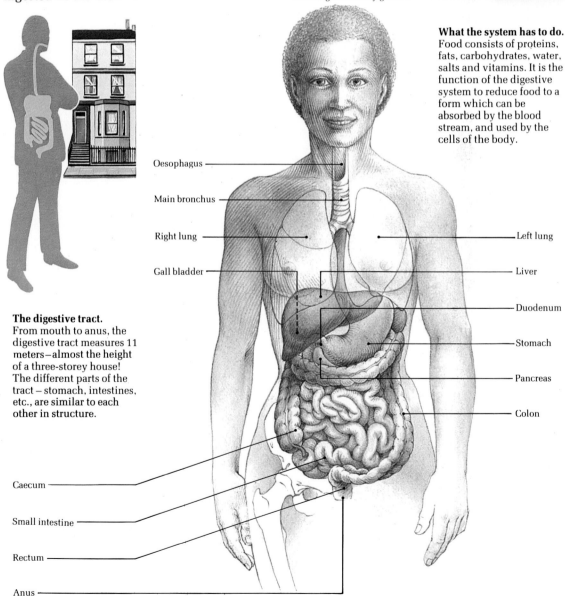

Oesophagus
Main bronchus
Right lung
Gall bladder
Left lung
Liver
Duodenum
Stomach
Pancreas
Colon
Caecum
Small intestine
Rectum
Anus

The digestive tract.
From mouth to anus, the digestive tract measures 11 meters—almost the height of a three-storey house! The different parts of the tract – stomach, intestines, etc., are similar to each other in structure.

32

The liver

The blood from the digestive tract flows into the portal vein which carries it to the liver. It contains dissolved products of digestion such as amino acids, fatty acids, glucose and vitamins. The liver can break these products down more, and can store glucose as glycogen for release when necessary. It also forms bile for digestion, releasing it into the gall bladder and thence to the duodenum.

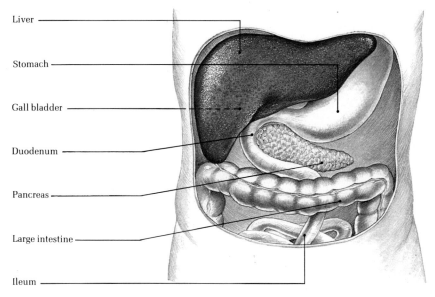

Liver
Stomach
Gall bladder
Duodenum
Pancreas
Large intestine
Ileum

WHAT HAPPENS TO YOUR FOOD

The stomach is that part of the alimentary canal, or digestive tract, which stores food before releasing it into the duodenum. It also churns and squeezes food (segmentation), partly digests it, and releases acids which destroy harmful bacteria. The illustration below shows **(1)** storage of food; **(2)** and **(3)** passing of food through the pyloric sphincter into the duodenum by peristalsis. This is a movement of the wall which occurs throughout the tract, making sure food is passed along. The movement consists of a wave of contraction followed by a wave of relaxation.

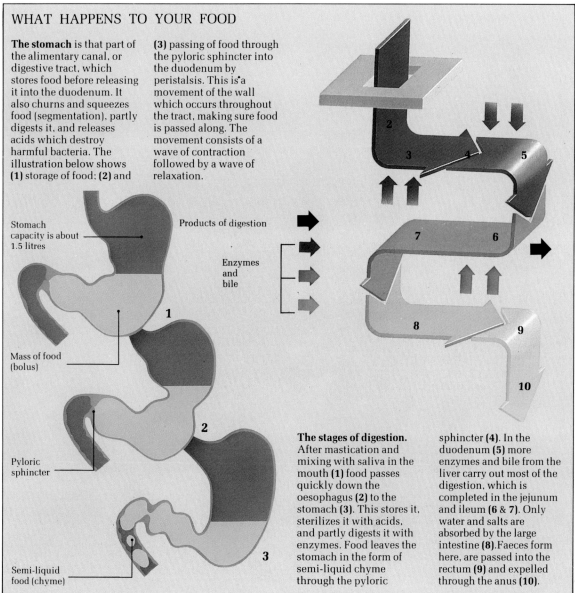

Stomach capacity is about 1.5 litres

Products of digestion

Enzymes and bile

Mass of food (bolus)

Pyloric sphincter

Semi-liquid food (chyme)

The stages of digestion. After mastication and mixing with saliva in the mouth **(1)** food passes quickly down the oesophagus **(2)** to the stomach **(3)**. This stores it, sterilizes it with acids, and partly digests it with enzymes. Food leaves the stomach in the form of semi-liquid chyme through the pyloric sphincter **(4)**. In the duodenum **(5)** more enzymes and bile from the liver carry out most of the digestion, which is completed in the jejunum and ileum **(6 & 7)**. Only water and salts are absorbed by the large intestine **(8)**. Faeces form here, are passed into the rectum **(9)** and expelled through the anus **(10)**.

Diverticulitis

Diverticulitis is an inflammation of the small pouches or bulges that sometimes form in the mucous membrane lining of the colon, or large intestine. The formation of these pouches is itself the result of a disorder called diverticulosis.

Diverticulosis is, in itself, not serious. From middle-age onwards, many people develop diverticula without any ill-effects. Their occurrence becomes more frequent with age; thirty per cent of men and women have such pouches when they are sixty or more. Those who suffer from chronic constipation and eat little roughage are the most vulnerable.

Physical symptoms

Roughage is the indigestible part of food in vegetables, fruits and bran. It provides the bulk for the motions. When your body passes a motion – that is, your bowels are opened – there is muscular pressure along the colon as well as in the rectum. The greatest back pressure is in the sigmoid colon and it is not surprising that this is the part where diverticula are most often found.

If your diet consists of food with hardly any roughage – white bread, eggs and milk, for instance – the muscles of the colon are constantly strained, as they try to push along a small amount of material upon which they can get no grip. In the end, after forty years of activity or more, the colon muscles become over-sized and ineffective, rather like those of a muscle-bound boxer.

Now, when the pressure inside the colon increases, weak places between the stiff, thick, muscle fibers bulge out, forming pouches made only of the slippery, lubricated mucous mem-

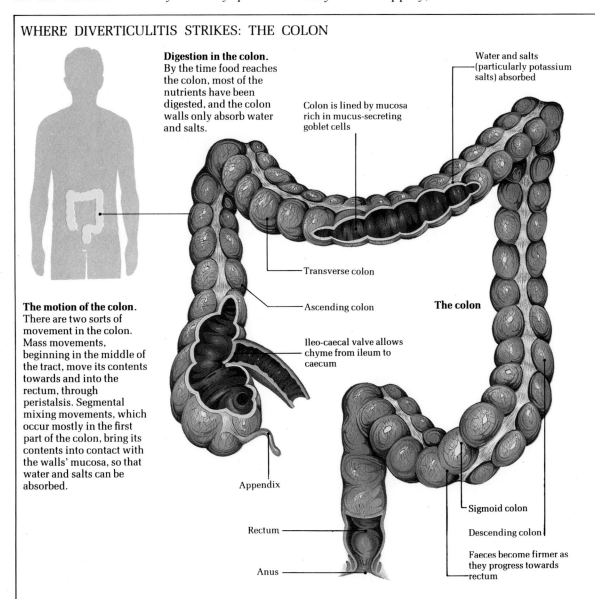

WHERE DIVERTICULITIS STRIKES: THE COLON

Digestion in the colon.
By the time food reaches the colon, most of the nutrients have been digested, and the colon walls only absorb water and salts.

Colon is lined by mucosa rich in mucus-secreting goblet cells

Water and salts (particularly potassium salts) absorbed

Transverse colon

Ascending colon

The colon

Ileo-caecal valve allows chyme from ileum to caecum

The motion of the colon.
There are two sorts of movement in the colon. Mass movements, beginning in the middle of the tract, move its contents towards and into the rectum, through peristalsis. Segmental mixing movements, which occur mostly in the first part of the colon, bring its contents into contact with the walls' mucosa, so that water and salts can be absorbed.

Appendix

Rectum

Anus

Sigmoid colon

Descending colon

Faeces become firmer as they progress towards rectum

brane and peritoneal covering. This is what happens in diverticular disease, or diverticulosis of the colon.

Naturally, as the waste material passes down your colon, bits of it tend to become lodged in any pouches there may be. As there is no muscle in the walls of the pouches, they may remain full when the rest of the bowel empties. In addition, more faecal material may well be pushed into them, where it becomes impacted.

If this happens, inflammation of one or more diverticula may occur. This is very like appendicitis. Waste and pus may be trapped in a pouch, or escape imperfectly, the result being diverticulitis. This is sometimes called left-side appendicitis when it is acute.

If you have simple diverticular disease – that is, without inflammation – you are likely to feel vague cramping pains on the left side of your abdomen and have irregular bowel movements. This is because of the awkward action of the over-sized muscles in the colon. There is no special pattern to the pain; nothing seems consistently to make it either better or worse.

If you develop acute diverticulitis – inflammation of the diverticula – you will have a raised temperature and also severe pain. This will be like appendicitis, but will be on the left rather than on the right side of your abdomen. You will be tender to touch over the colon.

Such an acute attack may subside completely; alternatively, you may be left with chronic diverticulitis, a low-key, but persistent, disorder. In this case, you will have continuing, but less severe, pain and tenderness on the left side of the abdomen. Your usual bowel habits may be upset and you are likely to pass some blood and jelly-like mucus with your faeces.

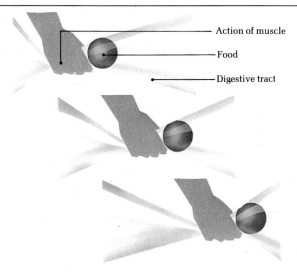

Action of muscle
Food
Digestive tract

Peristalsis.
The way in which food is moved along the alimentary canal is called peristalsis. The circular muscle fibers in the wall around the food contract behind it and relax in front of it. The longitudinal fibers squeeze it along. The effect is rather like that of a hand squeezing a ball along a rubber tube.

If there is not enough roughage in the diet, then the muscles of the colon have to work extra hard to move along the smaller amounts of faeces (below). Over a period of years, they will become too large and lose their efficiency.

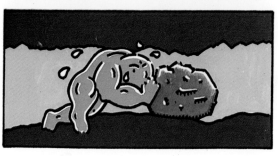

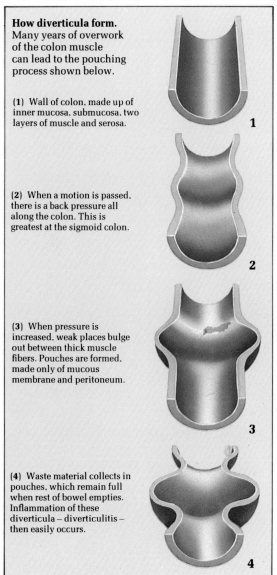

How diverticula form.
Many years of overwork of the colon muscle can lead to the pouching process shown below.

(1) Wall of colon, made up of inner mucosa, submucosa, two layers of muscle and serosa.

(2) When a motion is passed, there is a back pressure all along the colon. This is greatest at the sigmoid colon.

(3) When pressure is increased, weak places bulge out between thick muscle fibers. Pouches are formed, made only of mucous membrane and peritoneum.

(4) Waste material collects in pouches, which remain full when rest of bowel empties. Inflammation of these diverticula – diverticulitis – then easily occurs.

Diagnosis and treatment

A barium enema is the most useful investigation a doctor can carry out to establish the diagnosis. After the bowel has been thoroughly emptied, an enema of material that will show up on x-ray is passed into the rectum and colon via the anus. Not only will this indicate the characteristic signs of both diseases – pouches and the saw-tooth appearance of the large muscles – but it will eliminate others, such as CANCER OF THE COLON. Blood tests will show the usual inflammatory reaction – an increased number of white cells – in acute diverticulitis. Visual examination of the inside of the colon can be made with a sigmoidoscope.

Unless you have an acute attack of diverticulitis, the best treatment is simply to adjust your diet. This should include plenty of fruit, vegetables and wholewheat bread. You should take natural bran, increasing this to two tablespoons daily. This may make you more uncomfortable at first, but you will become accustomed to it after a fortnight. Your doctor may prescribe a mild sedative if you are inclined to be tense or nervous.

In an acute attack, you must rest in bed and adopt a liquid diet. Your doctor will prescribe a suitable antibiotic. If a pouch bursts or leaks, an operation is needed. This must be carried out as quickly as possible; perforation leads to peritonitis. Abscess, spasm or obstruction of the colon is equally serious.

If the symptoms are really troublesome over a long period, your doctor may suggest surgery in any case. The affected part of the bowel will be removed – a technique known as colonic resection. However, this is a major operation. It has dangers if you are elderly or overweight.

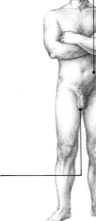

If the diverticula are not yet inflamed, bowel movements will be irregular, and there will be vague cramps in the left of the abdomen.
If inflammation has set in, the temperature will rise and the left of abdomen will be painful and tender.

If the condition is chronic blood and mucus will be passed with motions

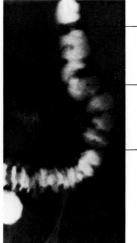

Colon

The grey areas show the wall "pouching" outwards, through an increase of pressure from inside the colon.

The dark lines show the folds in the colon.

With the aid of a barium enema the pouches and enlarged muscles characteristic of diverticular disease will show up on an X-ray.

PRESCRIPTION

Diagnosis
An X-ray following a barium enema will reveal the pouches characteristic of diverticular disease. A blood test will indicate the presence or otherwise of infection or inflammation (diverticulitis).

Treatment
Diverticulitis can normally be treated reasonably successfully with antibiotics. If the inflammation has not set in, simple adjustment of diet may prevent it, and gradually improve the condition of your intestines. What they have lacked is roughage, so gradually increase the amount of this in your food. There is plenty in wholewheat bread and fresh vegetables. If the inflammation has set in, you will need to take a more easily absorbed diet at first, then gradually adjust. Only in severe cases is removal of the part of the intestine affected by diverticulitis at all necessary.

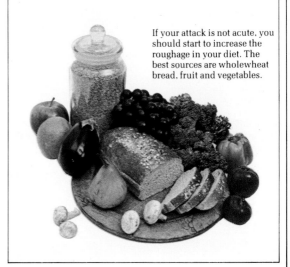

If your attack is not acute, you should start to increase the roughage in your diet. The best sources are wholewheat bread, fruit and vegetables.

Ulcerative Colitis

Ulcerative colitis is a severe, chronic, inflammation of the lining of the colon (large bowel), whose exact cause is unknown. The disease ranges in severity from mild, intermittent diarrhoea to profuse, severe diarrhoea and more widespread symptoms such as feverishness. The victim can temporarily recover, and then relapse without any apparent reason, this cycle continuing for years.

Physical symptoms

The disorder starts in the rectum, the final length of bowel before the anus. From there, it spreads backwards towards the caecum, the bulge at the beginning of the colon where the appendix is attached. There are signs of inflammation in the mucous membrane which lines the bowel, but the deeper part of the colon wall is not usually affected.

There are various theories as to the cause of the disease. Some doctors believe that infection is responsible, but no germ or other infective agent has been found consistently in ulcerative colitis. Others argue that it is an allergic disorder, but, except in a few cases where there is an allergy to milk, allergy does not seem to play an important role. A third theory is that the disease results from a failure of the body's autoimmune mechanism – the body is creating anti-bodies to attack the normal mucosa – but this is not proven. Anxiety and depression also seem to be causal factors and are often found in accompaniment to the disease. So, too, are bacterial infections – abscesses may form in the colon wall – but these are due to bacteria taking advantage of the weakened condition of the tissues rather than a cause of the disease.

Symptoms vary according to the severity of

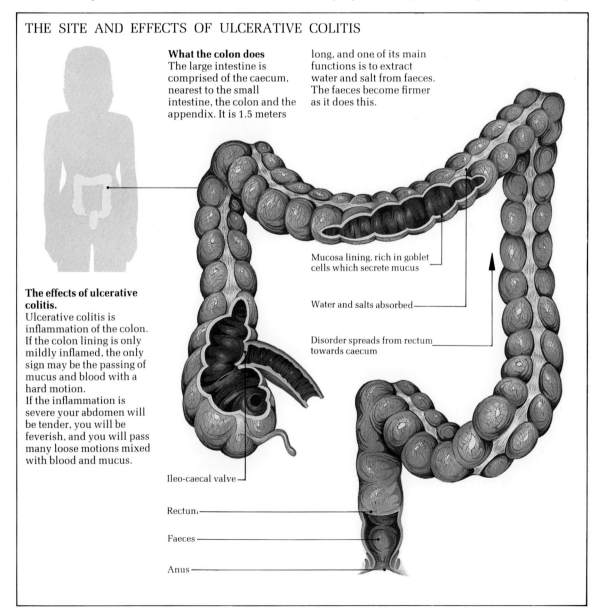

THE SITE AND EFFECTS OF ULCERATIVE COLITIS

What the colon does
The large intestine is comprised of the caecum, nearest to the small intestine, the colon and the appendix. It is 1.5 meters long, and one of its main functions is to extract water and salt from faeces. The faeces become firmer as it does this.

The effects of ulcerative colitis.
Ulcerative colitis is inflammation of the colon. If the colon lining is only mildly inflamed, the only sign may be the passing of mucus and blood with a hard motion.
If the inflammation is severe your abdomen will be tender, you will be feverish, and you will pass many loose motions mixed with blood and mucus.

Mucosa lining, rich in goblet cells which secrete mucus

Water and salts absorbed

Disorder spreads from rectum towards caecum

Ileo-caecal valve

Rectum

Faeces

Anus

the disease. You may simply pass some white, jelly-like mucus and bleed occasionally, with a hard, constipated motion. On the other hand, you may be severely ill, with fever, a fast pulse rate, a swollen, tender abdomen and up to twenty loose, unpleasant-smelling bowel movements daily. These may be mixed with blood and mucus. You will be anaemic through blood loss, become dehydrated through loss of fluid and will lose weight dramatically as the disease progresses.

Skin disorders, ARTHRITIS of the large joints and liver disorders may arise as possible complications. After many years – perhaps twenty, a CANCER OF THE COLON may develop if the whole of the large bowel is involved. In most cases, however, the disease remains mild and no more than a periodic nuisance, provided that it is promptly treated.

Diagnosis and treatment

In more than ninety-five per cent of cases, diagnosis can be made by rectal examination, using an instrument called a sigmoidoscope. The characteristic sign of ulcerative colitis is that the mucous membrane bleeds readily at the mere touch of a swab. Biopsies will be taken to confirm the diagnosis, while a barium enema allows the doctor to establish how far upwards the disorder extends.

Treatment can be medical or surgical. Hospitalization is essential if the disease becomes severe. You need rest and an adequate diet, avoiding milk and milk products in case they exacerbate the disease. Iron tablets and potassium supplements may be prescribed. You will also be given drugs to help control the diarrhoea. If your symptoms prove uncontrollable, an ileostomy will be performed.

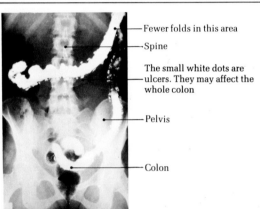

Fewer folds in this area

Spine

The small white dots are ulcers. They may affect the whole colon

Pelvis

Colon

Administering a barium enema highlights the colon on an X-ray. A blurred outline of the membrane indicates ulcerative colitis. Ulcers appear as white dots.

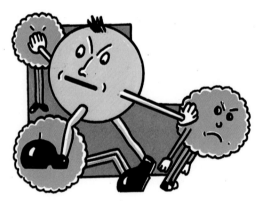

When the tissue of the colon is in a weakened condition, the bacteria which are always present in the colon can cause abcesses to form.

You may be feverish

Your pulse rate may be high

Your abdomen may be swollen

You may pass white jelly-like mucus with a hard motion.

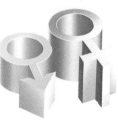

For every seven female sufferers from ulcerative colitis, there are five males

PRESCRIPTION

Diagnosis
Your doctor will examine the inside of your colon by means of a sigmoidoscope, introduced through the anus. The extent of the colitis will show up on an X-ray, after a barium meal.

Treatment
Most people need a fairly lengthy period of treatment after an attack of ulcerative colitis. The persistent diarrhoea leads to emaciation as well as dehydration in some cases, and anaemia is a normal result of an attack. A high roughage diet with plenty of foods like those below is sometimes useful, but can on occasion aggravate symptoms. It is best to work with your doctor on finding what best suits your particular case. Antibiotics are often used to keep the bacterial or other infection under control. As the emotional make-up of the patient is sometimes a contributory factor in the disease, psychotherapy may be recommended by your doctor. In a number of serious cases, the affected part of the intestine has to be removed.

Crohn's Disease

Crohn's disease is a chronic, progressive, inflammatory disease of the wall of the bowel. It can affect any part of the digestive tract, from the mouth to the anus, but it usually attacks the last part of the small intestine, or ileum. This is where it joins the large intestine, or colon.

While most sufferers develop the disorder in their teens or early twenties, there is a second, lesser, risk period from the age of sixty onwards. Then, the colon is more often affected than the ileum. While the disease is still relatively rare, it has become five times as common over the past ten years.

Physical symptoms

Nobody knows why Crohn's disease develops. It begins under the mucous membrane lining the affected part of the intestine; usually, short lengths of gut are affected, with healthy areas in between them. There may be ulcers – raw areas – inside the gut, or the whole tube may be constricted in part. The gut may be like a piece of string in one place, with normal intestine in between.

The disease usually starts off with bouts of abdominal pain, with diarrhoea, loss of weight and a general feeling of illness. You may have bouts of fever and may be tired and pale because of anaemia caused by lack of iron. This lack may be caused by the diarrhoea or failure to absorb iron properly through the unhealthy intestine wall. Your appetite will deteriorate, this adding to your under-nourished appearance. You may develop clubbing – curvature of your finger nails and a rounded enlargement of the terminal section of each finger. Sometimes the disease comes on with a sharp attack, then may clear completely.

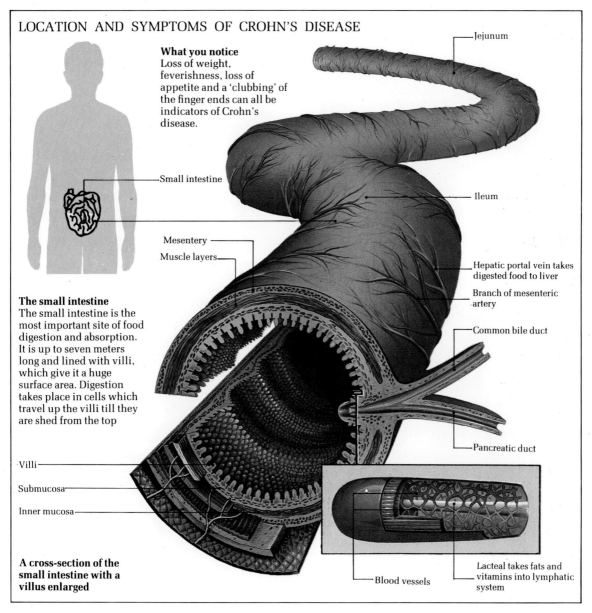

LOCATION AND SYMPTOMS OF CROHN'S DISEASE

Jejunum

What you notice
Loss of weight, feverishness, loss of appetite and a 'clubbing' of the finger ends can all be indicators of Crohn's disease.

Small intestine

Ileum

Mesentery

Muscle layers

Hepatic portal vein takes digested food to liver

Branch of mesenteric artery

The small intestine
The small intestine is the most important site of food digestion and absorption. It is up to seven meters long and lined with villi, which give it a huge surface area. Digestion takes place in cells which travel up the villi till they are shed from the top

Common bile duct

Pancreatic duct

Villi

Submucosa

Inner mucosa

A cross-section of the small intestine with a villus enlarged

Blood vessels

Lacteal takes fats and vitamins into lymphatic system

Diagnosis and treatment

The most useful form of investigation the doctor will employ is a barium follow-through. You are given a white fluid to drink, which is opaque to x-rays. This is observed as it passes through the last part of the ileum and down through the colon. Your doctor will also want to check your blood for anaemia, for signs of malabsorption of vitamin B12 and for lack of protein and folic acid.

A quarter of cases of Crohn's disease recover without any specific treatment. This is particularly likely if the disease developed very acutely in the first place. Troublesome pain and diarrhoea can be controlled by drugs, while you will need a highly-nourishing diet, with plenty of protein in it. Meat, fish, eggs, cheese and pulses are all suitable. Avoid excess milk and reduce roughage – that is, vegetables, fruit and bran. Iron, folic acid and perhaps vitamin B12 may be needed to combat anaemia, together with extra minerals to make up for losses in the motions.

If there is an acute flare-up of diarrhoea and pain, you will be hospitalized. Corticosteroids may be prescribed at first, though these will be replaced by other medicines as soon as practically possible. Antibiotics are useful if there is added infection.

In a certain percentage of cases, surgery may be necessary at some stage or other of the disease, though this figure is growing smaller as drug therapy becomes more advanced. The main reasons for operation are that the disease can narrow the bowel so much in one part that nothing can pass through it; and failure of medical treatment. Only surgery can relieve the pressure. Usually, an ileostomy is performed.

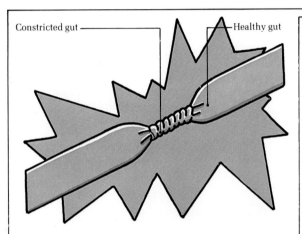

Constricted gut — — Healthy gut

What happens to the intestine. Crohn's disease normally takes the form of raw or constricted sections of gut separated by healthy sections. The restriction is only visible inside the intestine. Viewed from the outside the wall is thicker where constriction occurs.

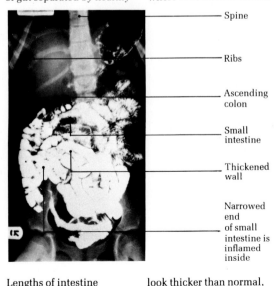

Spine

Ribs

Ascending colon

Small intestine

Thickened wall

Narrowed end of small intestine is inflamed inside

Lengths of intestine affected by Crohn's disease look thicker than normal, as the X-ray above shows.

PRESCRIPTION

Diagnosis
By giving you a blood test your doctor will be able to determine how your digestive processes are being affected. He or she will also send you for an X-ray, so that the condition of your intestine can be readily assessed

Treatment
If Crohn's disease comes on suddenly, then it is reasonably likely to disappear without having to be given any specific treatment. If it is painful, or if you have diarrhoea, then your doctor will be able to give you drugs to relieve these conditions. You will probably not feel like eating and, because of the condition of your intestine, you may become short of iron. When the worst is over, it will be important to build yourself up again with a highly nourishing diet. Proteins such as meat, fish, cheese and eggs are invaluable. Your intestines will not be able to cope with too much roughage, so cut down on that. If your bowel has become blocked through the disease, then surgery may be necessary.

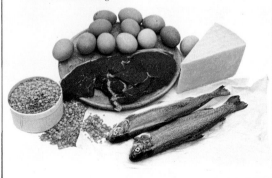

The most suitable diet for someone with Crohn's disease would be high in proteins – apart from milk – and low in roughage.

Colonic Cancer

Cancer of the colon and rectum happens when the growth rate of one type of cell in the large bowel gets out of control, crowding out other, normal cells and taking the nourishment from them. It is one of the commonest forms of cancer, affecting men and women in approximately equal numbers. Its incidence is at its highest where the incidence of STOMACH CANCER is at its lowest; thus, out of 100,000 people in the USA, approximately forty-five will have the disease, compared to twenty-five in the UK and seven in Japan.

Like most cancers, colonic or rectal cancer develop chiefly in middle age or later, the likelihood of their occurrence being greater after the age of fifty. Their exact cause is unknown, but it is thought that diet is an important factor. There may also be an hereditary tendency, while two other diseases in particular predispose to them. These are ULCERATIVE COLITIS and polyps in the rectum and colon. The latter are believed to be a major factor in colonic cancer. They are little lumps, like grapes, inside the colon, which bleed very slightly, but persistently, causing anaemia.

Physical symptoms
The large intestine consists of the colon, and the rectum, which empties waste material from the digestive system by the muscular contraction of a bowel movement. The colon itself consists of several parts: these are the caecum, where it starts; the ascending colon, going up the right side; the transverse colon, looping across from right to left; the descending colon, running down the left side; and the sigmoid colon, which is S-shaped (*sigma* is Greek for S) and joins the rectum. The rectum is more

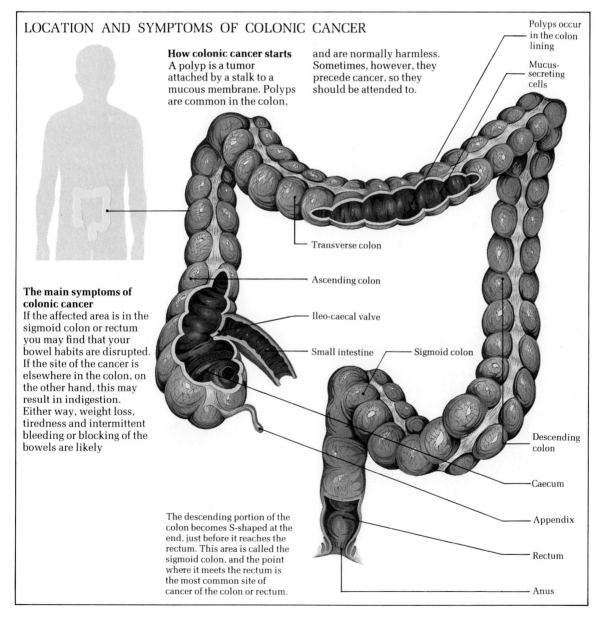

LOCATION AND SYMPTOMS OF COLONIC CANCER

How colonic cancer starts
A polyp is a tumor attached by a stalk to a mucous membrane. Polyps are common in the colon, and are normally harmless. Sometimes, however, they precede cancer, so they should be attended to.

Polyps occur in the colon lining

Mucus-secreting cells

Transverse colon

Ascending colon

Ileo-caecal valve

Small intestine

Sigmoid colon

The main symptoms of colonic cancer
If the affected area is in the sigmoid colon or rectum you may find that your bowel habits are disrupted. If the site of the cancer is elsewhere in the colon, on the other hand, this may result in indigestion. Either way, weight loss, tiredness and intermittent bleeding or blocking of the bowels are likely

Descending colon

Caecum

Appendix

Rectum

Anus

The descending portion of the colon becomes S-shaped at the end, just before it reaches the rectum. This area is called the sigmoid colon, and the point where it meets the rectum is the most common site of cancer of the colon or rectum.

sensitive than the other parts of the bowel; when waste material arrives there, it signals you to open your bowels.

Most cancers in this area probably start as polyps. The site where they most commonly arise is at the join between the sigmoid colon and the rectum. Thus, the illness is bound to upset your bowels. In other parts of the colon, the main symptom may be indigestion, but, wherever it is located, a cancer may cause intermittent bleeding or blocking.

If you are over fifty and find yourself unduly tired and that your bowel habits have changed for no particular reason, you should consult your doctor. You may feel that you want to pass a motion, but find yourself unable to produce much except mucus tinged with blood. Though you previously had a good digestion, you may find you are getting dyspepsia. Alternatively, the first thing you may notice can be that you are pale, anaemic and losing weight.

Diagnosis and treatment

After the usual form of physical examination, your doctor will carry out a rectal examination. This means feeling inside your anus with a gloved, lubricated finger. This does not hurt. He or she may also want to pass an instrument called a sigmoidoscope into your back passage, so that it can be examined visually. A barium enema – a special form of x-ray, which shows the outline of the large bowel – also helps establish a precise diagnosis.

Treatment is by operation; the affected part of the bowel must be removed. Unless the tumor is very low down, the diseased section can be cut out and the healthy ends joined. If this is impossible, a colostomy is performed.

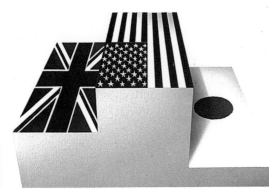

Investigating the colon
The straight sigmoidoscope can only examine a patient as far as the sigmoid colon. The colon itself is accessible to the fiber optic colonoscope, above.

Where the incidence of stomach cancer is high, that of colonic cancer tends to be low, and vice versa. Colonic cancer is seven times more common in the United States than in Japan.

PRESCRIPTION

Diagnosis
There are three main ways of examining the area. Your doctor may do this manually by passing a gloved finger into your anus. He or she may send you for an X-ray, preceded by a barium enema so that the outline of the bowel will be distinct, or carry out what amounts to a visual examination by means of a sigmoidoscope.

Treatment
A person can survive well with only a small proportion of the digestive tract intact. It is possible to cut out lengths of diseased tissue and knit together the remaining ends with very satisfactory results. Having said that, if the tumor is too close to the anus this will not be possible, and a false exit for waste material will have to be made. This is called a colostomy. The colon is brought to the surface so that the contents can discharge into a bag. Most people who use these bags find that they are rather less intrusive on their lives than they at first feared.

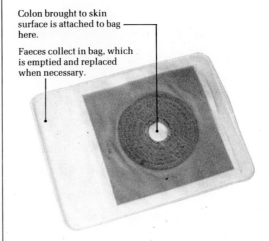

Colon brought to skin surface is attached to bag here.

Faeces collect in bag, which is emptied and replaced when necessary.

The colostomy bag (above) has a special attachment by which it is linked to a surgically produced exit from the colon. Faeces collect in the bag.

Gall Bladder Disease

The gall bladder is the reservoir for the bile continuously produced by the liver. It can be affected by two related diseases – cholecystitis (inflammation of the gall bladder) and cholelithiasis (stones within the bladder).

Cholecystitis can be acute – that is, a sudden, very severe attack, requiring immediate treatment – or chronic. In the latter case, the symptoms are milder, but keep recurring (there is seldom a chronic condition in which there is continuous pain). Cholelithiasis is caused by lumps or concentrations of material inside the gall bladder. Usually, these cause no trouble, but are always present in cases of cholecystitis.

Physical symptoms

Your liver produces about two pints (one liter) of bile daily; this is made more than ten times as concentrated in the gall bladder, where it is stored until it is needed. When you have had a meal – particularly one containing a good deal of fat – the gall bladder contracts like the bulb of a water pistol. Bile is ejected into the duodenum, where it is required for digestion.

If gall stones form, there is the risk that they may interfere with this process, though, in the majority of cases, they do not do so. If there is a big stone, or several smaller ones, however, you may get colicky pain after eating fatty foods. The gall bladder contracts and cannot squeeze the lumps out. The stone may block the exit duct, in which case cholecystitis is likely to develop; alternatively, it may lodge in the common bile duct, producing back pressure of bile in the liver. This, in turn, leads to yellow bile pigment getting into your circulation. The whites of your eyes and your skin turn yellow. This is a form of jaundice.

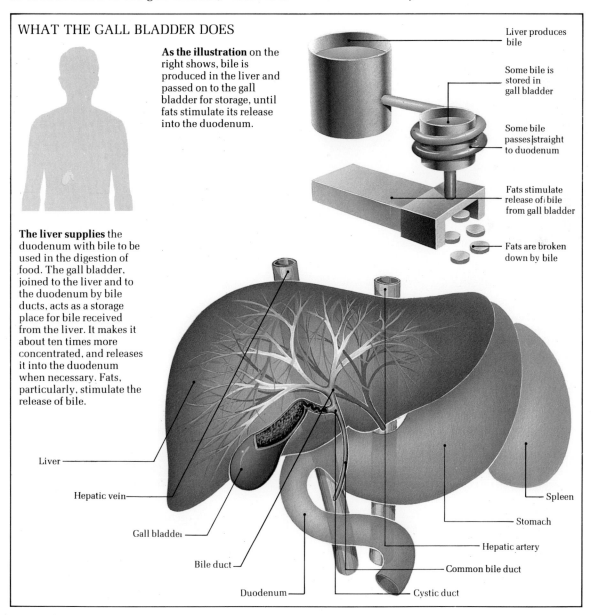

WHAT THE GALL BLADDER DOES

As the illustration on the right shows, bile is produced in the liver and passed on to the gall bladder for storage, until fats stimulate its release into the duodenum.

Liver produces bile

Some bile is stored in gall bladder

Some bile passes straight to duodenum

Fats stimulate release of bile from gall bladder

Fats are broken down by bile

The liver supplies the duodenum with bile to be used in the digestion of food. The gall bladder, joined to the liver and to the duodenum by bile ducts, acts as a storage place for bile received from the liver. It makes it about ten times more concentrated, and releases it into the duodenum when necessary. Fats, particularly, stimulate the release of bile.

Liver

Hepatic vein

Gall bladder

Bile duct

Duodenum

Spleen

Stomach

Hepatic artery

Common bile duct

Cystic duct

So-called 'silent' gall stones cause no symptoms and no trouble. At the other extreme, you may have an attack of acute cholecystitis, with sudden, agonizing pain in the upper part of your abdomen, usually on the right. You may also feel the pain in your right shoulder and shoulder blade, which share the same nerve roots. This is called referred pain. The abdomen will be tender where the gall bladder lies. You are likely to feel sick; usually, you become feverish. You may also be jaundiced, while your faeces may be unusually pale, since they contain no bile pigment.

Diagnosis and treatment

Clinical examination will include your chest as well as your abdomen, since your symptoms fit a number of diseases. A special investigation called a cholecystogram, will confirm the diagnosis (gall stones frequently do not show up on ordinary x-rays).

In acute cholecystitis, you will feel like lying very still. In all forms of the illness, you will find a hotwater bottle gives you some relief. In an acute attack, it is normal to wait for it to subside before embarking on treatment, though you will be given pain relievers by injection. You will not be allowed to eat any solid food and put on a liquid diet.

There are two forms of treatment. Chenodeoxycholic acid, which is taken by mouth, is only given if the stone is not opaque on x-ray and the gall bladder is functioning. Otherwise, an operation to remove the gall bladder is usually necessary. If you have a tendency to overweight – and other people in your immediate family have had gall stones – you would be wise to adopt a low-fat diet.

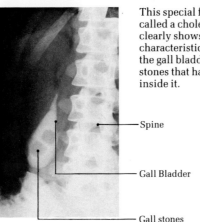

How pressure is created
Gallstones form from some of the constituents of bile. Sometimes they form in the bladder itself, and cause pain as it is prevented from emptying easily. Sometimes they form in the cystic duct and cause the bladder to become inflamed.

Sometimes, as represented here, they form in the common bile duct. This results in a diversion of pressure back onto the liver when the bladder attempts to squeeze bile into the duodenum, so that bile pigment is forced into the circulation. Jaundice is the result.

This special form of X-ray called a cholecystogram clearly shows the characteristic outline of the gall bladder, and the stones that have formed inside it.

Spine

Gall Bladder

Gall stones

PRESCRIPTION

Diagnosis
The main diagnostic tool in determining the presence of gall stones will be a type of X-ray called a cholecystogram.

Treatment
Most forms of gall stones are made partly from cholesterol, and a drug chenodeoxycholic acid can be given which dissolves these stones. This treatment is costly and time-consuming, and for these reasons not often used. If stones cause no trouble then they are normally left as they are. Standard treatment of troublesome ones involves removal of the gall-bladder. It is then impossible for gall-stones to form, as the bile is not allowed to become concentrated enough for this to happen. The main function of bile in the body is to dissolve fats, so it is wise to keep an eye on your intake of these if you have had gall bladder disease.

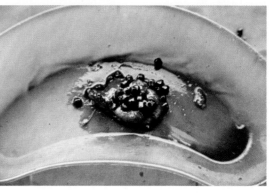

These gallstones, just removed from a bladder, give an idea of the varying sizes of stones.

Peptic Ulcers

A peptic ulcer is the general term used to describe the result of a hole being eroded in the mucous membrane that lines the stomach, the duodenum and other parts of the digestive tract. The type of ulcer produced is defined according to its site; hence, a peptic ulcer in the stomach is called a gastric ulcer, while one in the duodenum is called a duodenal ulcer.

Ulcers arise if the normally-resistant mucous membrane is severely damaged by inbalance between the combined action of the hydro-chloric acid and pepsin which are produced in the stomach to act on food to aid digestion. The commonest sites for such ulcers to develop are the stomach itself and the duodenum, since these are the parts usually exposed to the digestive fluids. Sometimes, however, the contents of the stomach – food, acid and pepsin – run back into the lower part of the oesophagus (gullet); if this happens, an ulcer can form there. There are normally two reasons for this – either pressure on the stomach, as in late pregnancy, or weakness of the ring of muscle at the entrance to the gullet from the stomach.

Three times as many people suffer from duodenal ulcers than gastric ones, while men are four times more likely than women to develop a duodenal ulcer. The highest risk period is between the ages of forty-five, and fifty-five, though about fifteen per cent of people in Western Europe and North America who develop a duodenal ulcer do so before they reach the age of forty.

Physical symptoms

Normally, several factors combine to prevent the acid and pepsin produced in the stomach destroying its lining and that of the duodenum.

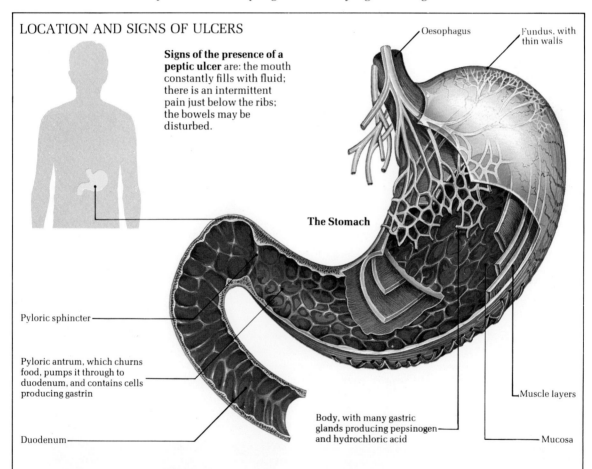

LOCATION AND SIGNS OF ULCERS

Signs of the presence of a peptic ulcer are: the mouth constantly fills with fluid; there is an intermittent pain just below the ribs; the bowels may be disturbed.

Oesophagus

Fundus, with thin walls

The Stomach

Pyloric sphincter

Pyloric antrum, which churns food, pumps it through to duodenum, and contains cells producing gastrin

Duodenum

Body, with many gastric glands producing pepsinogen and hydrochloric acid

Muscle layers

Mucosa

What happens in the stomach

The stomach has three main parts: the fundus, which acts mainly as a reservoir; the body which contains many gastric glands, and is the only place where these glands secrete acid; and the pyloric antrum, which has thick muscle and pumps food through the pyloric sphincter to the small bowel. The stomach only absorbs alcohol and glucose in any quantity, but the gastric glands of the fundus and body are lined by two main sorts of cells; peptic cells produce pepsinogen, which is converted by hydrochloric acid to pepsin and starts the breakdown of proteins; and oxyntic cells, which secrete hydrochloric acid. This also sterilizes, and makes calcium and iron suitable for absorption. Gastric glands in the antrum produce gastrin and alkaline mucus. Gastrin controls acid secretion. Intrinsic factor is also produced. This helps in the absorption of vitamin B12. Mucus cells produce mucus which helps to protect the wall.

The membrane is protected by an additional layer of mucus, while the acid mixture is not normally formed until there is food available to absorb it. The duodenum has an additional safeguard; it produces its own alkaline secretions to neutralize the mixture. The damage which is inevitably caused is speedily repaired by the body's own defences.

Ulcers occur when this natural cycle breaks down. The most important cause of duodenal ulcers is thought to be the excessive production of acid, particularly when the stomach is empty of food. This is probably the result of nervous tension, though irregular meals, excessive smoking and drinking and lack of sleep are all contributory factors. Gastric ulcers are thought to be the result of the stagnation of the digestive juices in the stomach, due to delays in emptying its contents and the regurgitation of bile into the stomach.

With either type of peptic ulcer, your main symptom will be pain just below the ribs, in the center of the body or slightly to the left. Occasionally, the pain may seem as though it is located on the left side of the chest. It comes and goes, with painfree periods between spasms; these can last for days, weeks, months and even years.

The pain rarely appears before breakfast, but usually develops in the late morning and gets worse towards evening. It may wake you at about two in the morning. Food may make it better or worse, but alkaline medicine usually eases it in about ten minutes.

Another common symptom is water brash – an increase in the production of saliva – which fills your mouth with fluid. This is a sympathetic reaction of one part of the digestive system

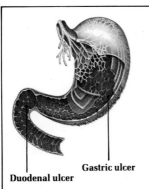

Gastric ulcer
Duodenal ulcer

Where peptic ulcers occur
A gastric ulcer is located in the stomach, a duodenal ulcer in the duodenum. The latter kind is the most common.
Peptic ulcers are caused by an excess of acid which makes a hole in the stomach or duodenal lining.
Acid is normally produced only when there is food in the stomach, and only in quantities sufficient to deal with a specific amount of food.
The duodenum produces alkalis which neutralize the acid received from the stomach, but if the stomach produces acid when it is empty, as seems to happen with a duodenal ulcer, all the acid received by the duodenum will not be neutralized.
Delayed emptying of the stomach and a resulting overproduction of acid or tendency to inflammation may well be linked with gastric ulcers.

How peptic ulcers may occur
In the case of a duodenal ulcer (top) acid passes through the pyloric sphincter to the duodenum, probably in the absence of food but in any case in unusually large quantities. The enzymes in the duodenum are insufficient to neutralize the acid received and the lining is worn away. In the case of a gastric ulcer (bottom) overproduction of acid may be associated with a delay in the passing of food through the pyloric sphincter to the duodenum. In these circumstances inflammation would be likely, and the digestive juices, sitting in the stomach longer than normal, could easily affect the lining.

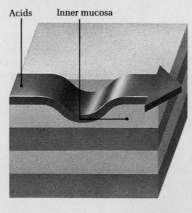

Acids   Inner mucosa

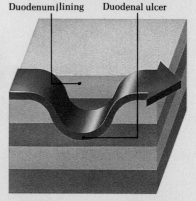

Duodenum lining   Duodenal ulcer

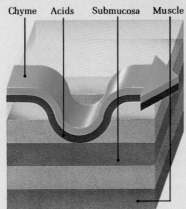

Chyme   Acids   Submucosa   Muscle

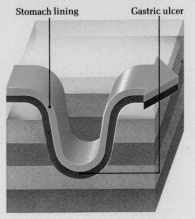

Stomach lining   Gastric ulcer

to another which is under attack. In the same way, you suffer from heartburn, a burning sensation in the gullet, in the chest, while your bowels may be disturbed with pain low in your abdomen.

Diagnosis and treatment

Physical examination will reveal mild tenderness when the doctor presses on the upper part of your abdomen. The clinching diagnosis will be made by barium meal.

The doctor may also carry out a more sophisticated investigation – endoscopy. Biopsies of the edge and surface of the ulcer may be taken to confirm the exact diagnosis and to check that you do not have cancer.

Most ulcers heal if you stop smoking and rest in bed for two or three weeks. Certain drugs can be prescribed to make bed rest unnecessary,

but, the latter is always better. Coffee and tea do no harm, as long as they are not taken on an empty stomach. Diet needs no restriction, except in the avoidance of excess.

There are two reasons for having surgical treatment. The first is if the ulcer shows no signs of healing after treatment or if there is the slightest suspicion of cancer. The other is if there is serious or persistent bleeding, perforation, or if swelling and inflammation of the tissues surrounding the ulcer block the entrance to the stomach.

Immediate side effects from ulcer surgery include diarrhoea, occasional vomiting, a feeling of fullness and faintness after taking food. However, these usually pass. In some patients, a long-term effect is anaemia, caused by poor absorption of vitamin B12. This is easily corrected by regular injections.

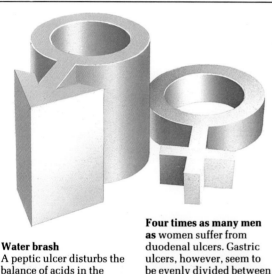

Water brash
A peptic ulcer disturbs the balance of acids in the stomach. Increased saliva production (right) may be a response to this.

Four times as many men as women suffer from duodenal ulcers. Gastric ulcers, however, seem to be evenly divided between the sexes.

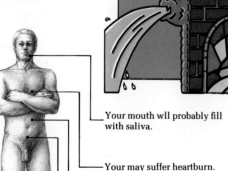

Your mouth wll probably fill with saliva.

Your may suffer heartburn.

You will feel a sporadic pain just below your ribs.

Abdominal pain may disturb your bowels.

PRESCRIPTION

Diagnosis
Your doctor will feel your abdomen to see if there are particularly tender areas.

An internal view can be obtained either by X-ray or by endoscopy. A specimen of tissue may be taken.

Treatment
Most symptoms of a gastric ulcer are caused by the acid produced in the stomach. These can be eased by antacids—that is, alkalis or similar chemicals which render the acid ineffective. Drugs can also be given which inhibit acid secretion. However, none of these get at the root cause of the trouble, and the most important treatment is rest, preferably in bed. The most important dietary consideration is that of quantity and frequency of food intake. Regular, small

meals are advisable. Light meals with a high nutritious content will assist general health.

If these methods fail, surgical treatment may be necessary. In the case of a gastric ulcer, the lower stomach, that produces most acid, might be removed. For a duodenal, an operation might be carried out to by-pass the duodenum. The vagus nerves which stimulate acid secretion may be cut. Anaemia caused by an ulcer bleeding may need separate treatment.

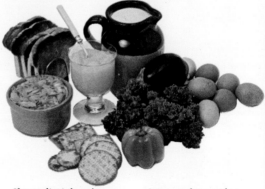

If your diet is based on heavy meals containing lots of fats and spices, it will probably help to alter

it to more frequent but much lighter meals containing milk and more bland foods.

Hernia

A hernia is the name doctors give to what happens when an organ from one part of the body protrudes into another. Laymen sometimes refer to this as rupture, but this is misleading, as nothing is, in fact, torn. The most usual form, for example, occurs when a loop of intestine and its immediate coverings bulge through a weakened part of the abdomen wall to form a lump under the skin. This need not be continuously present, as the loop can slip back into the abdomen.

Types of hernia are classified according to their site (for one of these, hiatus hernia, see p. 50). The commonest site is in the groin and the commonest type is inguinal hernia – four-fifths of all hernias are inguinal. Inguinal hernia nearly always occurs in males; it can happen in infants, or, more frequently, in middle-aged men and over.

Physical symptoms

Weakness of the muscle ring surrounding various abdominal openings in the groin, the upper inside thigh, or the navel is the underlying factor in all hernias. In inguinal hernia, for instance, muscular weakness is the root cause of both types – oblique and direct.

The former is the commonest. In it, the intestinal loop pushes its way down the inguinal canal. The direct type occurs when the loop of intestine forces its way between the fibers near the inguinal canal. Sometimes, a pouch is formed. In a femoral hernia, the weak spot is the femoral canal and ring.

The first thing you are likely to notice is a small lump or bulge in your groin (or at the navel or old abdominal scar, depending on the type of hernia). This need not always be present. If you are digging in the garden, say, or

THE DIFFERENT SORTS OF HERNIA

The structure of a hernia.
A rupture or hernia is a protrusion of gut or other abdominal contents through a weak portion of abdominal wall. It has three parts (see right): the hernial sac, a layer of peritoneum; the sac's contents, normally a loop of intestine; and the hernial coverings, made up of the wall through which

the gut has passed. The main sorts of hernia are: direct inguinal, indirect inguinal, femoral and umbilical. Indirect inguinal are the most common, affecting one woman for every twenty men. Direct inguinal hernias are very rare in women. Femoral hernias and umbilical hernias are more common in women.

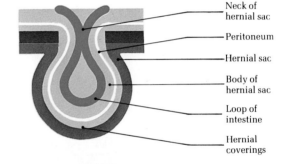

Neck of hernial sac

Peritoneum

Hernial sac

Body of hernial sac

Loop of intestine

Hernial coverings

Femoral hernias
The femoral canal is a weaker area where the abdomen meets the thigh. Peritoneum pushes through it, in the event of a femoral hernia. It shows itself as a swelling in the upper thigh.
A hernia is strangulated if the femoral ring constrains the blood vessels in a piece of bowel. This condition is serious and speedy surgery is important.

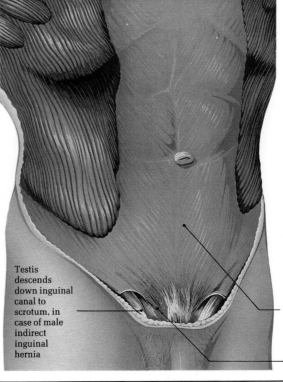

Femoral sheath

Inguinal ligament

Femoral ring

Femoral artery

Femoral vein

Femoral canal

Great saphenous vein

Testis descends down inguinal canal to scrotum, in case of male indirect inguinal hernia

Inguinal and umbilical hernias
In an indirect inguinal hernia – the most common kind of hernia – the sac body rests in the inguinal canal or scrotum, or, in the case of a woman, the labium majus.
The hernial sac of a direct inguinal hernia is restrained by the strong conjoint tendon. Old men with weak abdominal muscles are prone to this complaint.
Umbilical hernias of newborn children normally right themselves. In adults, the hernial sac protrudes at the linea alba near the navel and tends to gradually increase in size.

Linea alba, the site of umbilical hernias in adults

Inguinal ligament

have an acute coughing bout, you may feel the hernia descend; if you lie down for an hour or so, or go to bed at night, the hernia may temporarily disappear.

A hernia is likely to get bigger as it stretches and can reach a stage where it is present from the moment you get out of bed. Though it may drag and ache, you will have no real pain, unless it becomes strangulated. This is the chief danger in the disease. What happens is that the hernia becomes twisted, swollen or caught by a constricted muscle ring. As a result, the intestine is obstructed and, worse still, the blood supply is interrupted, with the resultant risk of gangrene unless prompt surgical action is taken. Physical symptoms are acute pain, with complete blockage of the bowels if there is an obstruction. The lump will be tender to touch and you will feel increasingly ill.

Diagnosis and treatment

If your doctor suspects you have a hernia, he or she will make you stand up and cough to see if there is an increase of pressure over the swelling as a result. Alternatively, this will make the hernia appear if it is not visible. If the bulge is there, he will want to find out if it is reducible – that is, if it can be pushed or eased back into the abdomen when you are lying down.

You can help by dieting and exercising if you are overweight. The main treatment, however, is surgical. The hernia and contents are returned to their rightful place inside the abdomen and the hole or split through which they escaped is sewn up. If the muscles and tissues of the abdominal wall are too fragile to repair effectively, grafts from another part of the body are used. A truss – a surgical belt with a pad to support the weak place—can be used.

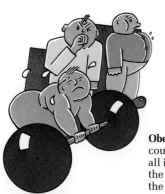

Obesity, extended coughing and heavy lifting all increase the pressure on the abdomen and increase the chances of a hernia.

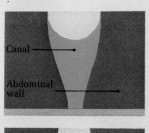
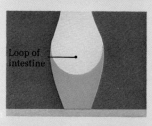
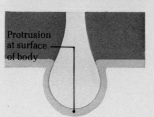

Canal

Abdominal wall

Loop of intestine

Protrusion at surface of body

Both inguinal and femoral canals are weak points in the abdominal wall down which a loop of intestine may travel (see left). The loop of intestine is shown in stages of advancement down a canal until it bulges into the abdominal wall. The femoral canal contains lymphatic vessels. The inguinal canal in men is the path by which the testes descend. In women it contains the ligament attached to the womb.

PRESCRIPTION

Diagnosis
The doctor will ask you to cough at the same time as he

or she feels the painful or swollen area. Any increase in pressure will be noted.

Treatment
Even if a hernia is no more than uncomfortable, the symptoms should be given attention, because of the danger of strangulation. The normal method of dealing

with the condition involves surgery. The parted muscle walls are brought together again. Care should obviously be taken for a long time afterwards with exercises such as lifting.

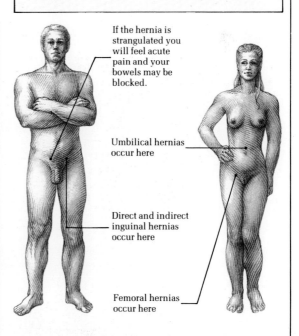

If the hernia is strangulated you will feel acute pain and your bowels may be blocked.

Umbilical hernias occur here

Direct and indirect inguinal hernias occur here

Femoral hernias occur here

The signs of a hernia.
The first sign of a hernia will probably be a bulge in the groin, or at the navel. It may then disappear, but is

more likely to increase in size. It will not be painful unless the blood supply to the hernial sac is restricted.

Hiatus Hernia

Hiatus hernia is a protrusion of a small part of the stomach through an opening – hiatus – in the diaphragm, a strong layer of muscle and ligamentous tissue separating the chest and the abdomen. The opening occurs at the junction between the oesophagus (gullet) and the stomach, the diaphragm's weakest point.

Hiatus hernia is extremely common, the likelihood of its incidence increasing with age. In five out of six cases, it is symptomless and the vast majority of cases cause no trouble. It is especially likely to strike the overweight; the chief victims are middle-aged, flabby women – three times as many women as men suffer from the disease – who often have borne children.

Physical symptoms

In eighty per cent of cases of hiatus hernia, the join of gullet and stomach protrudes upwards into the chest, taking with it an attached bag of stomach of variable size. In other cases, the gullet-stomach join remains in the right place at the level of the diaphragm, but a pouch of stomach pokes upwards into the chest next to it through the same gap.

Although many people ascribe all kinds of symptoms to the presence of hiatus hernia, there is no reason to think of it as anything more abnormal than sagging breasts or a bulging abdomen. The only reason for symptoms showing themselves is if there is reflux – backflow – of the acid contents of the stomach into the oesophagus.

The lining of the oesophagus is less resistant than that of the stomach itself to the effects of the acid and digestive juices that are mixed with food during the course of digestion. As a result, you may develop oesophagitis—inflam-

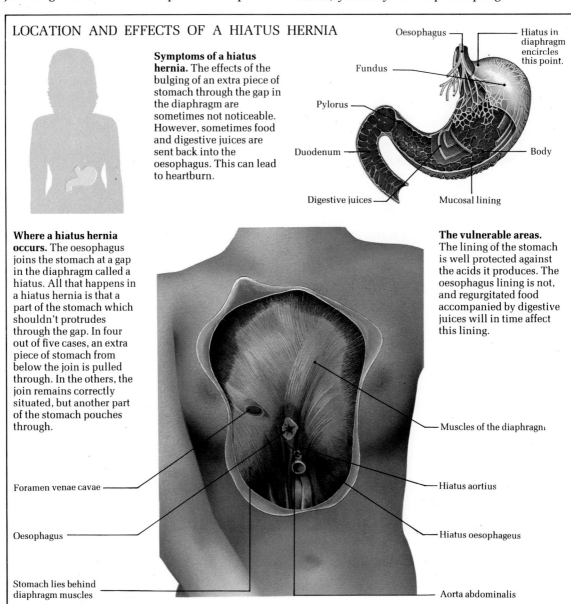

LOCATION AND EFFECTS OF A HIATUS HERNIA

Symptoms of a hiatus hernia. The effects of the bulging of an extra piece of stomach through the gap in the diaphragm are sometimes not noticeable. However, sometimes food and digestive juices are sent back into the oesophagus. This can lead to heartburn.

Oesophagus — Hiatus in diaphragm encircles this point.

Fundus

Pylorus

Duodenum

Digestive juices

Mucosal lining

Body

Where a hiatus hernia occurs. The oesophagus joins the stomach at a gap in the diaphragm called a hiatus. All that happens in a hiatus hernia is that a part of the stomach which shouldn't protrudes through the gap. In four out of five cases, an extra piece of stomach from below the join is pulled through. In the others, the join remains correctly situated, but another part of the stomach pouches through.

The vulnerable areas. The lining of the stomach is well protected against the acids it produces. The oesophagus lining is not, and regurgitated food accompanied by digestive juices will in time affect this lining.

Muscles of the diaphragm

Foramen venae cavae

Hiatus aortius

Oesophagus

Hiatus oesophageus

Stomach lies behind diaphragm muscles

Aorta abdominalis

mation of the lower end of the gullet – and, very rarely, a PEPTIC ULCER. Hot foods and alcohol make the symptoms worse.

Various vague symptoms may frequently be blamed on hiatus hernia without justification. If there is reflux, you may suffer from heartburn, a burning feeling in the gullet behind the breastbone and bring back acid material and food without vomiting. This happens if you stoop down or lie flat, especially on your right side, after a meal.

If you are developing oesophagitis, you may get pain, especially after irritating food and drink, low down behind the breastbone. If there is oozing of blood from the inflamed surface, you may become anaemic through loss of iron and feel tired. If there is swelling and scarring, you may develop a stricture which will cause difficulty in swallowing, but this is uncommon.

Diagnosis and treatment

Apart from making a careful general examination, your doctor will want you to have a special x-ray – a barium swallow and meal. You will be filmed as you swallow liquid that is opaque to x-rays to show up the presence of a hernia. Similarly, you will be asked to tilt your head down or the doctor will press on your abdomen to test for reflux. Sometimes, oesophagoscopy – passing a tube to look inside the gullet – is needed to clinch the diagnosis.

Most of the treatment is self-administered. If you are overweight, reduce by dieting carefully. Take only small amounts of food at any one time. Raise the head of your bed and, at the same time, put a bolster at the foot and use nonslip sheets and nightwear. Your doctor will supply antacids and other suitable medications. Rarely, surgery may be necessary.

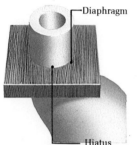
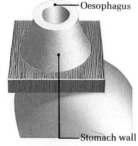

Diaphragm — Oesophagus — Hiatus — Stomach wall

The part of the stomach that forces its way through the hiatus in a hiatus hernia is normally that portion which meets the oesophagus, as the simple representation above shows.

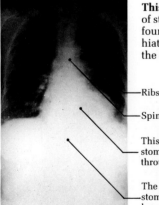

This X-ray shows a portion of stomach tissue that has found its way through the hiatus, the weakest part of the diaphragm.

Ribs

Spine

This 'D' shaped area of stomach has been pushed through the diaphragm.

The protruding area of stomach would normally be here.

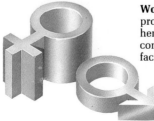

Women are three times as prone as men to hiatus hernia. Obesity is a common contributory factor.

PRESCRIPTION

Diagnosis
Your doctor will send you for a special X-ray which has to be preceded by your being given barium sulphate—a 'barium meal'—which shows up on X-rays. This will enable the hernia to be detected. He or she may also test to see if your stomach is throwing food back into your oesophagus, or even examine your oesophagus with a specially designed instrument.

Treatment
If you have a hiatus hernia you probably have a tendency towards obesity, and it is important to slim down. If the condition is causing indigestion, you should keep your meals small.

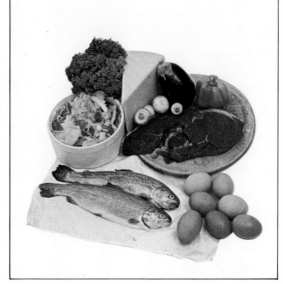

Appendicitis

Appendicitis is acute inflammation of the appendix, an earthworm-like organ extending from the caecum, the beginning of the large intestine in the right lower corner of the abdomen. Acute appendicitis, or a ruptured appendix, can lead to peritonitis, an acute inflammation of the membrane lining the abdomen and covering the viscera. This is a serious medical emergency, requiring urgent treatment.

Although appendicitis can occur at any age and in either sex, its peak period of incidence is between ten and forty. It is a particularly dangerous disease for children between the ages of ten and fourteen.

Physical symptoms

The appendix is a vestigial organ. Its original purpose was to help with the digestion of grasses, but it no longer plays any useful role in bodily functions. All it consists of is a narrow tube with a blind end; from this, it is easy to see how a hard fragment of waste material, a pip, or a fruit stone passing down the intestine may get stuck in the appendix.

Once the appendix is blocked, its wall swells up, making matters even worse. Infecting organisms settle and multiply in the part that is cut off, coming either from the bowel itself or via the blood stream.

A long appendix may get kinked or caught up in a band of peritoneum, the lining membrane of the abdomen. Whatever the cause of blockage, the results are the same.

The first physical sign of developing appendicitis is likely to be a cramping pain around the navel. You will not feel like eating, you will be likely to feel sick and may even vomit once or twice. A few hours later, the pain will shift

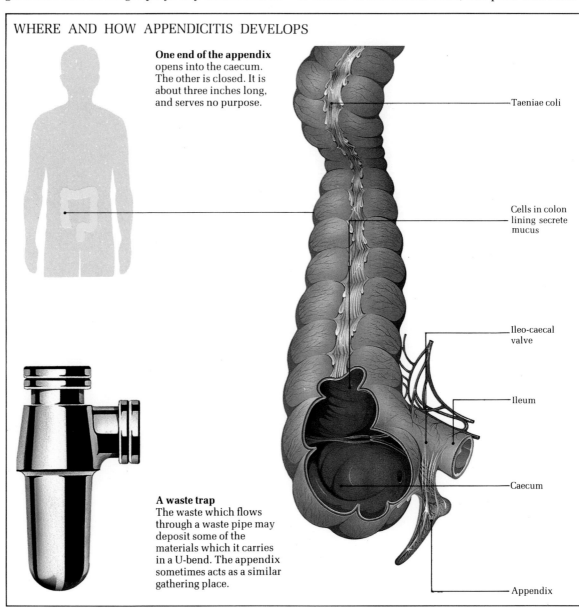

WHERE AND HOW APPENDICITIS DEVELOPS

One end of the appendix opens into the caecum. The other is closed. It is about three inches long, and serves no purpose.

Taeniae coli

Cells in colon lining secrete mucus

Ileo-caecal valve

Ileum

Caecum

Appendix

A waste trap
The waste which flows through a waste pipe may deposit some of the materials which it carries in a U-bend. The appendix sometimes acts as a similar gathering place.

52

to the lower part of the abdomen; this means that the peritoneum, which is sensitive to pain, has become inflamed over the appendix.

Later on, you may develop a mild fever – 37.5°C (99°F) on average – your tongue will be furred and you will be tender on the right side of the abdomen. Sometimes, if the appendix is running backwards, you may have the pain in the back instead of the abdomen. Wherever it lies, you may have constipation.

Diagnosis and treatment

Appendicitis is the commonest acute abdominal emergency and is sometimes difficult to diagnose. Children, in particular, find it difficult to say exactly where they feel the pain, while kidney infection, gastro-enteritis and some chest disorders may have similar symptoms and vice versa. There are no medical tests that your doctor can use to confirm the diagnosis, so he or she depends on physical examination plus what you are able to tell him.

The only safe treatment for appendicitis is surgical removal; rupture and peritonitis may result if the condition is left untreated. This does not involve much risk, especially below middle age. Bed rest and treatment with antibiotics is the only alternative, but the operation is always preferable. Many surgeons will remove the appendix if abdominal surgery is being carried out for other reasons – even if it is perfectly normal. The practice is controversial, but the reasoning is that, as the organ has no proven useful function, it is better to remove it.

Doctors today do not believe that there is such a condition as chronic appendicitis, or grumbling appendix; it is, however, possible to have repeated attacks.

The progress of appendicitis. These illustrations show how inflammation can follow a blocking of the appendix opening.

1. Waste matter passes by peristalsis through the colon. Nearly all the nutrients have been taken out. The appendix opens into the colon.

2. The hollow appendix serves no purpose but can be a source of danger if affected by bacteria.

3. Waste material caught up in the appendix and prevented from being expelled by a blockage will soon cause inflammation and build up of bacteria.

4. Inflammation and swelling can become severe. At this stage the pain will be great and treatment is imperative.

Waste matter passes into colon

Appendix

Peritoneum

The opening to the appendix becomes blocked by a piece of waste material

Infection settles in

Wall of appendix swells

Swelling of wall increases. Peritoneum may become inflamed. This will cause pain.

1   2   3   4

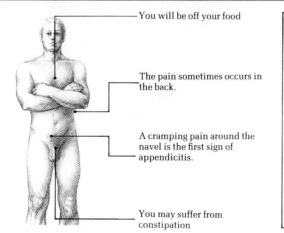

You will be off your food

The pain sometimes occurs in the back.

A cramping pain around the navel is the first sign of appendicitis.

You may suffer from constipation

PRESCRIPTION

Diagnosis
Your doctor will depend on your description of your symptoms and on feeling around the affected area to make a diagnosis.

Treatment
The need for surgery in appendicitis is extremely urgent, because of the danger that the appendix might burst. This could result in infection so widespread that the patient dies. Even if your doctor is not certain that your symptoms indicate appendicitis, he or she may recommend an operation. If it is not possible to operate on a patient, he is best kept half-sitting, so that infection only reaches those places where it can do least harm. He will not be allowed food, but will be given antibiotics.

Acute Gastro-enteritis

Acute gastro-enteritis, inflammation of the stomach and the intestines, is the second common group illness to affect the community. Colds and other acute respiratory infections hold first place. There are many different types of the disease, some being infectious and the others non-infectious. Infectious gastro-enteritis is the commonest; it includes summer diarrhoea, travellers' diarrhoea, gastric 'flu and infantile diarrhoea.

The disease is usually caused by bacteria, parasites or viruses, but toxins and allergies may be responsible too. Salmonella gastro-enteritis, for instance, is caused by the bacterial organism *Salmonella typhimurium*, which is responsible for seventy-five per cent of outbreaks of so-called food poisoning. What happens is that the food in question is contaminated by a human or animal carrier, bacteria being passed to their victim when the food is eaten.

Typhoid and paratyphoid fevers are caused by other types of Salmonella organisms, while all types of dysentery are viral infections. The severest of these is cholera, a tropical disorder; amoebic dysentery and giardiasis occur in hot countries from the tropics to Spain.

Non-infective gastro-enteritis can be the result of staphylococcal food poisoning and botulism. In this, bacterial toxins or poisons remain in the food, even though the organisms may have been killed by cooking or processing. Another non-infectious type is allergy – for instance, to shellfish, eggs or strawberries.

Physical symptoms

The main physical symptoms of gastro-enteritis are caused by the response of the digestive

WHERE AND HOW ACUTE GASTRO-ENTERITIS OCCURS

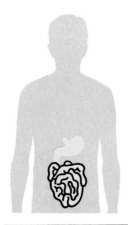

Causes and effects
In gastro-enteritis the stomach and intestine are inflamed. Vomiting and diarrhoea occur and there will be pains in the affected area. Eating food contaminated with bacteria and food allergies as well as virus infections are amongst the causes.

When eating abroad it is important to remember that local people may have built up a resistance which visitors do not have.

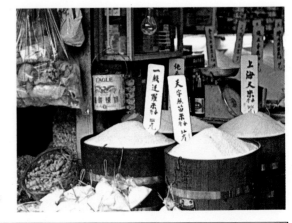

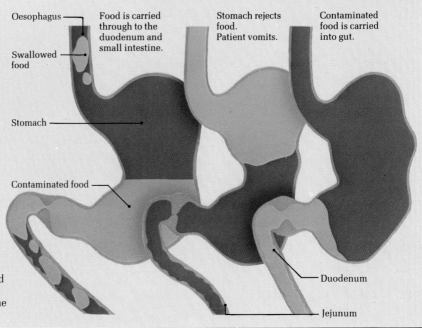

The digestive system reacts to contaminated food by attempting to remove it from the body via mouth or anus.

1. Harmful bacteria are carried in food into the stomach. Peristalsis begins, and some are carried into the small intestine.

2. The stomach detects the presence of the bacteria and expels its contents by causing vomiting.

3. The food that has passed into the small intestine is quickly expelled. It is not allowed to become firm in the colon, and is passed in the form of diarrhoea.

Oesophagus

Swallowed food

Stomach

Contaminated food

Food is carried through to the duodenum and small intestine.

Stomach rejects food.
Patient vomits.

Contaminated food is carried into gut.

Duodenum

Jejunum

system to poisons, a bacterial toxin, or infecting organisms inside it. If this happens, the system tries to expel them by vomiting and diarrhoea. The symptoms vary according to the seriousness of the attack; they can be so intense that you are in a state of collapse or so mild as to have only a nuisance value.

If you are suffering from infectious gastro-enteritis, you are likely to be feverish. You may have vomiting or diarrhoea or both together in either type, or vomiting first and diarrhoea a day later. Your abdomen may be distended and tender – you may have a severe cramping pain or merely an ache – while your faeces may contain blood, mucus or other abnormalities.

Diagnosis and treatment
If your case is part of an epidemic, your doctor will be aware of it. He or she will want to know if you have travelled abroad recently and may take a stool sample and a blood test.

Actual treatment depends on the severity of the attack. If specific antibiotic treatment is needed, it will be given, but antibiotics can be ineffective. If, as can happen in rare cases, the disease is highly infectious, you will be isolated in hospital until bacteriological tests prove negative three times running.

If you are in bed at home, avoid all solids until the acute symptoms have subsided. It is vital to keep up your fluid intake with fruit drinks (a teaspoonful of salt per pint may be added initially). You will need to rest in the warm. It is usually better to let the diarrhoea settle by itself, but a mild binding agent can be useful. When you can eat again, gradually work up to a highly-nutritious diet, with plenty of protein, sweet foods and vitamin supplements.

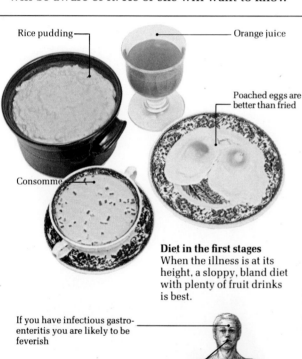

Rice pudding

Orange juice

Poached eggs are better than fried

Consomme

Diet in the first stages
When the illness is at its height, a sloppy, bland diet with plenty of fruit drinks is best.

If you have infectious gastro-enteritis you are likely to be feverish

Vomiting and diarrhoea are both possible

Your stomach will probably ache

The abdomen may be distended and tender

Loss of fluid may cause collapse

PRESCRIPTION

Diagnosis
Your blood and faeces may be tested . Your doctor will want to know if you have been travelling where you may have had no inbuilt resistance to local organisms.

Treatment
When the disease is at its most severe the patient will not be able to retain, or, for that matter, take in, anything but a very bland diet. Solids should be avoided altogether at first, but it is important to guard against the dehydration that can occur in severe cases, and keep up your fluid intake. When you are recovering you will need to build yourself up again. Foods with high protein and vitamin content will be important.

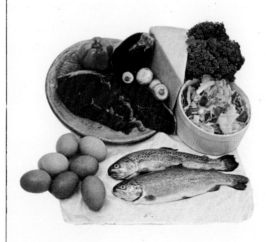

A nutritious diet with lots of proteins and vitamins is important once recovery is under way. The proteins will help to build up body tissue. They can sometimes be burnt for energy, but only if there are not enough 'energy' foods like bread, rice or potatoes. Vitamins are needed for chemical reactions of the body.

Cancer of the Stomach

Cancer of the stomach is a malignant tumor, which may form an ulcer, an outgrowth often near the entrance to the stomach, or a general thickening throughout the stomach lining. The disease is one of the commonest forms of cancer, second only to CANCER OF THE LUNG in men and CANCER OF THE BREAST in women.

In common with other cancers, there is more likelihood of stomach cancer developing in later life. It is twice as common in men as in women, occurring mainly after the age of fifty and reaching a peak in the seventies. Though its cause is unknown, it is thought that heredity and environment are both contributing factors. If you have a blood relation with stomach cancer, there is a more than average risk of you developing the disease. As far as environment is concerned, it is thought that diet is significant; Japan, for example, has one of the highest rates of stomach cancer in the world, while Japanese settled in the USA have a far lower incidence of the disease. This is probably because Western diets contain elements missing from the native Japanese one.

Higher risk can also stem from medical causes. People with blood group A seem more susceptible to the disease than others; so, too, do sufferers from pernicious anaemia and achlorhydria (the absence of hydrochloric acid in stomach secretions).

Physical symptoms

The symptoms of stomach cancer can be often hard to detect until the disease has reached a fairly advanced stage. You are likely to go off your food and feel uncomfortably full after even a small meal. You will feel lethargic and you may lose weight – cancer causes weight

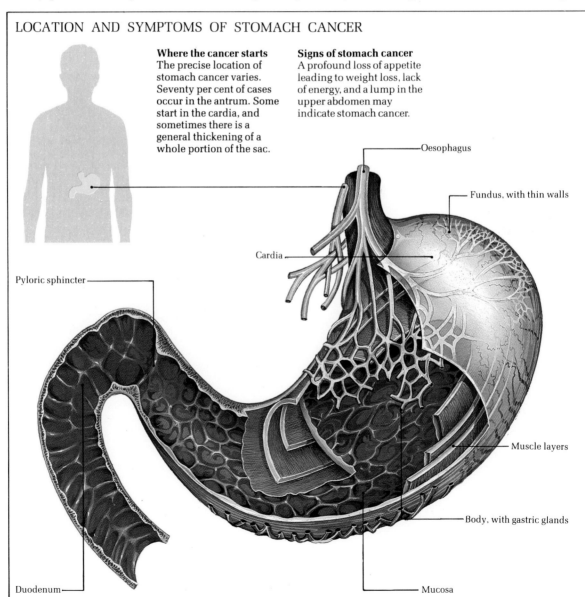

LOCATION AND SYMPTOMS OF STOMACH CANCER

Where the cancer starts
The precise location of stomach cancer varies. Seventy per cent of cases occur in the antrum. Some start in the cardia, and sometimes there is a general thickening of a whole portion of the sac.

Signs of stomach cancer
A profound loss of appetite leading to weight loss, lack of energy, and a lump in the upper abdomen may indicate stomach cancer.

Oesophagus

Fundus, with thin walls

Cardia

Pyloric sphincter

Muscle layers

Body, with gastric glands

Duodenum

Mucosa

loss *and* distinct loss of appetite. The first medical symptom may be anaemia. You may have difficulty in swallowing, as people do with gullet problems; alternatively, if you are thin, the first physical sign of the disease may be a lump in the upper abdomen.

Diagnosis and treatment

Though in theory stomach cancer should be easy to treat, early diagnosis is all-important. If the cancer is allowed to reach an advanced stage, the prognosis is extremely poor. A barium meal, as prescribed for PEPTIC ULCER, will usually reveal the presence of a stomach tumor, but, if there is any doubt, a gastroenterologist – a physician with particular expertise in this field – will examine you internally and take samples (biopsies) with an instrument called an endoscope. Blood tests may show

anaemia, lack of protein and other characteristic abnormalities associated with the disease.

Prevention, however, is far better than early diagnosis and cure. Careful control of diet can help. Vomiting is an important symptom, as are other stomach upsets. Sufferers from benign gastric disturbances should take particular care, especially after the age of fifty; benign symptoms can sometimes mask the outset of disease.

In some cases, surgical removal of part of the stomach is the best treatment, followed by radiotherapy and/or chemotherapy. The former kills the cancer cells directly by radiation; the latter kills them by interfering with their metabolism. Both these forms of treatment may make you feel temporarily sick. The outlook varies, depending more on the type of tumor cell than on how long you have had it.

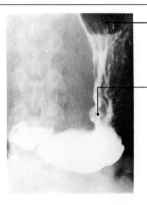

Black area indicates air in the top of the stomach.

The crater is the cancer growth. The crater has raised edges

The raised edges around the crater indicate that the patient has cancer rather than, say, an ulcer.

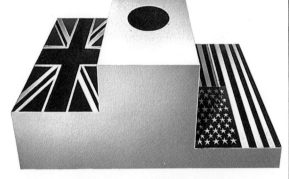

Stomach cancer is more common in Japan than in the UK or USA. Diet may partly explain this.

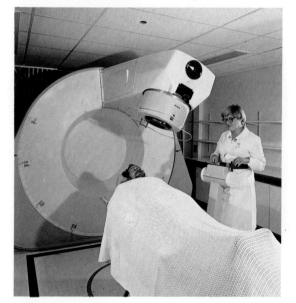

Radiotherapy
If it is necessary to remove part of the stomach this treatment will be followed by radiotherapy or chemotherapy to kill remaining cancerous cells and so prevent recurrence.

PRESCRIPTION

Diagnosis
Your doctor will send you for a blood test, and an X-ray, which will be preceded by a barium meal. Endoscopy—internal examination by means of a lighted tube, which allows your stomach to be seen directly—may also be used.

Treatment
The best chance of a permanent cure is still afforded by surgical treatment. The cancer, along with any tissue that it may have affected, is removed. Radiotherapy or chemotherapy will probably be necessary. This treatment is designed to destroy cancer cells. Both have side-effects of making the patient feel unwell, but these effects wear off. Your doctor will inform you of any dietary requirements made necessary.

Nervous/Introduction

The nervous system's working tissue comprises cells called neurones. Such cells transmit impulses to other cells. The central system, that is the brain and spinal cord, contains the cell bodies. These bodies are attached to fibers or axons which conduct messages. Some axons are very long – from the spine to the foot, for example. A nerve is a bundle of these fibers, some of which conduct impulses towards the brain (sensory), some of which conduct them from the brain (motor). Most fibers are coated in a myelin sheath, which gives them a white appearance. Those that are not – the very thin fibers – are grey. All the nerves branch from 31 pairs arising in the spinal cord and 12 cranial nerves arising in the brain. The autonomic nervous system, connected in the brain with the central system, regulates such reflex activities as digestion, respiration and blood circulation.

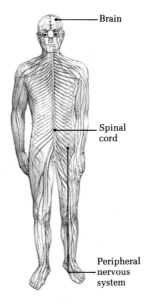

Brain
Spinal cord
Peripheral nervous system

The nervous system is concerned with the acquisition of information from and the sending of instructions to all parts of the body. The brain and spinal cord form the central part of the system. The central system receives, processes and acts on the information received from the peripheral nervous system. The afferent nerves in the peripheral system transmit sensory information. The efferent motor nerves carry instructions.

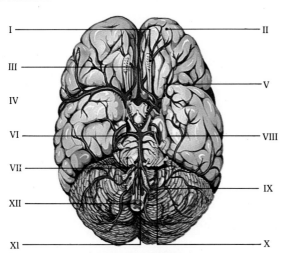

I
III
IV
VI
VII
XII
XI
II
V
VIII
IX
X

The cranial nerves
The head, neck and major organs of the body are supplied by the twelve cranial nerves which lead into the underside of the brain. Their functions are as follows:
I Sense of smell (sensory);
II Optic nerve (sensory);
III, IV & VI Eye muscles (sensory and motor);
V Chewing and facial sensations (sensory and motor);
VII Facial expression; taste in front two thirds of tongue (sensory and motor); VIII Auditory (sensory) and vestibular (concerned with balance); IX Muscles of swallowing; taste and sensation in back of tongue (sensory and motor);
X Chest and abdominal organs; parasympathetic (sensory and motor); palate and larynx;
XI Neck muscles (motor);
XII Tongue movement (motor).

How nerve signals are transmitted.
The electrical signal travels down the axon surface until it reaches the synapse with the muscle at the muscle end plate. A chemical is released from the nerve axon and travels over to the muscle. When enough of the chemical (called a transmitter) has arrived at the muscle a new electrical signal starts. This is then transmitted within the muscle to start contraction.

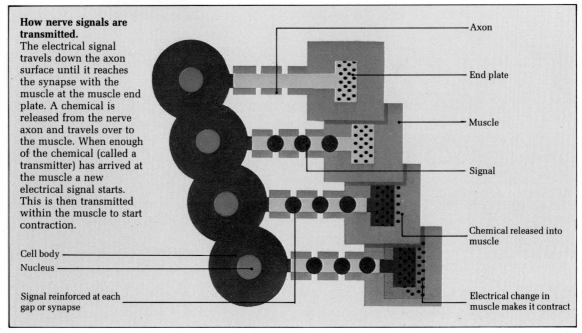

Axon
End plate
Muscle
Signal
Chemical released into muscle
Electrical change in muscle makes it contract

Cell body
Nucleus
Signal reinforced at each gap or synapse

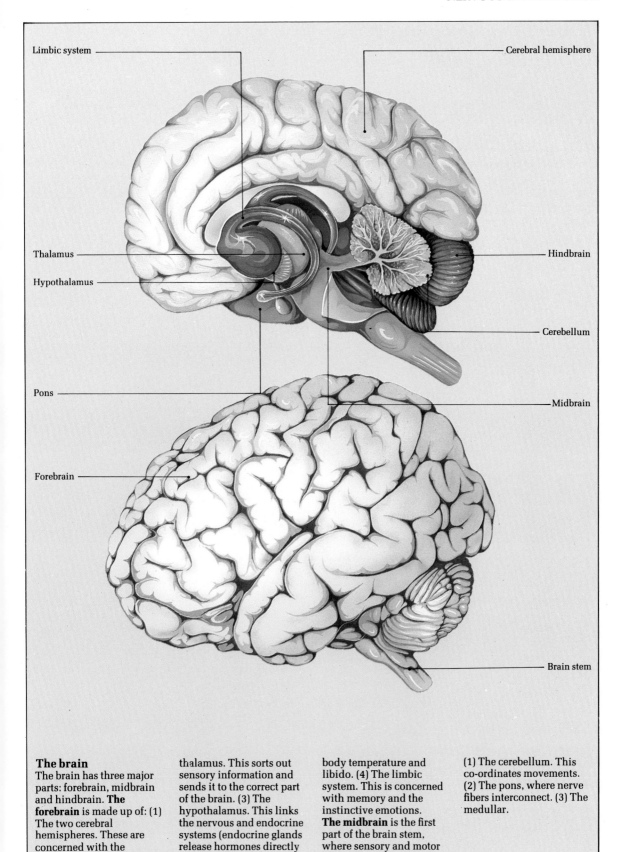

Limbic system

Cerebral hemisphere

Thalamus

Hypothalamus

Hindbrain

Cerebellum

Pons

Midbrain

Forebrain

Brain stem

The brain

The brain has three major parts: forebrain, midbrain and hindbrain. **The forebrain** is made up of: (1) The two cerebral hemispheres. These are concerned with the 'higher' mental functions involving logic and creativity. (2) The thalamus. This sorts out sensory information and sends it to the correct part of the brain. (3) The hypothalamus. This links the nervous and endocrine systems (endocrine glands release hormones directly into the blood stream) and it contains centers to control appetite, thirst, body temperature and libido. (4) The limbic system. This is concerned with memory and the instinctive emotions. **The midbrain** is the first part of the brain stem, where sensory and motor nerve fibers cross to supply opposite sides of the body. **The hindbrain** contains: (1) The cerebellum. This co-ordinates movements. (2) The pons, where nerve fibers interconnect. (3) The medullar.

Multiple Sclerosis

Multiple sclerosis is a mysterious disease. It can last on and off for many years, acute attacks being followed by periods of remission. Its exact cause is unknown, though some doctors think it is caused by a slow-acting virus to which the victim's body has an inbuilt lack of immunity. The disease affects the outer covering of the nerve fibers around scattered small areas of the brain, the nerve leading directly from it and the nerves of the spinal cord. In extreme cases, the areas involved can be destroyed and replaced by scar tissue (scleroses); the nerves involved cease to function. The results may be noticeable anywhere in the body – hence the old name for the disease was disseminated sclerosis.

Physical symptoms
To understand what happens in multiple sclerosis, it is essential to understand something of the workings of the nervous system. This consists of two parts – the central nervous system and the peripheral nervous system. The former comprises the brain, the brain stem and spinal cord, together with the cranial, or head, nerves, including the optic nerve. The latter consists of the nerve fibers running through your limbs and skin, which are ultimately dependent on cells in the central nervous system. If the central nervous system is damaged in any way, the peripheral nerves may be put out of action; if a peripheral nerve is damaged, however, this affects only the local area which that nerve serves.

Thus, although it is the central nervous system which is affected by multiple sclerosis, the results can be seen in the peripheral nervous system as well. The central system con-

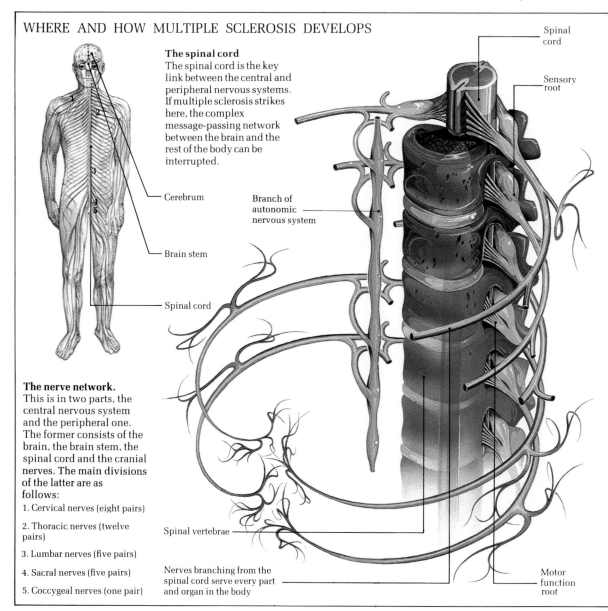

WHERE AND HOW MULTIPLE SCLEROSIS DEVELOPS

The spinal cord
The spinal cord is the key link between the central and peripheral nervous systems. If multiple sclerosis strikes here, the complex message-passing network between the brain and the rest of the body can be interrupted.

Cerebrum

Brain stem

Spinal cord

The nerve network.
This is in two parts, the central nervous system and the peripheral one. The former consists of the brain, the brain stem, the spinal cord and the cranial nerves. The main divisions of the latter are as follows:

1. Cervical nerves (eight pairs)

2. Thoracic nerves (twelve pairs)

3. Lumbar nerves (five pairs)

4. Sacral nerves (five pairs)

5. Coccygeal nerves (one pair)

Branch of autonomic nervous system

Spinal vertebrae

Nerves branching from the spinal cord serve every part and organ in the body

Spinal cord

Sensory root

Motor function root

sists of nerve cells, with long fibers growing out of them. These are coated with individual sheaths of a protective, insulating material called myelin. If these myelin sheaths are destroyed by disease, or deteriorate, the nerves cannot work properly and scars form in the nervous tissue. At this stage, when the myelin is actively breaking down, the symptoms of multiple sclerosis are at their worst; they become less, or disappear altogether, when a scar has formed.

What the symptoms of multiple sclerosis are depends upon where in the central nervous system the myelin is deficient and to what extent it has become so. The disease may not cause any symptoms at all and its victim may feel perfectly healthy. However, any function of the nervous system – sensation, movement, emotions – can be upset. One symptom may reveal itself in one part of this system only, or the effects may be scattered.

Usually the optic nerve, the nerve of your eye, is the first to be noticeably affected. You feel pain in or around one eye and your sight in that eye becomes progressively dulled over a week or so. After that time, however, your sight begins to improve and, in most cases, it is back to normal within two or three months after the initial attack.

Other early symptoms may include double vision or giddiness. These are the result of scarring in the brain stem; like the eye symptoms, these almost always disappear after a time. You may find your muscular co-ordination affected, making writing, say, difficult or even impossible.

If plaques of multiple sclerosis have formed in your spinal cord, you may notice that one of

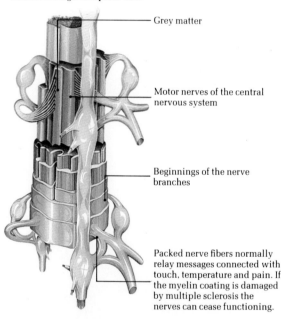

Section through the spinal cord

Grey matter

Motor nerves of the central nervous system

Beginnings of the nerve branches

Packed nerve fibers normally relay messages connected with touch, temperature and pain. If the myelin coating is damaged by multiple sclerosis the nerves can cease functioning.

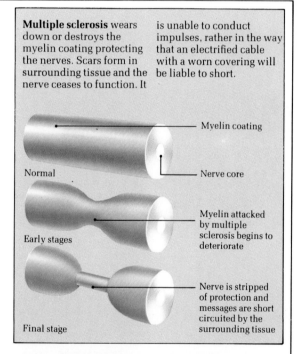

Multiple sclerosis wears down or destroys the myelin coating protecting the nerves. Scars form in surrounding tissue and the nerve ceases to function. It is unable to conduct impulses, rather in the way that an electrified cable with a worn covering will be liable to short.

Myelin coating

Normal

Nerve core

Myelin attacked by multiple sclerosis begins to deteriorate

Early stages

Nerve is stripped of protection and messages are short circuited by the surrounding tissue

Final stage

The cause of multiple sclerosis is unknown, though it is suspected that it is caused by a virus to which the body has a natural lack of immunity. Its incidence varies according to climate, age and sex. It is almost unknown in the tropics, but is at its most prevalent in temperate zones. More than three times as many women as men catch the disease, the chief risk period being between twenty and forty, with a peak age of thirty. It is highly unusual for anyone over fifty to be affected.

The proportion of sufferers from multiple sclerosis is two females to one male.

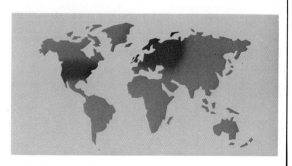

your legs is dragging, particularly after you have taken a lot of exercise. Alternatively, your sensations may be affected. A feeling of numbness may spread upwards from your feet to your waist, or upwards from one of your hands through the arms. Occasionally, you may find it difficult to articulate clearly – this is called dysarthria—or find it hard to control your bladder. You may also find that you are more easily emotionally aroused than usual, laughing and crying for what seem to be trivial reasons. This is termed emotional liability

Attacks of the disease come in spasms. You may, for instance, have an attack affecting your eyes, from which you completely recover. Following this, you may not suffer from symptoms of multiple sclerosis for years, if at all. A sequence of attacks often leads to residual weakness, however; in the most extreme cases,

walking may eventually become impossible.

Diagnosis and treatment

If your doctor suspects that you are suffering from multiple sclerosis, the first step will be to examine the inside of your eyes with an ophthalmoscope, a special kind of torch adapted for this purpose. The tell-tale indication of multiple sclerosis is the appearance of the optic disc. This is the head of the optic nerve lying at the back of your eye in the retina, from which it collects the messages which make up sight and conveys them to the optic computer at the back of the brain. In multiple sclerosis, the optic disc will have a particular appearance, which doctors call temporal pallor.

A more sophisticated test for multiple sclerosis is called the Visual Evoked Response test. In multiple sclerosis, the results shown by

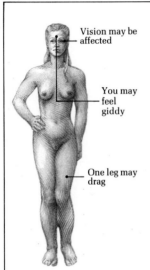

Vision may be affected

You may feel giddy

One leg may drag

What you notice.
The symptoms of multiple sclerosis depend very much on the part of the central nervous system that is affected. If the brain stem is scarred, for example, you may have spells of giddiness or double vision; if the spinal cord, you may find that one leg drags. The optic nerve is most commonly affected first. This results in pain around one eye, and dulled sight which improves after a couple of weeks. Emotions, speech and bladder control can also suffer. Symptoms may be single or scattered.

The effects of multiple sclerosis
If a part of the central nervous system is damaged the part of the peripheral system which it monitors can be put out of action. If a part of the peripheral system is damaged then the effect is normally localized. Multiple sclerosis is a disease of the central nervous system which affects the functioning of the peripheral system. If the myelin sheath round a central nerve deteriorates then the nerve cannot function properly. The myelin cannot be replaced as only the peripheral system contains the Schwann cells which manufacture it.

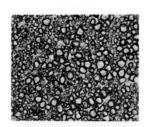

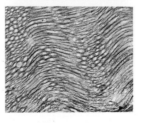

A cross section of a nerve showing the axons (top) magnified 300 times. A longitudinal view (×120) is shown above.

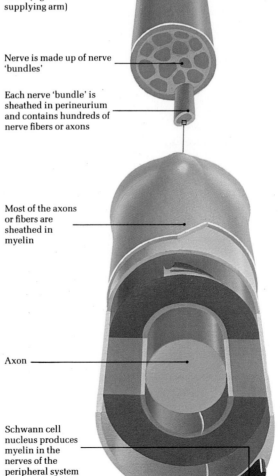

Epineurium sheath surrounds peripheral nerve (e.g. radial nerve supplying arm)

Nerve is made up of nerve 'bundles'

Each nerve 'bundle' is sheathed in perineurium and contains hundreds of nerve fibers or axons

Most of the axons or fibers are sheathed in myelin

Axon

Schwann cell nucleus produces myelin in the nerves of the peripheral system the test are often slower than normal. This is because the nerves from the eye cannot work as efficiently as usual if their myelin sheathes have been damaged.

Blood tests will show the presence of characteristic antigens; the presence of these is not conclusive, however, as they occur in other disorders as well. A sample of cerebrospinal fluid – the fluid which surrounds your spinal cord and brain – may be taken by lumbar puncture. This, too, will show abnormalities.

If the symptoms are centered in your spinal cord, the doctor will check to see whether or not you have a neurofibroma. This is a tumor of the spinal cord which can be removed by operation. Its presence is detected by a special form of x-ray technique called myleography; in this, a substance that will show up on x-ray is intoduced into the cerebrospinal fluid through a needle. If a tumour is present, it will appear as a block on the x-ray film.

Specific treatment for general symptoms will be prescribed – for instance, a two-week course of injections speeds up relief from an acute attack. Further treatment will be directed towards particular symptoms; drugs may be prescribed to aid you if you are suffering from painful spasms, difficulty in controlling your bladder, or stiffness, while physiotherapy is invaluable if there is muscular weakness.

You should avoid heavy exertion and take care of yourself if you have any infection. Multiple sclerosis is aggravated by other illnesses. You may well find that hot baths make the symptoms worse. Pregnancy, however, is not a problem, though a relapse is more likely in the period immediately following the birth of a child.

Physiotherapy.
A physiotherapist's job is to treat illness by means which can be regarded as physical as distinct from chemical or surgical. Nerve injuries and strokes commonly render a number of muscles inactive. Muscles directly affected must be treated and those indirectly rendered unusable because they are dependant on these must be kept in good shape. The physiotherapist on the right is helping to maintain the patient's hip, abdomen and thigh muscles.

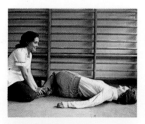 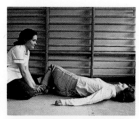 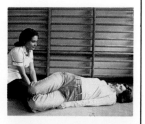
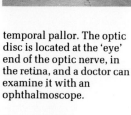 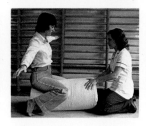 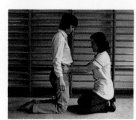

Making the diagnosis
One indication that a patient probably has multiple sclerosis is a change in the appearance of the optic disc known as temporal pallor. The optic disc is located at the 'eye' end of the optic nerve, in the retina, and a doctor can examine it with an ophthalmoscope.

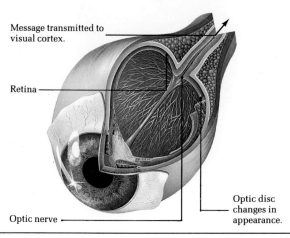

Message transmitted to visual cortex.

Retina

Optic nerve

Optic disc changes in appearance.

PRESCRIPTION

Diagnosis
As the only nerve that can be directly observed is the optic nerve, your doctor will look through your eye with an ophthalmoscope. The speed at which your nerves are conducting messages may also be tested.

Treatment
There is no known cure for multiple sclerosis, but the disease often disappears of its own accord. Treatment tends at the moment to be in the form of drugs that relieve the symptoms. With the aid of a physiotherapist you can do a great deal to keep your muscles well toned and useful. However, you should take care not to over-exert yourself, especially if you have contracted some other infection. Any part of you that is dependant on the working of the nervous system can be affected, so you may find that you are very emotionally sensitive.

Strokes

A stroke is a sudden interruption of the blood supply to part of the brain. The effects of this vary from case to case; a stroke can lead to loss of consciousness, permanent or temporary paralysis, depending on the degree of oxygen deprivation, and, in extreme cases, death.

Strokes can occur in any one of three ways. One cause is a thrombosis, or clotting, in an artery, which means that part of the brain is completely cut off from its blood supply. A second is an embolism, in which a wandering blood clot, bubble of air, or lump of fat settles in an artery and chokes the blood supply. The third is by haemorrhage, that is, bleeding from a ruptured blood vessel. By far the commonest underlying cause is ATHEROSCLEROSIS, which affects the vessels in the brain in particular. The disease is most common after middle age; the typical victim is elderly, what doctors term atherosclerotic, diabetic and suffering from high blood pressure.

Physical symptoms

Strokes stem from problems with the blood circulation in the brain. This has an extremely generous blood supply, as befits such a vital organ. Not only do the two vertebral arteries combine to form the basilar artery, but the internal carotid arteries also enter the skull. A central feature is the Circle of Willis. This is a ring of blood vessels into which blood flows, with many branches. These, in turn, join up with each other, so that if one branch gets blocked the others can take over its function.

The usual preliminary to a stroke is the gradual blocking of an atherosclerotic vessel in the brain. There may be warning signs of this in the form of what are called mini-strokes; the

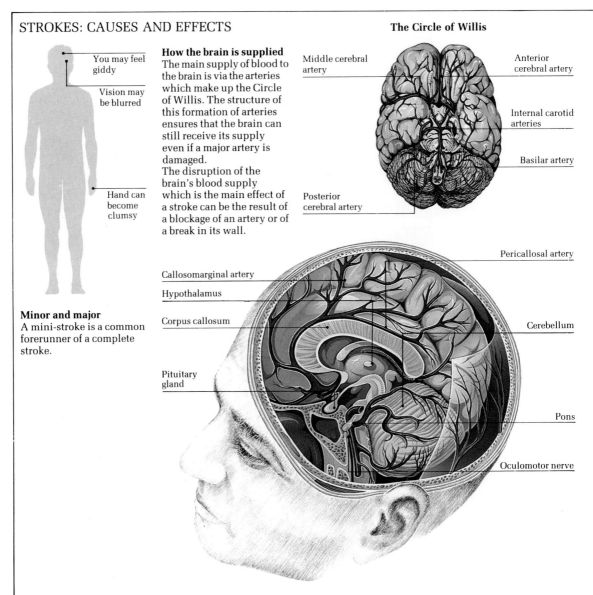

STROKES: CAUSES AND EFFECTS

You may feel giddy

Vision may be blurred

Hand can become clumsy

Minor and major
A mini-stroke is a common forerunner of a complete stroke.

How the brain is supplied
The main supply of blood to the brain is via the arteries which make up the Circle of Willis. The structure of this formation of arteries ensures that the brain can still receive its supply even if a major artery is damaged.
The disruption of the brain's blood supply which is the main effect of a stroke can be the result of a blockage of an artery or of a break in its wall.

The Circle of Willis

Middle cerebral artery

Anterior cerebral artery

Internal carotid arteries

Basilar artery

Posterior cerebral artery

Pericallosal artery

Callosomarginal artery

Hypothalamus

Corpus callosum

Cerebellum

Pituitary gland

Pons

Oculomotor nerve

are passing attacks of weakness or clumsiness in one hand and giddy turns and falls, in which, though you do not lose consciousness, you may suffer from disturbance of vision lasting a few minutes and brief loss of memory. Though any of these symptoms may have other causes, their persistence may indicate arterial failure.

Completed stroke occurs when the blood supply is completely cut off – either by clotting in a blocked vessel, embolism, or breaking of a blood vessel because the wall is damaged. Subarachnoid haemorrhage is one particular form of cerebral haemorrhage. This occurs when a small blister, or aneurysm, on the Circle of Willis bursts; the blister is either present from birth or has developed as a result of atherosclerosis.

Whatever is the cause of the stroke, symp-toms will vary depending on the part of the brain being deprived of blood. If the artery involved is the middle cerebral or the internal carotid artery, for instance, any of the following symptoms can occur. You may be unable to produce the word you want to say due to interference with the word store in the brain. There will be weakness of the face – a tic, for example—of the arm and, less often, of the leg on the left, while there may be impairment of sensation on the right side of your body.

If the right side of your brain is affected, your speech will remain practically normal, but your sense of direction may be impaired and you may lose awareness of the left of your body. If the front of your brain is involved, you may temporarily revert to the reflexes you had as a baby. If the basilar artery is in jeopardy, your sight will be affected.

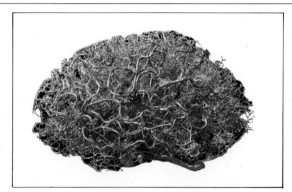

These arteries have been treated so that the brain's supply network can be easily observed.

Valve disease
Disease of the heart can sometimes result in small pieces of a damaged valve being transmitted through the blood stream to the brain arteries. A blockage here will cause a stroke.

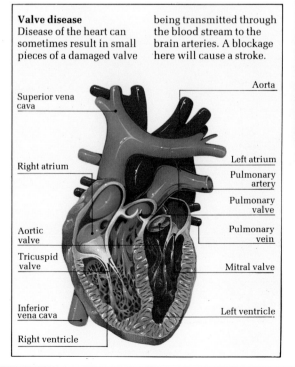

Superior vena cava

Right atrium

Aortic valve

Tricuspid valve

Inferior vena cava

Right ventricle

Aorta

Left atrium

Pulmonary artery

Pulmonary valve

Pulmonary vein

Mitral valve

Left ventricle

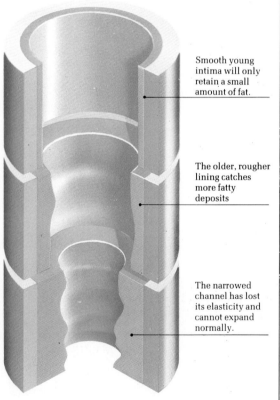

Smooth young intima will only retain a small amount of fat.

The older, rougher lining catches more fatty deposits

The narrowed channel has lost its elasticity and cannot expand normally.

The main cause
A condition of the arteries called atherosclerosis makes strokes more likely. This tends to occur when arteries have lost their elasticity, and are thus unable to cope with extra blood flow requirements. Their linings become rough and encourage deposits to accumulate. This is especially likely if the patient is a heavy smoker. The result is that extra blood which might be required under conditions of normal exertion cannot be supplied: the arteries are too hard to expand, and narrowed by fat.

Though a stroke seems grim just after it happens, the outlook is surprisingly good. The eminent French scientist Louis Pasteur (1822–1895), for instance, made many of his major discoveries after he had suffered numerous strokes, including one which led his doctor to despair of his life.

Diagnosis and treatment

It is normally fairly easy to diagnose what has caused a stroke; usually, your blood pressure and/or the state of your arteries is basically at fault. In a few cases, however, SYPHILIS – a venereal disease—of the arteries may be the primary cause; one of three special types of blood test is used to settle whether or not this is the case. Another type of blood test – the erythrocyte sedimentation rate (ESR) – will eliminate or confirm the possibility of cranial arteritis. This is an inflammation of the blood vessels which recovers well with treatment. A progressive stroke may be the result of poly-cythaemia vera, an abnormal increase in the number of red blood cells. This is revealed by a blood count.

The doctor may also check for DIABETES MELLITUS through a glucose tolerance test. Though diabetes is not a direct cause of stroke, it is frequently an associated disease. The amount of cholesterol and other lipids (fats) in your blood will also be measured, if you are unduly young to have a stroke.

Examination of the heart should also be made. This is because heart disease, particular-ly mitral stenosis (see RHEUMATIC HEART DIS-EASE) can lead to a stroke. Fragments from a damaged heart valve can block a small brain artery and starve the brain of blood.

The symptoms of a stroke depend on which part of the brain has been deprived of blood. The most commonly affected area is the territory of the left internal carotid artery. Disruption of the blood flow here can produce paralysis, usually of the right side. Sensitivity in a side of the face is lost, as well as the use of the limbs. Speech and swallowing can also be affected.

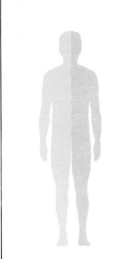

Limbic system — Cerebral hemisphere

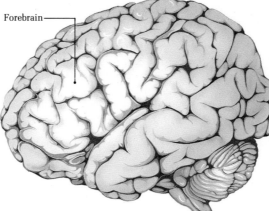

Pons

Hypothalamus

Thalamus

Forebrain

If the right side of the brain is affected the sense of direction can suffer and awareness of one side of the body can be lost. Speech is unlikely to be affected if the effects are confined to the right side. Deprivation of supply to the frontal lobe can result in reversal to infantile reflexes

Hindbrain

Cerebellum

Midbrain

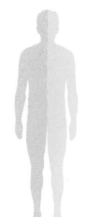

If the left side of the brain is affected, symptoms are often quite distinct. Thrombosis of the left internal carotid can produce paralysis in one side, normally the right. Speech is likely to be impaired if the left half of the brain is affected. Disabling of the basilar artery can result in a worsening of vision.

Where there is doubt about exactly what is going on inside the brain, a CAT scan – CAT means computerized axial tomography—will usually provide the answer. This is a special type of x-ray, which shows head and brain as if they were cut into slices.

However, there is no magic involved in treating a stroke. Mostly, it is a matter of reinforcing nature's own tendency to recovery. The patient must be nourished, though precautions must be taken if there is difficulty in swallowing, and then encouraged and helped to move as much as possible. Physiotherapists, sometimes using electrical treatment, will keep the muscles in good order, until the patient is able to direct them again. Occasionally, a technique called bio-feedback is useful in helping you to regain control over the muscles; this is a method by which a machine indicates whether you are making the right muscle move. Speech therapy is useful. Not only does it help to overcome the physical problem, but it also encourages a stroke victim to cope with the frustrating stage of inability to remember the right word.

Recovery from stroke continues for as long as twelve months and so must the efforts to aid it. If you have mitral stenosis, it is important that you remain on anticoagulants to prevent further attacks. Aspirin is thought by some doctors to be a help in preventing mini-strokes, though it is by no means certain whether they can help prevent major ones.

If you have raised blood pressure – a common cause of stroke – you can help yourself in addition to receiving help from your doctor. Reduce your weight if it is above the right amount for your height.

Finding the fault.
If the symptoms of a stroke are not of a sort to give a clear-cut indication of precisely what part of the brain is affected, then a CAT scan can resolve the issue. It involves taking a series of cross-sectional X-ray photographs across the head and brain so that the affected area is revealed. The normal appearance of a scanned head is shown

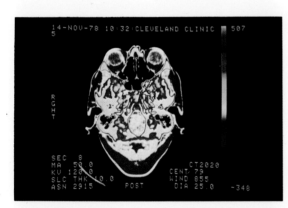

If you think that someone is having a stroke, put him on his side so that the fluids can drain from his throat and mouth. If he comes round, he will be able to hear even if he cannot speak, so do not shout but reassure him gently.

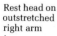
Rest head on outstretched right arm

Draw up left arm

Draw up left leg

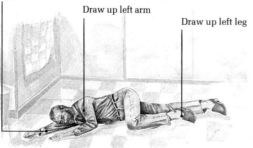

PRESCRIPTION

Diagnosis
Some sort of disease of the arteries is by far the most common cause of a stroke, but factors related to rheumatic heart disease, diabetes or other less serious complaints will also have to be discounted. A CAT scan will determine which part of the brain is affected.

Treatment
Recovery from a stroke is a steady but gradual process. All the disabled parts of the body—the muscles, the speech—need to be brought back into use by the appropriate form of therapy, and until such time as therapy can begin, unused muscles must be kept in good shape. Bio-feedback is a useful way of re-learning muscle control. Obesity will put unnecessary strain on your heart and circulation.

Getting better.
During the time that a person cannot move his own muscles a physiotherapist must manipulate them to prevent atrophy. The physiotherapist is taking the patient through exercises related to standing and sitting (1 & 2) and in the bridging and rolling exercises (3 & 4) she is developing muscles less frequently used.

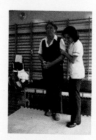
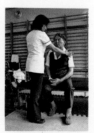
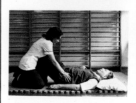
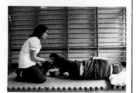

Shingles

Shingles is an acute virus infection of the sensory nerves, with the accompanying characteristics of pain along the infected neural path and a rash. The disease is most likely to occur if you are run down for any reason, or if the affected nerve roots have been damaged. It can strike at any age from childhood onwards.

The virus concerned is also responsible for chicken pox and there is a well-established link between the two diseases. A grand-parent with shingles, for instance, can give chicken pox to a child who has not previously contracted the disease. However, unlike chicken pox, second attacks of shingles are not rare.

Physical symptoms

What is likely to happen in a case of shingles is that, after an attack of chicken pox, the virus is not destroyed. Instead, it lies dormant in the body, remaining inactive until conditions are favorable for it to multiply and attack you.

This is exactly what happens in herpes simplex, the common 'cold blister' on the lips. In this, the virus remains latent in cells at the junction of the skin and the mucous membrane of the lips and nose, ready to emerge and cause an outcrop of blisters when your resistance is lowered through physical or psychological stress. In shingles, or herpes zoster, the affected ganglia become inflamed and swell up.

The first thing you will notice is pain on one side of your chest, abdomen or face, plus a mild fever. Though the pain is often extremely severe, there are no obvious visible symptoms at this stage. It normally extends half way around the body. After about four days, the characteristic rash appears in the form of minute blisters along the line of a nerve; these,

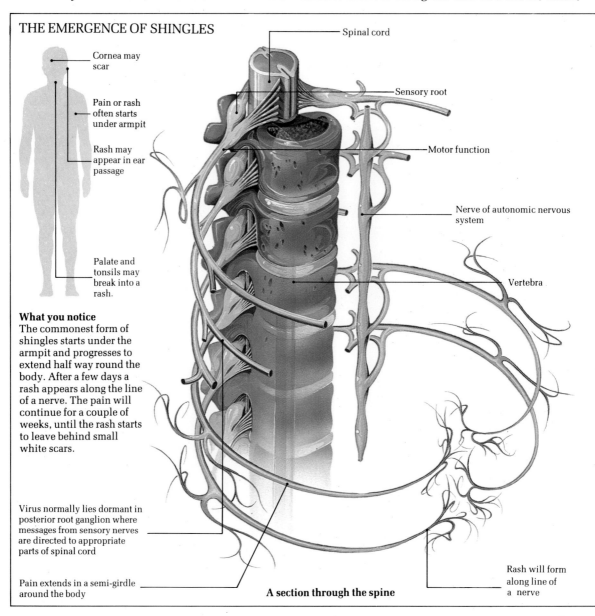

THE EMERGENCE OF SHINGLES

Spinal cord

Cornea may scar

Pain or rash often starts under armpit

Rash may appear in ear passage

Palate and tonsils may break into a rash.

Sensory root

Motor function

Nerve of autonomic nervous system

Vertebra

What you notice
The commonest form of shingles starts under the armpit and progresses to extend half way round the body. After a few days a rash appears along the line of a nerve. The pain will continue for a couple of weeks, until the rash starts to leave behind small white scars.

Virus normally lies dormant in posterior root ganglion where messages from sensory nerves are directed to appropriate parts of spinal cord

Pain extends in a semi-girdle around the body

A section through the spine

Rash will form along line of a nerve

however, remain localized within two or three skin segments in the chest or abdomen.

The skin around the blisters may be red and tender, while the pain continues intensely until the rash begins to fade in a week or so. Tiny white scars are left behind the blisters; you will find that these are insensitive to pin pricks. In the young, there are usually no other after effects; in the elderly, however, pain may persist in the place of the rash as post-herpetic neuralgia. This is not as acute as the original shingles pain, but it is persistent and wearing. The sensation in the skin – where your clothes rub, for instance – is unpleasant.

Diagnosis and treatment
Apply the usual homely remedies of rest, plenty of fluid and painkillers, such as soluble aspirin. Use calamine lotion to soothe your skin. Your doctor may prescribe drugs – some to help you cope with the irritation and some to enable you to relax.

You will recover from the actual illness within two or three weeks, so the main aim of any special treatment is to prevent the long-lasting residual effects of post-herpetic neuralgia. Your doctor may prescribe steroids if there is a risk of this.

If the neuralgia becomes established, you are likely to have developed a depressive illness as well. Your doctor will treat this with an anti-depressant, which, as well as affecting your mood, should have the effect of reducing the pain to more tolerable proportions.

At all costs, resist the natural inclination to protect the painful, hypersensitive areas by covering them with a bandage or plaster. This only makes matters worse.

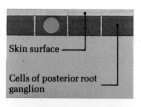

The virus emerges
1 The zoster virus can lie dormant in the body.

Skin surface

Cells of posterior root ganglion

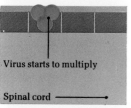

2 When the carrier is particularly run down the virus will be able to start multiplying.

Virus starts to multiply

Spinal cord

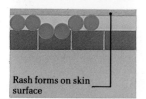

3 The infection will show itself on the surface in the form of a rash which spreads along the line of a nerve.

Rash forms on skin surface

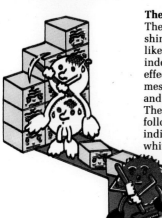

The virus responsible.
The virus that causes shingles is shaped rather like a brick, and it does indeed form a barrier to the effective transmission of messages along a nerve and into the spinal cord. The swelling which follows its becoming active indicates the arrival of white blood cells.

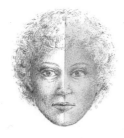

If the geniculate ganglion of the facial nerve is affected the rash will appear in the ear passage. It may spread to the motor part of the nerve, and affect the ophthalmic branch of the trigeminal nerve. This may scar the cornea.

PRESCRIPTION

Diagnosis
Your doctor will ask you about the pain, may take your temperature, and will look to see if the rash has yet appeared.

Treatment
There is no known way of either dealing with chicken pox so that the virus cannot lie dormant, or of killing the dormant virus, or of preventing the disease from running its course once it has started. Treatment, then, is aimed at making the patient as comfortable as possible, allowing the disease to run its course, and making sure complications do not arise. Rest is important, and good diet: the attack may have occurred because you were run down. Take lots of drinks, and ease the pain with aspirins, soothing the affected skin area with a traditional remedy such as calamine lotion.

Migraine

Migraine is a common disease, likely to start after puberty and disappear after the age of fifty. Sometimes, it does not develop until you are over forty, but, from this age onwards, other causes for severe headache need to be considered, such as high blood pressure or ATHEROSCLEROSIS. Women more frequently suffer from the disease than men, roughly in the ratio of seven to three.

Physical symptoms

Migraine headaches are almost always idiopathic – that is, they cannot be traced to one specific cause. What you experience is a disturbance of vision, for instance, and the various headache symptoms of migraine. The head pain is undoubtedly due to a reaction in the arteries of the scalp, eye sockets, face and/or the base of the brain. At the height of the attack, the surface arteries may be seen to be swollen, together with the surrounding tissues. They are also tender to touch.

Migraine can be triggered off by a substance called tyramine, contained in such foods as cheese, red wine or chocolate. Alternatively, substances made by the body itself may be the cause. Though you may not always suffer from the full range of symptoms, what usually happens is that you start by feeling particularly well. You may notice a slight bloating due to fluid retention. The effects on vision are like a shimmering heat haze; this first affects half your field of vision and then spreads. This may develop into patches of blurring or distortion.

You may also – or instead – have numbness or tingling, usually affecting one hand and extending up the arm into the face, including the mouth and tongue. Less frequently, the

RESTRICTING THE BRAINS BLOOD SUPPLY

What you see
The first signs of the onset of a migraine attack are normally visual. Half of your field of vision may appear to be covered by a shimmering haze. You may see zig-zag lights and flashes or part of your visual field may be blurred or distorted. Numbness may extend from one hand up the arm to the face.

Migraine commonly affects only one side of the head. The head pain which is its main characteristic is caused by events in the arteries inside and outside the skull, notably those of the scalp, eye sockets, face, and base of the brain. After the visual symptoms (left), speech may be impaired through the blood supply to the word store being diminished. A headache following this symptom will always be on the left side. Headaches do not always follow these visual disturbances, but if they do, it is normally within about 20 minutes.

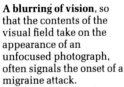
A blurring of vision, so that the contents of the visual field take on the appearance of an unfocused photograph, often signals the onset of a migraine attack.

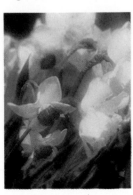

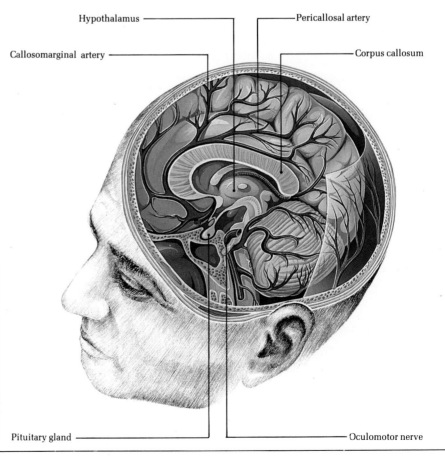

Hypothalamus

Pericallosal artery

Callosomarginal artery

Corpus callosum

Pituitary gland

Oculomotor nerve

advance symptoms can affect your speech.

These early symptoms last about twenty minutes. Then, the headache starts, though this is not always the case, as, sometimes, the symptoms actually constitute the attack. The main characteristic of the headache is its severity. At its height, you may vomit and be unable to bear the light. It may last for hours; the sign of it coming to an end is passing a large quantity of urine.

Diagnosis and treatment

There is usually no difficulty in recognizing migraine for what it is. Your doctor will want to know whether other members of your family suffer from it and, if you are a woman, whether you are taking the oral contraceptive pill. This sometimes produces migraine as a side effect. If you are over forty, he will take your blood pressure and probably test your cholesterol level and thyroid function to check that the supply pipes to your brain are functioning well.

If particular kinds of food or drink bring on a migraine, avoid them. Stress is often a factor, so try to come to terms with it, as deliberately avoiding it is often even more frustrating. If you suffer from recurrent migraine, your doctor will prescribe drugs to help you, but, even if you can get only fifteen minutes sleep after an attack has begun, this will greatly improve the situation. This applies even if you wake with a migraine in the morning.

Bio-feedback training can also be useful. In this, you are taught to alter the blood flow to your hands and, secondarily, to your head. Learning this is time-consuming initially, but it can be an effective preventative.

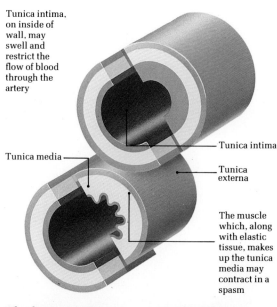

Tunica intima, on inside of wall, may swell and restrict the flow of blood through the artery

Tunica media

Tunica intima

Tunica externa

The muscle which, along with elastic tissue, makes up the tunica media may contract in a spasm

What happens in the artery

Migraine symptoms are the result of dilation of the arteries which supply the brain, so that parts of the brain are deprived of oxygen and other necessities. This constriction can be the result of a spasm of the muscle in the wall of the artery or, more commonly, of a swelling of the wall itself. Both events cause the passage to narrow.

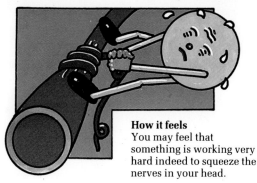

How it feels
You may feel that something is working very hard indeed to squeeze the nerves in your head.

PRESCRIPTION

Diagnosis
Your description of your symptoms will normally be sufficient for diagnosis.

Treatment
Blood pressure tests, investigation of possible effects of a contraceptive pill, or checks on blood composition and thyroid activity are all possible checks your doctor will make. It is possible that migraine is associated with some routine factor in your life such as stress or diet. Learning how to sleep before an attack, bio-feedback techniques, cutting out substances such as chocolate, and coming to terms with those things in your life which make you anxious, are possible paths to relief. Below: While stress is undoubtedly a contributory factor in the onset of a migraine attack, certain substances manufactured by the body, or eaten, are also under suspicion.

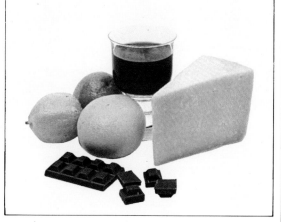

Parkinson's Disease

Parkinson's disease is a common disorder caused by wear and tear in a particular group of brain cells. The result is difficulty with movements and a characteristic muscular tremor. The disease gets its name from the London physician James Parkinson, who called it the 'shaking palsy'.

The disease is neither hereditary nor contagious. It usually strikes people over fifty, affecting about one in two hundred of the elderly across the world, irrespective of race. Men are slightly more liable to it than women.

Physical symptoms

The precise cause of Parkinson's disease is unknown, but it is thought to involve the degeneration of cells in the brain stem. These cells – those of the *substantia nigra* (black stuff) and the *locus coeruleus* (blue place)

produce a substance called dopamine, one of the chemicals necessary for conveying messages along the nerve fibers. Dopamine is chiefly concerned with muscle movement. In Parkinson's disease, there is a shortage of dopamine, the effects being very like those of a battery running down.

The disease develops extremely gradually. Probably the first thing that you will notice is that your hand trembles when it is resting on your lap. The tremor is usually a rhythmic movement of your bent fingers against your thumb. This happens quite slowly, as though you were powdering a meat extract cube. If you are anxious or upset, the tremor gets worse; when you want to do something active, such as combing your hair, it stops. It also ceases completely when you go to sleep.

While your hands and arms are the first parts

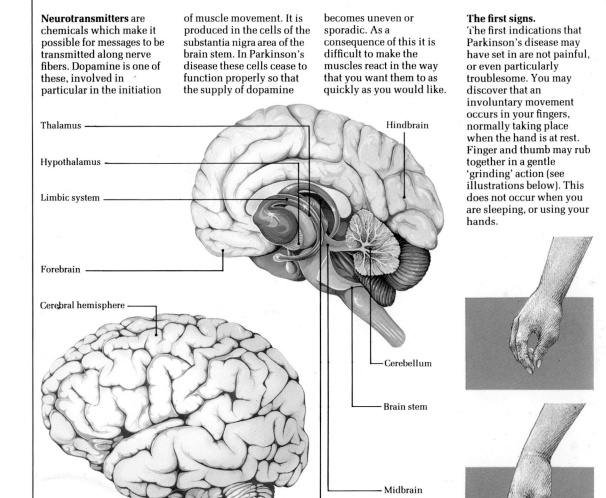

INTERRUPTED DOPAMINE SUPPLY

Neurotransmitters are chemicals which make it possible for messages to be transmitted along nerve fibers. Dopamine is one of these, involved in particular in the initiation of muscle movement. It is produced in the cells of the substantia nigra area of the brain stem. In Parkinson's disease these cells cease to function properly so that the supply of dopamine becomes uneven or sporadic. As a consequence of this it is difficult to make the muscles react in the way that you want them to as quickly as you would like.

The first signs.
The first indications that Parkinson's disease may have set in are not painful, or even particularly troublesome. You may discover that an involuntary movement occurs in your fingers, normally taking place when the hand is at rest. Finger and thumb may rub together in a gentle 'grinding' action (see illustrations below). This does not occur when you are sleeping, or using your hands.

Thalamus

Hypothalamus

Limbic system

Forebrain

Cerebral hemisphere

Hindbrain

Cerebellum

Brain stem

Midbrain

Substantia nigra where dopamine is produced

of your body to be affected, your head and feet may become involved later. You may also notice that your muscles become stiff, though not painful; this is most noticeable in your neck, shoulder and hip. You tend to take up a bent posture, leaning forward slightly. This affects the way you walk and makes you vulnerable to a fall. You may become depressed. Muscle reactions also slow.

Diagnosis and treatment

There are no specific tests for Parkinson's disease, but your doctor may time the tremor. This has a typical rhythm of four to six movements per second. You will be asked about any medicines you may have been taking and whether you have ever had a brain infection.

Treatment is now largely by a drug called L-dopa (Levadopa), which has revolutionized the treatment of the disease since its introduction in 1967. It is taken by mouth, in a combined form with an anti-enzyme, and is converted to dopamine in the brain to make up for the deficiency. The anti-enzyme is to prevent the L-dopa being metabolized before it can reach the brain. The doctor will watch the dosage carefully in case of side effects. Other drugs can also be used.

Physiotherapy may help you to use your muscles more effectively, while in extremely severe cases – these are very rare – an operation on the affected part of the brain can be performed.

As with all chronic, progressive disorders, do not give up any activity a moment before you must. In the meantime, take the sensible precaution of building up a reserve of less stressful hobbies and occupations.

In short supply.
If the supply of water from the containers is unreliable and irregular, the wheel will only be able to turn fitfully. In a similar way, the breakdown of the substantia nigra cells, and consequent irregular supply of dopamine, has an adverse effect on the initiation of movement in the muscles.

(1) Water is supplied steadily, enabling wheel to turn regularly.

(2) Water supply is interrupted and becomes sporadic. Wheel ceases to turn smoothly.

(3) Providing the brain with the dopamine it is lacking is like re-establishing the water supply.

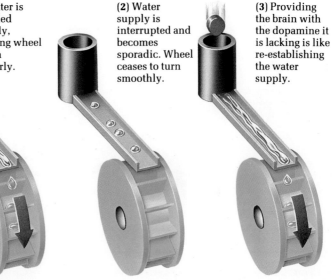

Treatment made effective
Dopamine deficiency can now be made good by treatment with levodopa, which is converted into dopamine by the brain.

Nearly all the levodopa taken by mouth would be metabolized before reaching the brain, so an anti-enzyme is added to inhibit this process.

Levodopa without anti-enzyme is broken down in gut, liver and kidneys.

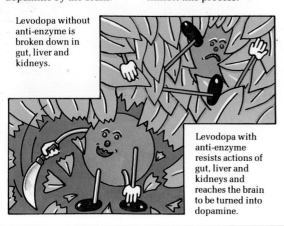

Levodopa with anti-enzyme resists actions of gut, liver and kidneys and reaches the brain to be turned into dopamine.

PRESCRIPTION

Diagnosis
Your doctor will diagnose Parkinson's disease through its effect on the muscles. He or she will want to know about any loss of control.

Treatment
Two sorts of drug can be used to combat Parkinson's disease. One sort has an inhibiting effect on movement altogether. The tremor is relieved, but complete control is not regained. L-dopa has the much more satisfactory effect of appearing to replace the lost dopamine, so that muscle control is regained. Where drugs cannot be used, or are ineffective, brain surgery has had markedly good results.

Circulatory/Introduction

All the body's cells apart from those of the liver and spleen receive their nutrients and oxygen from and pass out wastes into the tissue fluid. The tissue fluid in turn receives nutrients from and passes waste into the blood capillaries. So a constant blood flow keeps all the cells alive. The blood collects oxygen from the lungs and nutrients from the liver and intestine. Waste is filtered from it by the kidneys. The two pumps which make up the heart circulate it. The right side of the heart pumps blood from the veins into the lungs, where it collects oxygen. The left side receives blood from the lungs and sends it into the first artery, the aorta. Some is then diverted through the liver and intestine or kidneys. The rest flows through the dividing network of arteries which ends with the capillaries. The return journey through larger and larger veins then begins.

The circulatory system. The arteries divide and subdivide, gradually diminishing in thickness. The aorta, which leaves the heart, is about as thick as its owner's thumb. The capillaries, at the 'outskirts' of the system, are about 1mm long and $\frac{1}{100}$mm thick. It is here that the blood performs its function of nutrient/waste exchange. Capillaries permeate all living tissue apart from cartilage and the transparent tissue of the eye. At the artery end of a capillary oxygen and nutrients pass into the surrounding tissue. At the vein end, lower blood pressure allows fluid carrying waste to enter.

Blood cells make up about half of the total volume of the blood. Red cells (below left) contain oxygen-carrying haemoglobin. The much less numerous white cells (below right) defend against disease.

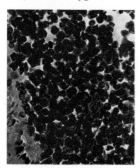
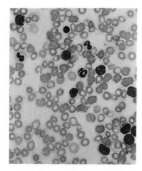

Arteries and veins: construction
The arterial walls are thicker than the walls of the veins, mainly because of a thicker muscle and elastic layer. This enables them to cope with the higher pressures to which they are subjected, and to smooth out the flow of blood by expanding with each heartbeat. This expansion is felt as a pulse where the arteries come close to the surface.

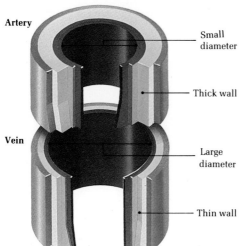

Artery

Small diameter

Thick wall

Vein

Large diameter

Thin wall

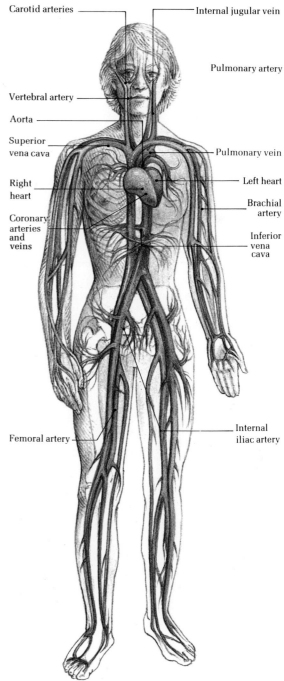

Carotid arteries

Internal jugular vein

Pulmonary artery

Vertebral artery

Aorta

Superior vena cava

Pulmonary vein

Right heart

Left heart

Brachial artery

Coronary arteries and veins

Inferior vena cava

Femoral artery

Internal iliac artery

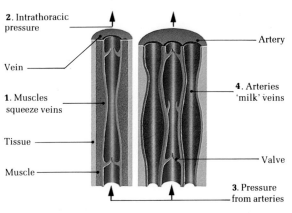

2. Intrathoracic pressure

Vein

1. Muscles squeeze veins

Tissue

Muscle

Artery

4. Arteries 'milk' veins

Valve

3. Pressure from arteries

Blood flow in the veins.
Effective venous return is vital. Blood reaches the venous system from the arteries by way of the capillaries, bringing waste which has been exchanged for nutrients. Pressure in the veins is low, and blood moves slowly. It relies for movement on: **1**. Surrounding muscle. Leg muscles are especially important. When they contract, blood is forced through the valves towards the heart. **2**. Intrathoracic pressure. This is due to the expansion of the lungs when a person inhales, and has the effect of sucking blood into the thorax. **3**. The 'cardiac pump'. This is the pressure from the arteries which is carried across the capillary network. **4**. Deep veins are often wrapped around the arteries. The pulsation of these arteries has a 'milking' effect on the veins around them.

The network of blood vessels.
The main arteries and veins responsible for the continuing fresh blood supply to the whole of the body are shown right.

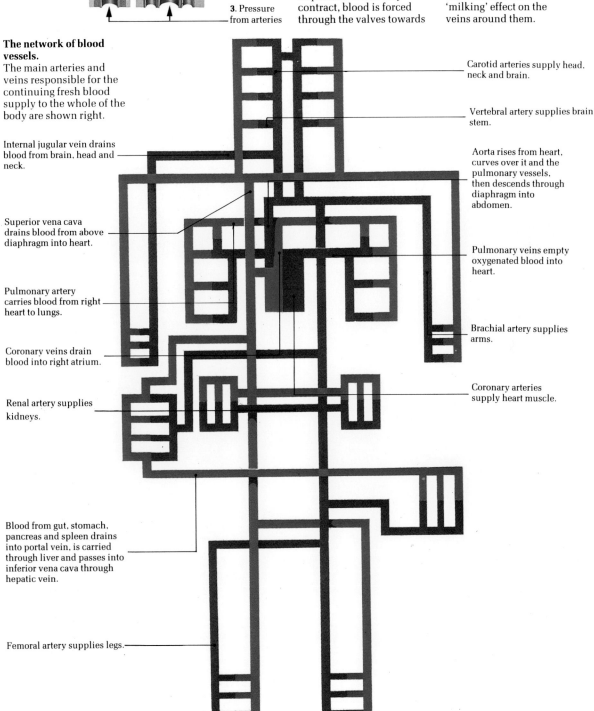

Internal jugular vein drains blood from brain, head and neck.

Superior vena cava drains blood from above diaphragm into heart.

Pulmonary artery carries blood from right heart to lungs.

Coronary veins drain blood into right atrium.

Renal artery supplies kidneys.

Blood from gut, stomach, pancreas and spleen drains into portal vein, is carried through liver and passes into inferior vena cava through hepatic vein.

Femoral artery supplies legs.

Carotid arteries supply head, neck and brain.

Vertebral artery supplies brain stem.

Aorta rises from heart, curves over it and the pulmonary vessels, then descends through diaphragm into abdomen.

Pulmonary veins empty oxygenated blood into heart.

Brachial artery supplies arms.

Coronary arteries supply heart muscle.

To understand the action of the heart, it is necessary to understand that each chamber has two phases, systole, or contraction, and diastole, or relaxation. The right atrium and left atrium both undergo these phases at the same time, as do the left ventricle and right ventricle. So in atrial systole, blood empties under pressure from the right atrium into the right ventricle, and from the left atrium into the left ventricle. In ventricular systole – which occurs when the ventricles have filled with blood – blood empties under pressure from the left ventricle into the aorta, and thence to the rest of the body, and from the right ventricle into the pulmonary artery, and thence to the lungs. The atria, at low pressure, can receive blood from the lungs (left atrium) or the rest of the body (right atrium). The heartbeat consists of two sounds, one made by the closing of the valves between the atria and the ventricles, and another higher sound made by the closing of the valves at the exit from either ventricle.

The blood is made up of red cells, white cells, and a fluid called plasma in which they float. The red cells collect oxygen from the lungs and carry it round the body. Each cell has a thin shell. People with shells of similar structure belong to the same blood group. Cells from foreign blood groups introduced into a person's blood are destroyed. The white cells of the blood proliferate in response to infection. They can increase three- or four-fold. The plasma is a solution of salt, proteins, glucose and other substances in water. It carries waste and nutritious substances from and to the tissues. Plasma makes up just over half the blood volume, cells just under half.

THE ACTION OF THE HEART

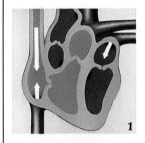

A heart beat
The moment of highest blood pressure is called systole, that of lowest pressure diastole. In atrial diastole (left) blood flows from the systemic system into the right atrium and from the pulmonary into the left.

1

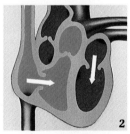

During this time the ventricles have been expelling blood. When they stop, the valves between atria and ventricles open and impulses are sent to the atria causing atrial systole: blood is pumped into the dilated ventricles.

2

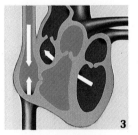

Electrical impulses then initiate ventricular systole: the mitral and tricuspid valves snap closed, and the pressure in the ventricles rises sharply. Papillary muscles and chordae tendinae prevent the valves from inverting into the atria.

3

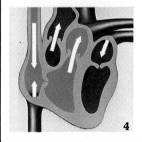

When the pressure in the ventricles is greater than that in the aorta and pulmonary artery the semilunar valves are forced open and blood streams through. As the pressure falls in the ventricles these valves close and they refill.

4

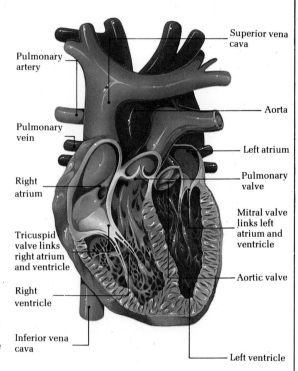

Pulmonary artery

Pulmonary vein

Right atrium

Tricuspid valve links right atrium and ventricle

Right ventricle

Inferior vena cava

Superior vena cava

Aorta

Left atrium

Pulmonary valve

Mitral valve links left atrium and ventricle

Aortic valve

Left ventricle

What the heart does.
The contracting action of the heart is the main driving force behind the circulation of the blood. The organ is essentially two pumps. The left heart pumps oxygenated blood which it has received from the lungs into what is called the systemic circulation – that is, the whole system of arteries and veins excluding that to and from the lungs. The pulmonary circulation carries blood from the right heart to the lungs via the pulmonary artery and brings it from the lungs to the left atrium via the pulmonary veins. Thus, the atria on either side of the heart receive blood from the veins, the ventricles pump it into the arteries. The left ventricle does most of the work, pumping blood into the aorta, the main systemic artery. It is accordingly the largest chamber.

Varicose Veins

Varicose veins are swollen and distorted veins visible as knotty bulges just under the skin. They usually occur in the legs — these contain the saphenous vein, the longest in the body – as a result of the veins involved being over-full of blood. This is, in itself, a consequence of faults in the valves which govern the flow of blood in the veins.

After the age of forty, varicose veins occur in the legs of about a quarter of the male population and half the female one. Though there is an hereditary tendency to the disease, varicose veins can also be brought on by a collection of circumstances. Chief amongst these is some form of pressure at the upper end of the vein; causes of this range from over-tight underwear to pregnancy and just plain fat in the abdomen. People who spend a great deal of their time standing or sitting are more at risk than those whose jobs involve physical activity.

Varicose veins also arise at the exit from the back passage, where they are called piles or haemorrhoids, and in the testicles, where they form a varicocele. Piles are more likely to appear if you are constipated. They are also common in pregnancy, where there is both constipation and generally increased pressure inside the abdomen. Varicoceles can be made worse by strain – as in heavy lifting – and by constipation. They are more likely to occur in the left testicle than the right; the left testicular vein comes under pressure from the colon when you are constipated.

Physical symptoms
Since veins do not have to withstand the same pressure as arteries, they have much thinner, weaker walls. Inside these walls, there are

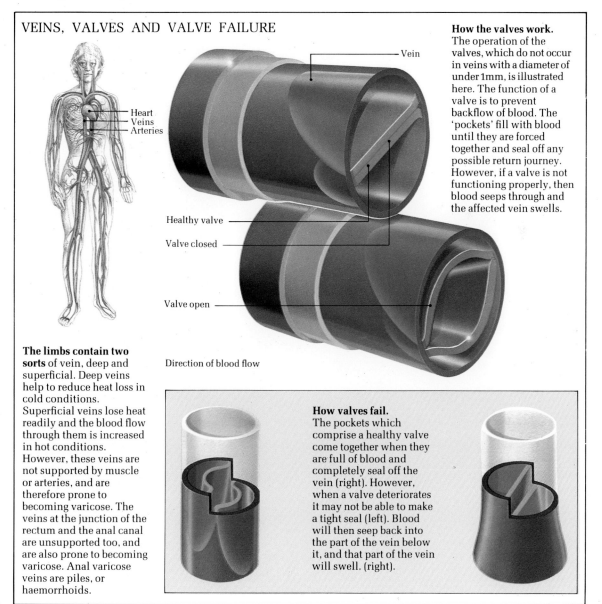

VEINS, VALVES AND VALVE FAILURE

Heart
Veins
Arteries

Vein

Healthy valve

Valve closed

Valve open

Direction of blood flow

How the valves work.
The operation of the valves, which do not occur in veins with a diameter of under 1mm, is illustrated here. The function of a valve is to prevent backflow of blood. The 'pockets' fill with blood until they are forced together and seal off any possible return journey. However, if a valve is not functioning properly, then blood seeps through and the affected vein swells.

The limbs contain two sorts of vein, deep and superficial. Deep veins help to reduce heat loss in cold conditions. Superficial veins lose heat readily and the blood flow through them is increased in hot conditions. However, these veins are not supported by muscle or arteries, and are therefore prone to becoming varicose. The veins at the junction of the rectum and the anal canal are unsupported too, and are also prone to becoming varicose. Anal varicose veins are piles, or haemorrhoids.

How valves fail.
The pockets which comprise a healthy valve come together when they are full of blood and completely seal off the vein (right). However, when a valve deteriorates it may not be able to make a tight seal (left). Blood will then seep back into the part of the vein below it, and that part of the vein will swell. (right).

valves designed to help stop the blood from running backwards, as would otherwise be likely – back to the foot instead of up to the abdomen, for instance. In normal conditions, these valves are like small pockets; they fill up if the blood is running slowly and meet in the middle of the vein to stop the backflow. If, however, the valves are not perfectly formed, the blood leaks and the vein swells up.

This problem does not arise with the body's deep veins. These are supported by the muscles they run through, while they also lie close to the arteries and so have the support of the same sheath of connective tissue. The veins just under the skin, however, have no such support. In piles or a varicocele, similar conditions apply.

Varicose veins are noticeable as bluish swellings in your leg. They usually start below the knee, but extend above it as they become worse. Your legs ache, especially in hot weather; if you have to stand for long, your ankles may swell. Thrombosis – clotting of the blood in the vein while it is flowing sluggishly – will give you pain over a small area. You can usually feel the clotted vein as a hard, tender cord, while the surrounding tissue is hot and red. This is not dangerous in itself, but it is a warning that you should seek treatment.

Untreated varicose veins can lead to varicose ulcers, which are very slow and difficult to heal. Basically, this is caused by a breakdown of the skin, where it has not been properly drained of used blood because of the varicose vein. Usually, this starts with an accidental knock that would normally have no ill effects.

A varicocele looks and feels like a bag of worms, although in fact the dilated veins run in a network over the testicle's surface. Piles

Deep and superficial veins. The arrangement of the veins of the legs into deep and superficial is useful in controlling the temperature of the body. In the deep veins there is a tendency to absorb heat from the surrounding arteries and retain it in the body. If the conditions are cold the flow through the deep veins is increased. In hot conditions, heat can be lost by increasing the blood flow near the surface. The main disadvantage of this arrangement is that it is relatively easy for surface veins to start swelling – if a person has to stand for long stretches at a time, for example. The deep veins are kept in shape and assisted in their function of blood transportation by the action of the leg muscles. But for the superficial veins muscle support is scarce. If the valves allow them to overfill with blood, then they easily spread and become distorted in shape.

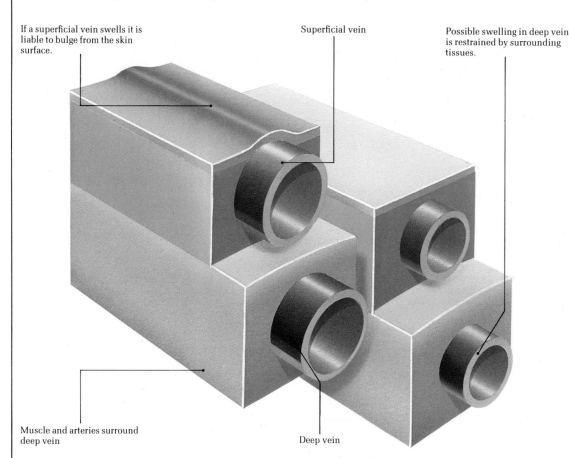

If a superficial vein swells it is liable to bulge from the skin surface.

Superficial vein

Possible swelling in deep vein is restrained by surrounding tissues.

Muscle and arteries surround deep vein

Deep vein

usually first become noticeable when you find blood on the toilet paper; this can be quite considerable if a swollen rectal vein breaks.

Piles may be just inside the rectum or outside the anus, the exit from the rectum. External piles can clot; this makes sitting down or passing faeces extremely painful. You can feel the hard, swollen vein like a pea at the anal aperture.

Diagnosis and treatment

Since varicose veins are always what are termed superficial tissues, they can be diagnosed by sight and touch. Only if your doctor suspects an important cause of increased pressure inside the abdomen will special investigations be made. Protoscopy – passing a protoscope into the back passage – may help to assess how serious are your piles.

Varicoceles are treated by operation to remove the dilated vein which is causing pressure and damage to the testicle. Small veins, which are less subject to swelling, take over. The basic treatment for piles is to avoid constipation through attention to diet and the use of a laxative. If the piles are inflamed, suppositories will make you more comfortable. If piles are persistently troublesome, the doctor may prescribe a local operation to remove them or injections to make them clot and shrivel up.

The best form of treatment is specific. A small, isolated vein can be dealt with by injection, which makes it clot once and for all. Otherwise all the veins involved can be removed under general anaesthetic. You will take about three weeks to recover from this, until the deep veins take over fully the work of the veins which have been removed.

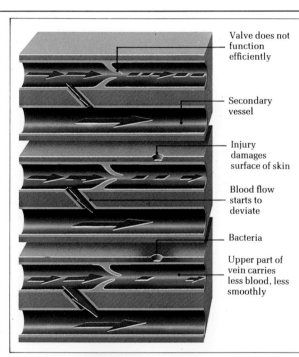

Valve does not function efficiently

Secondary vessel

Injury damages surface of skin

Blood flow starts to deviate

Bacteria

Upper part of vein carries less blood, less smoothly

Varicose ulcers.
In the normal course of events the body deals with infections of the skin surface after injury by bringing extra nutrients and anti-bacterial agents in the blood, and carrying away the waste. A varicose vein may impede this process so that the effects of an injury linger.
Below: 1 A defective valve makes for inefficient blood flow. 2 A secondary vessel widens to carry blood which the affected vein cannot cope with. An injury occurs in the isolated area. 3 Bacteria thrive in the isolated area. The skin cannot knit together.

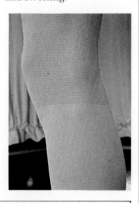

Supporting stockings do not cure varicose veins but they relieve discomfort and swelling.

How valves help.
If the valves in the legs do not work, then the blood has a tendency to succumb to the pull of gravity, rather like the exhausted athletes in the picture. If there were knots in the rope, they might be able to stop for a breather, and continue upwards slightly refreshed.

PRESCRIPTION

Diagnosis
Diagnosis is usually a fairly simple matter. The veins are normally visible, or tangible, just below the skin surface. However, your doctor may want to check that a blockage in a deep vein is not causing overloading.

Treatment
Relief from discomfort is given by supports such as elastic stockings or bandages. The only lasting treatment will be surgical. If the affected veins are small, they can be effectively isolated from the system of venous return, by an operation that closes off the blood flow through them. If they are large, they can be removed altogether. If this operation is successful, then the blood is soon diverted through the deep veins.

Atherosclerosis

Atherosclerosis is a condition in which fats and other substances are deposited in the inner linings of the arteries, which silt up like a river as a result. The consequence is that the supply of blood to the body's various organs is restricted to a point where it may become inadequate for their needs. The condition is extremely serious, since the arteries carry the oxygen and nourishment vital for life to every part of the body, including such key organs as the brain, heart and kidneys.

No one is immune from atherosclerosis; in some degree, it develops in everybody as they grow older. If it develops prematurely, however, it can be a killer disease. It is a major cause of death in both the USA and the UK, for instance; in the former, more than a million people die each year from causes directly related to the condition. You are particularly at risk around the age of fifty – especially if you are overweight, eat rich food stuffed with fattening carbohydrates, consume excessive amounts of alcohol and smoke heavily. Sufferers are also likely to lead a sedentary life.

Physical symptoms

Your arteries are flexible, muscular tubes, with a smooth, delicate lining called the intima. As you grow older, this tends to get thicker and show signs of wear and tear. In particular, its surface may become roughened.

This is where the trouble may start. If the blood moves around sluggishly and is laden with fat, this may get caught on the sides, particularly at a bend or fork. A small obstruction collects more, just like silt in a river.

One of two things can then happen. Bits may break loose and get carried along until,

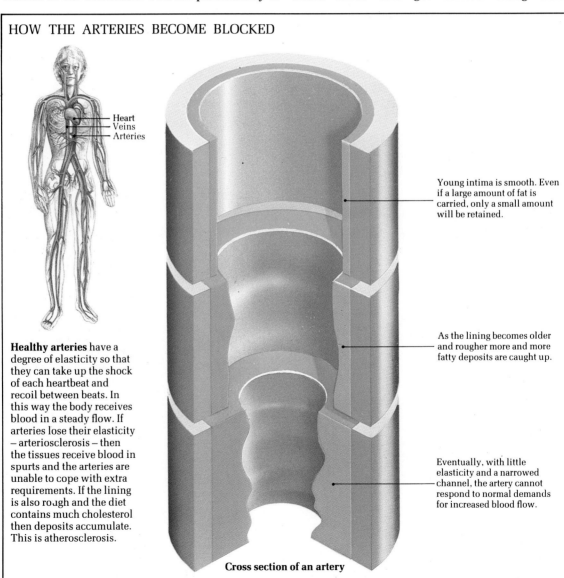

HOW THE ARTERIES BECOME BLOCKED

Heart
Veins
Arteries

Healthy arteries have a degree of elasticity so that they can take up the shock of each heartbeat and recoil between beats. In this way the body receives blood in a steady flow. If arteries lose their elasticity – arteriosclerosis – then the tissues receive blood in spurts and the arteries are unable to cope with extra requirements. If the lining is also rough and the diet contains much cholesterol then deposits accumulate. This is atherosclerosis.

Young intima is smooth. Even if a large amount of fat is carried, only a small amount will be retained.

As the lining becomes older and rougher more and more fatty deposits are caught up.

Eventually, with little elasticity and a narrowed channel, the artery cannot respond to normal demands for increased blood flow.

Cross section of an artery

perhaps, they stick in a smaller, half-blocked blood vessel, completely cutting off the blood supply to the tissues depending on that artery. This is called embolism and can happen extremely quickly. More frequently, however, the artery narrows until the blood is moving slow enough to clot. This is thrombosis.

What you notice depends on which of your arteries is feeling the strain most. If they are your coronary arteries, you may develop angina – that is, pain in the heart muscle because it is not getting enough blood to work properly. This may lead to a heart attack. If your brain is affected, your memory may lose its reliability and your intelligence deteriorate. You may get passing feelings of dizziness or one-sided weakness. The danger is of stroke. Threat to the kidneys means high blood pressure.

If your limbs are involved, symptoms will first develop in your legs. Your calves may ache when you walk because the muscles are starved of blood. Your feet will be ice cold.

Diagnosis and treatment

General and specific examinations will be carried out. Your eyes will certainly be examined with an ophthalmoscope to assess the state of the blood vessels, arteries and veins running across the retina. Blood pressure and the state of the heart will be measured, while a simple test will assess the state of your leg arteries. Blood tests will detect THYROID DISORDERS and DIABETES MELLITUS. Both these diseases are associated with atherosclerosis.

Treatment will vary according to what parts of the body are involved. You can help yourself by keeping your weight down and exercising daily.

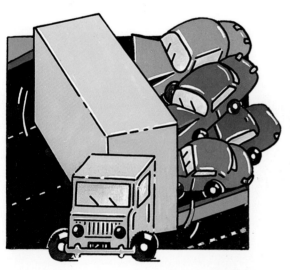

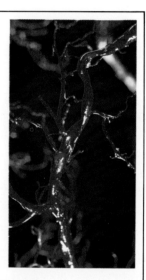

A diet too high in animal fat or refined sugar, lack of exercise and high blood pressure may all make for thick, hard arteries like these.

The blood flow through a narrowed artery is so slow that there is a tendency for it to clot. In a similar way if part of a road is impeded, the danger of further collisions is increased so that traffic may soon be brought to a complete halt.

The importance of diet
There is a good deal of statistical evidence to show that an excess of fats in the blood contributes to atherosclerosis. Animal fats produce this excess. Vegetable oils, on the other hand, seem to have a beneficial effect.

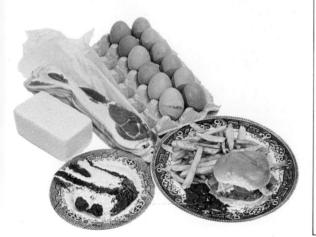

PRESCRIPTION

Diagnosis
Your doctor will look through your eyes. This is the only way a direct sight of the state of your blood vessels is possible. Your blood will be tested and its pressure measured.

Treatment
Sometimes drugs are given which cut down the amount of cholesterol in the blood, but there is no consensus on their effectiveness. Short-term precautions against blood-clotting may be taken by administering anti-coagulants. Surgery is sometimes undertaken to replace badly affected arteries. But alter the habits which contribute to atherosclerosis—lack of exercise, high cholesterol diet, stress, smoking, overdosing on sugar.

Coronary Heart Disease

Coronary artery disease results in a dangerous shortage in the blood supply to the heart muscle. Any extra strain on the muscle produces chest pain as a result.

Since the commonest cause of the disease is ATHEROSCLEROSIS, the person most likely to suffer from it is the type of person doctors define as atherosclerotic. The main risk factors are the amount of fatty acids in the blood, high blood pressure, diabetes and excessive cigarette consumption.

Physical symptoms

A heart attack can mean an artery has closed, cutting off the supply of blood and therefore of oxygen to a section of heart muscle, which dies as a result. This is called necrosis. Unless a very large area is involved, the rest of the heart muscle carries on functioning, limping at first;

in due course, the dead muscle is replaced by scar tissue. To make up for the failed arteries, small, previously unimportant, vessels gradually enlarge and may take over their functions.

The first warning of coronary heart disease often comes with unaccustomed physical exercise. Pain in the heart muscle is deep, constricting, gripping and sometimes stabbing; it may extend down your left arm or upwards into your throat and lower jaw. Note, however, that all or any of these symptoms can be caused by simple anxiety, so do not jump to the worst conclusion at first.

With progressive coronary disease, less and less exertion brings on the pain – even the effort of eating a meal, for instance. Emotional upsets become dangerous.

For a few weeks before a heart attack, you may feel vaguely unwell or tired. If you already

DEPRIVING THE HEART OF ITS BLOOD SUPPLY

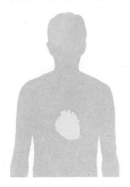

The coronary arteries are the first to branch from the aorta. They spread throughout the myocardium – the heart muscle – so that if one is blocked a portion of the heart will be starved of blood and oxygen.

An artificial pacemaker below delivers small, regular electric shocks to the heart. It makes sure the heart keeps beating, if there are interruptions in its conducting system.

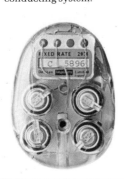

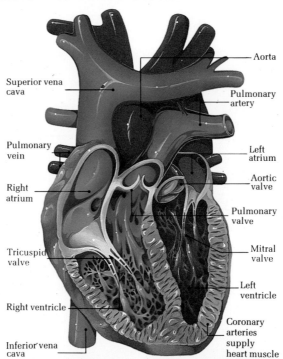

- Aorta
- Superior vena cava
- Pulmonary artery
- Pulmonary vein
- Left atrium
- Aortic valve
- Right atrium
- Pulmonary valve
- Tricuspid valve
- Mitral valve
- Left ventricle
- Right ventricle
- Coronary arteries supply heart muscle
- Inferior vena cava

How the pain is caused. If the heart has to work harder than usual supplying the body with an increased flow of blood then it will use up more oxygen and form more carbon dioxide. If the coronary arteries are unable to dilate further, but the heart is still short of oxygen, then a severe pain develops. This is called angina and is the main symptom of a coronary thrombosis. What distinguishes angina due to coronary thrombosis from angina with other causes is the fact that with a coronary thrombosis the pain does not go away if you rest.

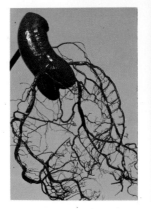

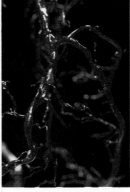

The picture on the far left shows the coronary arteries with their normal thickness. For a thrombosis to occur the arteries must be lined with greasy deposits and thickened as in the picture on the near left. A blockage here will mean that part of the heart muscle is starved of its blood. Severe narrowing, too, can be sufficient to deprive a portion of the heart of blood.

have angina, this may get worse. The attack itself comes on rapidly when you are upset, making a physical effort, have eaten a heavy meal, or the weather has suddenly turned cold. Normally, the chest pain is so intense that you literally feel you are dying. You sweat and find it difficult to breathe. Occasionally, however, there are no symptoms.

Diagnosis and treatment

In the event of a heart attack, sit in a chair and wait for medical help. If you are in acute pain and distress, the doctor will deal with this promptly by emergency treatment. Special investigations include electrocardiography to detect irregularities of rhythm, shortage of blood, and the presence and position of an infarct. Your progress to recovery can be monitored by repeat tests. A chest x-ray is also

necessary to check for any other abnormality in the chest, while a series of blood tests will indicate the extent of the damage. Your cholesterol level will also be measured.

Cardiac catheterization is an essential preliminary to surgery, in which the blocked artery is bypassed by a vein graft, so reestablishing the blood supply to the heart muscle. An electronic pacemaker may also be inserted into your chest to help your heart keep a regular rhythm.

If you have simple coronary disease, the treatment may well be purely medicinal. During a coronary attack, standard medical treatment is to remain in bed for two days or so, taking the prescribed drugs to relieve the condition. After recovery, take all the obvious dietary and other precautions: don't overeat; avoid fatty foods; avoid stress; don't smoke.

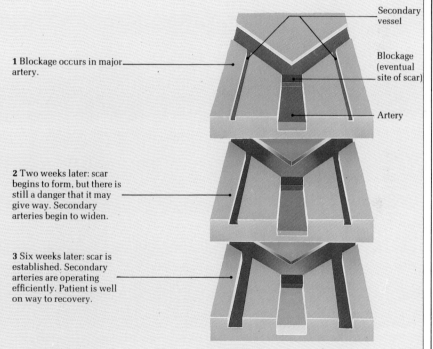

How a thrombosis occurs. The term coronary thrombosis describes a condition in which fatty deposits and a deteriorating lining have caused a blockage in a coronary artery. The effect of this is to suffocate part of the heart muscle – a condition termed myocardial infarction. Although the first attack of this sort can be fatal, most people do in fact recover. This is possible because secondary arteries widen to carry blood which cannot now pass down the blocked artery. There is a danger period during which the scar at the point of the thrombosis may give way, but if this is survived then it will establish itself and remain harmless.

1 Blockage occurs in major artery.

2 Two weeks later: scar begins to form, but there is still a danger that it may give way. Secondary arteries begin to widen.

3 Six weeks later: scar is established. Secondary arteries are operating efficiently. Patient is well on way to recovery.

Secondary vessel

Blockage (eventual site of scar)

Artery

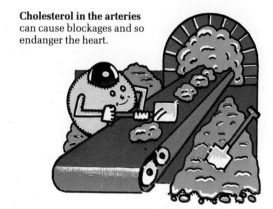

Cholesterol in the arteries can cause blockages and so endanger the heart.

PRESCRIPTION

Diagnosis
The doctor may want to confirm his or her diagnosis by electrocardiogram tests.

Treatment
Complete rest is vital. The scar must be given time to establish itself. There is a danger of a second attack, so during the first three weeks, the minimum of exertion must be taken. After six weeks, the scar in your heart should be established. Stress, high-fat diet and smoking all contribute to the disease, so a careful eye must be kept on all these. Surgery may relieve a restricted supply.

Aneurysm

An aneurysm is a bulge or swelling which forms in a weak area of arterial wall, which cannot resist the pressure of the blood pumping along the artery. There are two main types – a true aneurysm and a false aneurysm. In true aneurysm, only the inner lining of the artery gives way, with the result that the swelling is contained by the outer wall. In false aneurysm, the artery is completely ruptured.

Aneurysms can develop in any artery. Some are the result of congenital weakness, but most are a consequence of disease of the arteries. Many small ones are symptomless; the main cause of problems is if they are in the aorta – the body's largest artery – or the brain.

Physical symptoms

The most typical form of congenital aneurysm – that is, one you are born with – is one linked to the Circle of Willis, the ring of vessels which supply blood to most of the brain. A 'berry' aneurysm here shows as a little swelling where a branch artery leaves the ring. These are uncommon and usually cause no problems.

Aneurysm can also occur if the wall of an artery is accidentally damaged – by a bullet, for instance, or during a surgical operation. This can happen anywhere in the body.

The likeliest cause of aneurysm, however, is atherosclerosis. This most frequently affects the descending aorta, the main vessel carrying blood to the abdomen and legs. The physical results of this are often obvious. A bulge in such a large artery usually produces a sizeable swelling in the abdomen, with a characteristic pulsation that you can see and feel with each heart beat. Sometimes, too, an aneurysm is formed if blood gets under the lining of the

A WEAKNESS OF THE ARTERY WALL

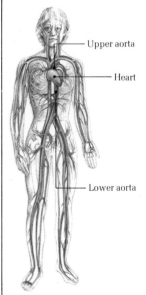

- Upper aorta
- Heart
- Lower aorta

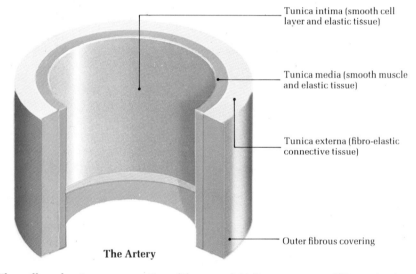

The Artery

- Tunica intima (smooth cell layer and elastic tissue)
- Tunica media (smooth muscle and elastic tissue)
- Tunica externa (fibro-elastic connective tissue)
- Outer fibrous covering

Causes and sites
Atheroma – deposits of cholesterol in the artery lining – has overtaken syphilis as the main cause of aneurysm. The main affected site has in turn shifted from the upper aorta to the lower aorta.

The weak spot in an artery wall, like a weak spot in an inflatable rubber tube, may well burst.

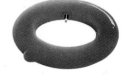

The walls under stress
The walls of the arteries must be strong to withstand the pressures created by the pumping action of the powerful left ventricle. If there is a weak spot in an artery then it will soon start bulging. This bulge is called an aneurysm. If it remained stable it would not be dangerous, but once it has developed there is a chance that it might burst.

Congenital aneurysms
Most aneurysms are caused by conditions that develop over time such as atheroma, but sometimes the defect in the arterial wall is congenital. The small aneurysms that sometimes occur in the arteries leading off the Circle of Willis, for example, are probably present from birth. They are not usually noticeable till later in life, but they may then cause a stroke.

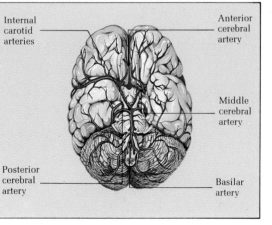

- Internal carotid arteries
- Anterior cerebral artery
- Middle cerebral artery
- Posterior cerebral artery
- Basilar artery

aorta, with the same physical results.

Aneurysm of the aorta is likely to cause you pain in the upper part of your abdomen. You may also have pangs like indigestion, or backache. The throbbing bulge will not necessarily be noticeable to you, but your doctor will probably detect it during physical examination. Treatment is essential; the chief danger with aneurysms is that they may leak or rupture without attention, in which case emergency medical measures are necessary. If an aneurysm leaks inside the skull, for instance, the result will be a STROKE. The main indication of this is a sudden, extremely severe, headache at the back of the head.

Diagnosis and treatment

If your doctor suspects aortic aneurysm, he will x-ray your chest and abdomen. An electrocar-

diogram will confirm that the symptoms are not due to a coronary attack.

If your doctor suspects you have a leaking brain aneurysm, you will be immediately admitted to hospital. If there is any doubt, you will have a lumbar puncture. The doctor takes a sample of cerebrospinal fluid by passing a long, hollow needle between two vertebrae in the lower part of your back under local anaesthetic. If an aneurysm is leaking, there will be blood in the fluid.

To avoid trouble from aneurysm, you should take the same remedial actions described for ATHEROSCLEROSIS and stroke. The usual form of treatment is surgical. A graft can be sewn inside an aneurysm to strengthen it and so avoid the risk of its bursting. Alternatively, the affected vessel can be tied off, the blood flow thus being re-routed to a healthy vessel.

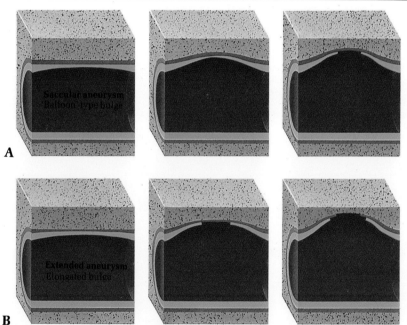

Types of aneurysm
If an aneurysm bulges in a balloon shape (**B**) it is called saccular. It will probably be a relatively simple task to remove it. But most aneurysms extend along an artery (**A**). This variety is much more difficult to treat. If the artery is minor it can be sealed above and below the aneurysm, and other vessels will be able to supply the area. Methods of treating major arteries include replacement of the affected segment with a tube of synthetic fabric, and grafting on of a non-essential vein.

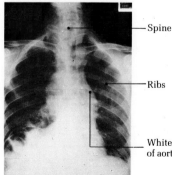

Spine

Ribs

White area shows enlargement of aorta

The bulging area on the aorta is clearly visible on the above X-ray as an extended white area.

PRESCRIPTION

Diagnosis
Your doctor will want to make sure that you have not had a coronary attack. He or she will do this through an electro-cardiogram test.

Treatment
Urgency of treatment depends on the location of the aneurysm. If it is in the brain supply network, you will be sent into hospital and a sample of the fluid around your brain will be taken and tested. Two sorts of surgery are used on aneurysms: the artery can be strengthened, or the blood flow diverted through another artery.

Rheumatic Heart Disease

Rheumatic heart disease is an illness in which the valves of the heart become damaged and distorted, so that they cannot open and close properly. The disease can strike at any age, but it most commonly has its roots in childhood as a consequence of rheumatic fever. Caused by a class of germ called streptococci, this illness develops two to three weeks after an initial sore throat and cold in the nose. What happens is that the body over-reacts to the infection, so that the antibodies it is producing attack the joints, tendons, heart valves and heart muscle.

Chronic rheumatic heart disease, however, may not appear until two to fifty years after the initial attack of fever; indeed, half the adults later diagnosed as having the disease are not aware of having had the fever in the past. Nevertheless, the sort of person who develops rheumatic heart disease is likely to be one who has had rheumatic fever as a child – perhaps more than once. The chance of this happening is much more frequent in women than in men, although the fever affects both sexes equally. The symptoms may become obvious only when there is an extra strain on the heart – in pregnancy, for instance – or after the accumulated wear and tear of middle age.

Physical symptoms

Rheumatic heart disease can affect either valve of the left ventricle—the mitral, which stops blood flowing back into the atrium, and the aortic, which guards the exit from the left ventricle into the main artery of the body, the aorta. If rheumatic heart disease affects either valve, they may become stiff and stuck together, so that it is more difficult to drive the blood past them. This is mitral or aortic

INCAPACITY OF THE HEART'S VALVES

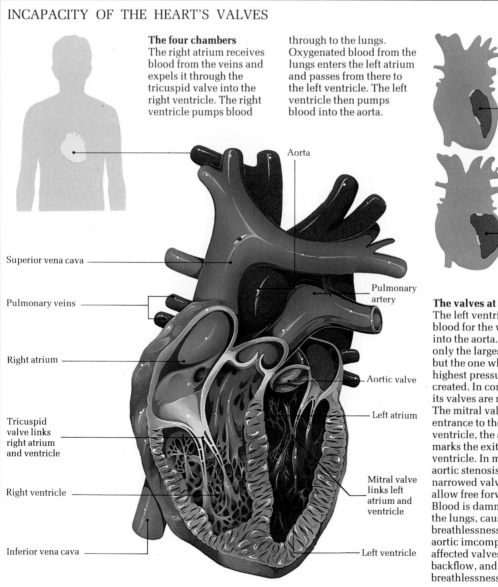

The four chambers
The right atrium receives blood from the veins and expels it through the tricuspid valve into the right ventricle. The right ventricle pumps blood through to the lungs. Oxygenated blood from the lungs enters the left atrium and passes from there to the left ventricle. The left ventricle then pumps blood into the aorta.

Aorta

Superior vena cava

Pulmonary veins

Right atrium

Tricuspid valve links right atrium and ventricle

Right ventricle

Inferior vena cava

Pulmonary artery

Aortic valve

Left atrium

Mitral valve links left atrium and ventricle

Left ventricle

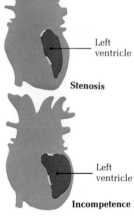

Left ventricle

Stenosis

Left ventricle

Incompetence

The valves at risk
The left ventricle pumps blood for the whole body into the aorta. So it is not only the largest chamber, but the one where the highest pressures are created. In consequence, its valves are most at risk. The mitral valve marks the entrance to the left ventricle, the aortic valve marks the exit from this ventricle. In mitral or aortic stenosis the narrowed valve does not allow free forward flow. Blood is dammed back in the lungs, causing breathlessness. In mitral or aortic imcompetence the affected valves allow backflow, and breathlessness increases.

stenosis. They may not work at all, so that the blood flows the wrong way. This is mitral or aortic incompetence.

With mitral stenosis, you are likely to develop shortness of breath, palpitations, frequent bronchitis, cold hands and cold feet. You may spit blood. You will feel constantly tired and may have a high color over your cheek bones. This is a second-stage sign of mitral incompetence, too; in this, shortness of breath is increased still further.

With aortic stenosis, you may remain symptomless until old age. Alternatively, you may get chest pains – angina – with exercise, shortness of breath and fainting turns. With aortic incompetence, these symptoms get worse.

Diagnosis and treatment

Chest x-ray is the main diagnostic tool, together with electrocardiogram and echocardiogram. Cardiac catheterization – passing a tube into the heart via a vein or artery, depending on the side affected – provides an on the spot assessment of how well the various parts of your heart are working. This is usually considered essential when heart surgery is being planned.

There is little you can do for yourself, except to live within the limits of your heart's capability. If you develop a throat infection or are due to have dental treatment, you will be given antibiotics to lessen the risk of infection.

Irregular heart beat can be helped by drugs, which are a major part of treatment for other conditions which may develop as well. Surgery can be very effective. It is possible to replace many defective valves or, in mitral stenosis, the symptoms can be relieved by cutting the tight, stiff ring of valvular tissue.

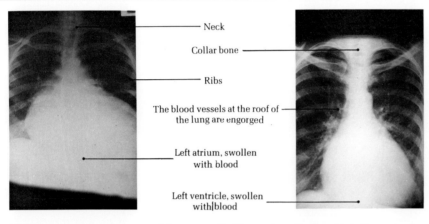

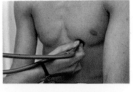

Neck

Collar bone

Ribs

The blood vessels at the roof of the lung are engorged

Left atrium, swollen with blood

Left ventricle, swollen with blood

Through the stethoscope. The heart makes two distinct sounds. The first, lower sound is made by the sudden closure of the atrio-ventricular valves; the second, higher-pitched sound is made by the closing of the semilunar valves – one of which is the aortic. Irregular beating such as can be heard if the atria beat faster than the ventricles can occur in rheumatic heart disease.

The X-ray above left shows mitral stenosis. The mitral valve between left atrium and left ventricle is faulty, and the left atrium – the white area on the X-ray – is enlarged. The X-ray above right shows aortic stenosis. The aortic valve through which blood passes from the heart into the systemic circulation is faulty, and the left ventricle – again the white area – is greatly enlarged.

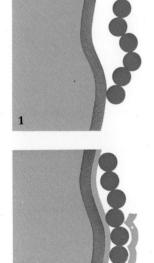

1

2

Like an allergy. In rheumatic fever an invasion of organisms called streptococci can in some people produce antibodies which, as well as attacking the organisms, affect the heart valves and the tissues of the larger joints. The joints become inflamed, stiff and painful. If the condition is not treated it may increase susceptibility to heart disease.

1. Streptococci attack bodily tissue

2. Tissue produces antibodies which attack streptococci but also affect heart valves and larger joints of body

---

PRESCRIPTION

Diagnosis
After listening to your heartbeat your doctor will probably send you for an X-ray and E.C.G. Inspection by cardiac catheterization is unpleasant but gives valuable information.

Treatment
If the heartbeat is not regular, the first treatment may be in the form of drugs administered to regularize it. If surgery is necessary this will be undertaken either to make existing valves efficient again, or to replace the faulty ones altogether. It should be remembered that heart disease is a complication of rheumatic fever—and usually a complication that only arises after many years. More effective treatment of rheumatic fever has been possible since the anti-bacterial drugs called sulphonamides were discovered in the 1930s. Early treatment of rheumatic fever seems to be the most effective way of combating the disease.

Raynaud's Disease

Named after the French physician M. Raynaud (1834–81), Raynaud's disease is a condition in which spasms of the arteries supplying blood to the fingers or toes causes them to become white then blue then red, as well as numb, on exposure to cold. Often only one or two fingers are affected when the cause is an emotional upset. Attacks vary in length from minutes to hours. Eventually, painful small blisters can develop.

The disease chiefly affects women. Primary Raynaud's is common in young women. Secondary Raynaud's affects older age groups who are occupationally prone to it, are very thin or have abnormal blood vessels.

Physical symptons
Raynaud's disease has many causes. There may be damage in the arteries. It can be the result of a disorder of the endocrine or nervous system, sensitivity to substances such as tobacco, exposure to cold, emotional crisis or associated with another general circulatory disorder. The commonest immediate cause is cold.

What happens is that the arteries react over-vigorously to a drop in temperature. Normally, when you are cold, the muscles in the walls of the arteries supplying your skin, hands and feet contract. This stops you getting even colder as the result of too much blood reaching the surface of the skin.

If, however, the arteries to your fingers are squeezed tightly by the muscles in their walls, blood cannot pass along them. Your fingers become white, instead of their normal pinkish colour. Because the nerves have no blood supply, you are unable to feel anything with the white fingers.

AN OVER-REACTION OF THE ARTERIES

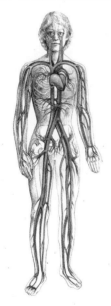

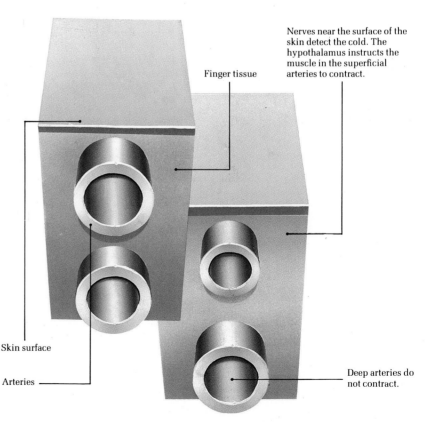

How Raynaud's Disease occurs.
In cold or emergency conditions, when heat or oxygen is at a premium, a nervous mechanism can come into play whereby the arteries at the extremities are constricted, and so the blood flow through them is decreased. Those areas where it is needed most receive correspondingly more. In Raynaud's disease this useful reaction is distorted, so that the response is out of all proportion to the stimulus. A relatively small amount of cold, or a little anxiety can result in the muscles of the artery walls cutting off some of the supply to the fingers. The arteries serving the fingers are at varying distances from the surface. Fortunately it is only those near the surface that respond in this way.

The muscle within the arteries is under the control of the sympathetic nervous system. This in turn is under the control of the hypothalamus in the brain.

Finger tissue

Nerves near the surface of the skin detect the cold. The hypothalamus instructs the muscle in the superficial arteries to contract.

Skin surface

Arteries

Deep arteries do not contract.

There may also be a stage when your fingers become cyanotic – that is, they turn bluish. This is because the circulation in them has slowed down to such an extent that the oxygen in the tiniest blood vessels (the capillaries) has been used up. As a result, the blood changes colour from red to a purplish blue.

If your hands get cold – even if other people find the weather quite warm – your fingers may thus grow white or blue and numb. When you warm them up, they gradually turn red and are painful as they come back to life. If you have Raynaud's disease, any infection – for instance, around the nails of your fingers – will take longer to heal. You will also stand a more than average risk of what doctors term toxemia of pregnancy. This is a potentially serious set of complications which can occur if you are pregnant. However, these can be dealt with.

The heightened reaction to cold can also cause chilblains, or pernio. These also affect young women more than others.

Diagnosis and treatment

The nature of the disorder is so obvious that no special tests are needed for the doctor to make his or her diagnosis. For both Raynaud's disease and chilblains, there is no permanent cure, so it is best to plan your life accordingly. You should avoid cold and keep your hands and feet warm with thick gloves and socks. You should also give up smoking.

Pain from ulceration can be relieved by sedatives, while alcohol rubs sometimes help to prevent the spasms. In severe cases, sympathectomy – cutting the appropriate sympathetic nerves – will produce immediate relief, but this only lasts a year or so.

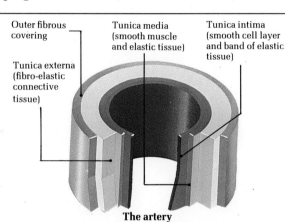

Outer fibrous covering

Tunica media (smooth muscle and elastic tissue)

Tunica intima (smooth cell layer and band of elastic tissue)

Tunica externa (fibro-elastic connective tissue)

The artery

In the larger arteries the tunica media is predominantly elastic tissue which distends with each heartbeat and recoils during diastole. In this way the flow of blood is smoothed out. However, as the arteries become smaller the proportion of muscle in their walls increases. This means that the effect of constriction of the arteries in the hands or feet can be more extreme, in terms of the proportion of normal blood flow that is stemmed.

Raynaud's disease is like a bottleneck of the fingers. The channel along which the blood is flowing is suddenly constricted, so that access is severely limited.

PRESCRIPTION

Diagnosis
From the symptoms you describe, it should be clear to your doctor that you are suffering from Raynaud's disease.

Treatment
It is best to try to avoid bringing on the symptoms, so do not subject your fingers, if you can avoid it, to unusually severe levels of cold. Smoking makes this complaint worse. Cutting the nerves that serve the arteries is not always successful, because the responsibility for the disorder often lies within the arteries. Drugs can be given that help to keep the arteries open.

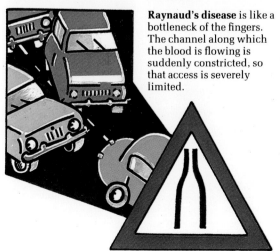

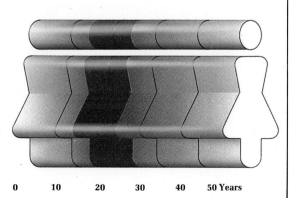

| 0 | 10 | 20 | 30 | 40 | 50 Years |

Girls between the ages of 14 and 24 are most liable to Raynaud's disease. By the time a sufferer has reached her forties she will probably have outgrown it.

Urinary/Introduction

Urine is formed in the kidneys, from which it drains into the ureters. These 25cm-long tubes move it by peristalsis (muscle contractions in their walls) to the bladder. It is retained here by the internal sphincter until it is emptied through the urethra. In forming urine, the kidneys regulate the amount of water and salt in the body, and the acidity of its fluids. They are essentially filters – or rather one million filters called nephrons. Everything in the blood apart from cells and proteins passes into the nephrons; that is: water, salts, amino-acids (which build up the proteins), and waste products. Most but not all water and most nutrients are reabsorbed into the blood. Salt is passed into the urine in proportions up to 2%. And waste products – mainly urea, formed when the body breaks down proteins – are, in large part, passed out in the urine.

The filtration process
The job of filtering the blood and regulating its make-up is carried out by tiny tubules in the kidney called nephrons. Each kidney has about a million of these. At the top of each is Bowman's capsule, which surrounds tufts of capillaries called glomeruli. Plasma is allowed through the walls of the glomeruli, but blood cells and protein molecules are too large and so pass the kidneys by. Much of the filtrate is reabsorbed into capillaries which surround the upper nephron, the proximal convoluted tubule. Wastes remain in the tubule. The loop of Henle in the medulla of the kidney and the distal convoluted tubule back in the cortex regulate the re-absorption of sodium and water and control the acid-alkali balance of the body. Collecting ducts take away urine containing unwanted salts, urea and water.

Blood cells and protein molecules

Plasma

Bowman's capsule

Sodium, water, salts, glucose and amino-acids reabsorbed

Sodium and water

Urine

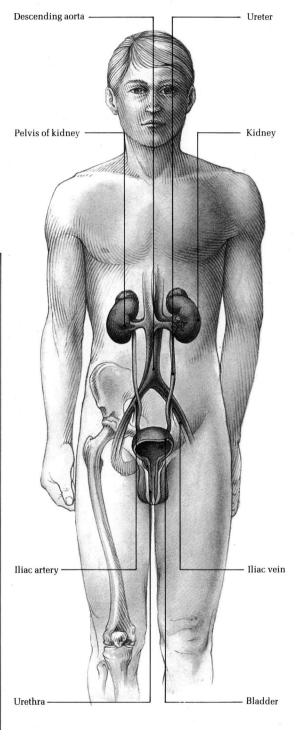

Descending aorta

Ureter

Pelvis of kidney

Kidney

Iliac artery

Iliac vein

Urethra

Bladder

The urinary system
The kidneys are next to the spinal cord, just under the cover of the lowest ribs. The renal artery brings blood to the kidneys and the renal vein takes it away. The kidney processes the blood and filters it, producing urine. This collects in the pelvis of the kidney and is taken away in the ureter. The bladder stores it, and it is finally expelled through the urethra.

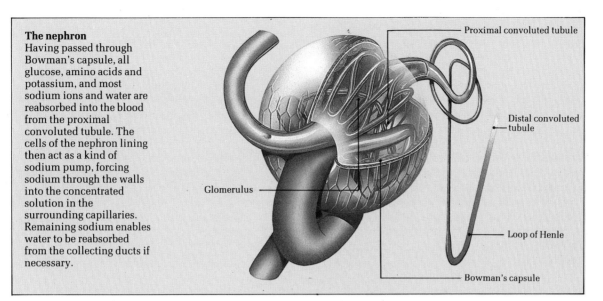

The nephron

Having passed through Bowman's capsule, all glucose, amino acids and potassium, and most sodium ions and water are reabsorbed into the blood from the proximal convoluted tubule. The cells of the nephron lining then act as a kind of sodium pump, forcing sodium through the walls into the concentrated solution in the surrounding capillaries. Remaining sodium enables water to be reabsorbed from the collecting ducts if necessary.

Proximal convoluted tubule

Distal convoluted tubule

Loop of Henle

Bowman's capsule

Glomerulus

The Kidney

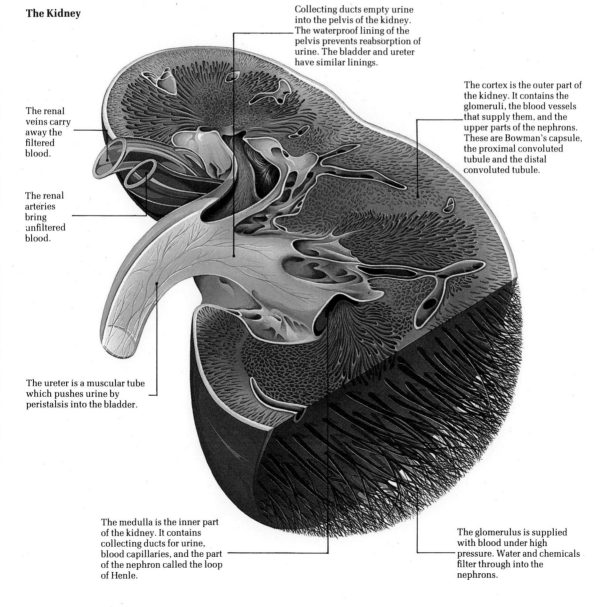

Collecting ducts empty urine into the pelvis of the kidney. The waterproof lining of the pelvis prevents reabsorption of urine. The bladder and ureter have similar linings.

The cortex is the outer part of the kidney. It contains the glomeruli, the blood vessels that supply them, and the upper parts of the nephrons. These are Bowman's capsule, the proximal convoluted tubule and the distal convoluted tubule.

The renal veins carry away the filtered blood.

The renal arteries bring unfiltered blood.

The ureter is a muscular tube which pushes urine by peristalsis into the bladder.

The medulla is the inner part of the kidney. It contains collecting ducts for urine, blood capillaries, and the part of the nephron called the loop of Henle.

The glomerulus is supplied with blood under high pressure. Water and chemicals filter through into the nephrons.

91

Cystitis

Cystitis is inflammation of the urinary bladder. It can occur at any age and in either sex; it is generally found more frequently in women than in men, though men over fifty with ENLARGED PROSTATE glands are also particularly prone to cystitis. The disease is usually the result of bacterial infection, though a virus or fungus can also bring on the ailment in some cases. The commonest cause, however, is a rod-shaped bacterium called *Escherichia coli*. Normally, this lives in the intestine, but, after a bowel movement, it can be wiped onto the urethra. Germs travelling down the tubes from the kidneys can also cause the disease, while another common cause is the gonococcus, the coffee bean-shaped germ of the VENEREAL DISEASE gonorrhea.

Some chemicals and drugs may also lead to cystitis, while a well-known form is popularly termed 'honeymoon cystitis'. As its name implies, inexperienced women can contract this by sexual intercourse and it is frequently the cause of early marital quarrels and misunderstandings when it occurs. However, structural abnormalities, associated with cystitis and leading to stagnation and then infection of the urine, are more common in children and men.

Physical symptoms

In cystitis, the lining of the bladder becomes inflamed and red, while its surface may bleed and pus can form. The chief symptom is a continuous dull pain low in the abdomen, which becomes acute when you pass water. You may notice a burning feeling when you urinate, which you may want to do more frequently than usual. Your urine itself may be cloudy with pus or blood, or smell unpleasant.

INFLAMMATION OF THE BLADDER

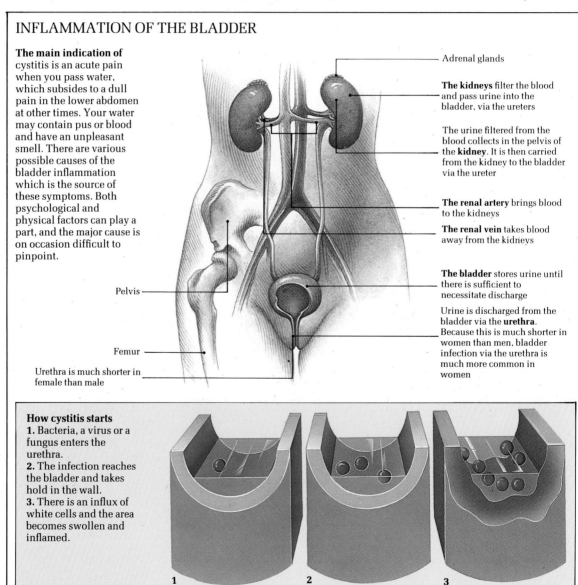

The main indication of cystitis is an acute pain when you pass water, which subsides to a dull pain in the lower abdomen at other times. Your water may contain pus or blood and have an unpleasant smell. There are various possible causes of the bladder inflammation which is the source of these symptoms. Both psychological and physical factors can play a part, and the major cause is on occasion difficult to pinpoint.

Adrenal glands

The kidneys filter the blood and pass urine into the bladder, via the ureters

The urine filtered from the blood collects in the pelvis of the **kidney**. It is then carried from the kidney to the bladder via the ureter

The renal artery brings blood to the kidneys

The renal vein takes blood away from the kidneys

The bladder stores urine until there is sufficient to necessitate discharge

Urine is discharged from the bladder via the **urethra**. Because this is much shorter in women than men, bladder infection via the urethra is much more common in women

Pelvis

Femur

Urethra is much shorter in female than male

How cystitis starts
1. Bacteria, a virus or a fungus enters the urethra.
2. The infection reaches the bladder and takes hold in the wall.
3. There is an influx of white cells and the area becomes swollen and inflamed.

1   2   3

Diagnosis and treatment

In all cases, examination of a midstream specimen of urine – what is known as an MSU – is required. Apart from showing the proportions of blood and pus cells, and the protein contained in the urine, it will also indicate to the doctor which organism is responsible for the infection and which antibiotic will be most effective in dealing with it.

In children and men, x-ray examinations must also be made. This is because a substantial proportion of such cases have some form of abnormality in the urinary system, which needs treatment as well as the physical disease. In the first technique, an intravenous urogram, the patient is given an injection then an x-ray. The second, micturition cystography, is carried out only under certain circumstances.

It is both comforting and helpful to keep warm and to take plenty of watery drinks. The doctor will prescribe a suitable antibiotic. On average, treatment need last no longer than a week and you should be feeling better within twenty-four to forty-eight hours.

After the acute episode has subsided, any underlying cause, such as an enlarged prostate or a narrow part in the male urethra, must be dealt with surgically. For women whose cystitis is related to sexual intercourse, one dose of a suitable anti-bacterial drug after coitus usually solves the problem. Some people need to take a nightly tablet of one of the antibiotics.

Although tiresome and depressing, cystitis is not a dangerous disease. It should be treated effectively when it occurs, however, as otherwise it can become chronic and disabling. It can also lead to pyelonephritis if the kidneys or urinary tract are abnormal.

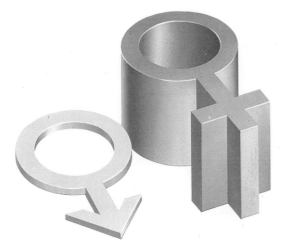

For every man with cystitis there are approximately twenty women. However, men are more prone to complications.

PRESCRIPTION

Diagnosis
Your doctor will want to test your urine to find out what sort of infection is causing the symptoms. In the case of men or children contracting cystitis, it may be necessary to take special x-rays.

Treatment
Keep warm, rest, and if an infection is causing the cystitis, take the antibiotics prescribed by the doctor. An attack of cystitis is often associated with occasions of sexual activity. If this is the case, an antibiotic taken after intercourse may prevent the onset of any infection. A sexual partner should be helped to understand the causes of the disorder so that he (or she) can be as helpful and considerate as possible. Increased anxiety brought on by an uncomprehending partner can obviously make things worse.

If the cystitis is caused by a restricted urethra, then surgery may be necessary.

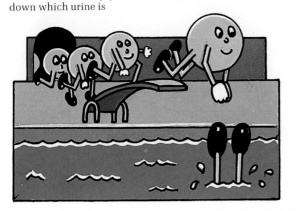

The bacteria or other organisms which cause the bladder to inflame normally reach it by the urethra. This is the pipe down which urine is expelled. It is shorter in women, which partly accounts for the higher incidence of cystitis among them.

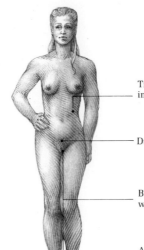

Treatment is important, as infection can spread.

Dull pain in lower abdomen.

Blood or pus may be passed in water.

Acute pain when water is passed.

Venereal Disease

Venereal diseases are endemic – that is, they are always present in the community – and are found throughout the world. They are usually contracted during sexual intercourse with an infected partner. They include gonorrhoea and non-specific urethritis (NSU), which are very common but easy to treat, and syphilis, which is rare but extremely serious if left untreated.

Physical symptoms

Both gonorrhoea and NSU affect men more obviously than women. It is known that gonorrhoea is caused by an organism called the gonococcus, but the infecting organism of NSU has not been identified – hence its name. The symptoms are similar in either case. It usually takes between two and ten days of incubation after infection for gonorrhoea to reveal itself. The usual effect in a male is urethritis –

inflammation of the urine tube – with irritation and a discharge which turns white or yellow after about twenty-four hours. If intercourse has been oral, a sore throat may be the result, while in women and passive male homosexuals, a mild discharge from the vagina or rectum may pass unnoticed. NSU produces similar effects.

In either sex, untreated gonorrhoea may cause sterility. If treatment is neglected, ARTHRITIS, septicaemia, meningitis or heart disease may result. Newborn babies may be infected by their mothers, with consequential blindness.

Apart from the congenital form, acquired before birth, syphilis presents itself in three distinct stages. These are primary, secondary and tertiary. The first two stages last for about two years, during which time the victim is infectious. The tertiary stage lasts for the rest of

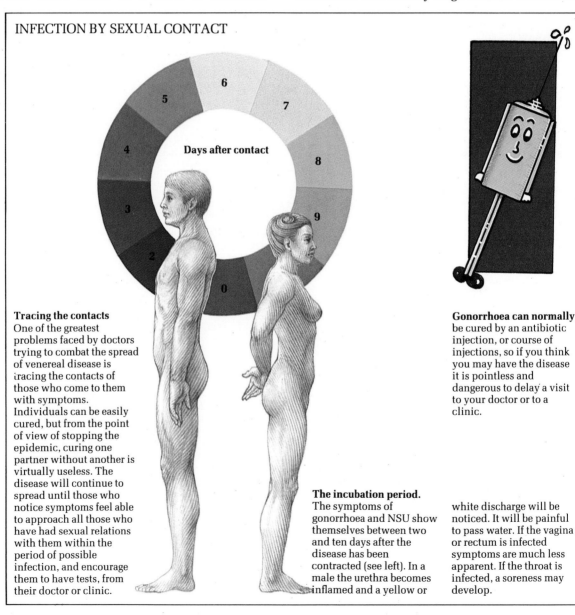

INFECTION BY SEXUAL CONTACT

Days after contact

Tracing the contacts
One of the greatest problems faced by doctors trying to combat the spread of venereal disease is tracing the contacts of those who come to them with symptoms. Individuals can be easily cured, but from the point of view of stopping the epidemic, curing one partner without another is virtually useless. The disease will continue to spread until those who notice symptoms feel able to approach all those who have had sexual relations with them within the period of possible infection, and encourage them to have tests, from their doctor or clinic.

The incubation period.
The symptoms of gonorrhoea and NSU show themselves between two and ten days after the disease has been contracted (see left). In a male the urethra becomes inflamed and a yellow or white discharge will be noticed. It will be painful to pass water. If the vagina or rectum is infected symptoms are much less apparent. If the throat is infected, a soreness may develop.

Gonorrhoea can normally be cured by an antibiotic injection, or course of injections, so if you think you may have the disease it is pointless and dangerous to delay a visit to your doctor or to a clinic.

the victim's life, but there is now no danger to others.

The first hard evidence of syphilitic exposure comes between nine and ninety days after exposure to the disease. It consists of a hard, painless sore, with enlarged, painless lymph glands in the groin. The sore, called a chancre, is usually found on the penis in a man; in both women and homosexual males, however, the sore may be hidden in the vagina or the rectum.

Unless you have treatment, the secondary stage of the disease follows between six to eight weeks later. A rose-pink rash develops and, later, little lumps, or papules, appear in the skin. You may have a fever. The tertiary stage appears between three and ten years after this. Any system or organ in your body can be damaged – most disastrously, the brain – as the disease progresses.

Diagnosis and treatment

In gonorrhoea, a smear from the affected area is taken so that the gonococcus can be identified microscopically. Since one of the greatest dangers is that syphilis has also developed, a test for this must be made a month later. These tests are made on the blood. If syphilis is present, you can only be regarded as cured after two years of clear blood tests.

A ten-day course of injections is enough to cure most cases of gonorrhoea. Tetracyclines are often the best treatment for NSU. In the early stages of syphilis, there is a ninety-seven per cent cure rate in a ten to twelve day course.

One of the greatest problems facing those attempting to stem epidemics of venereal disease is the difficulty of tracing contacts. Your doctor or clinic will ask you to try to persuade possible candidates to be tested,

The stages of syphilis
The first symptoms of the disease show after a period between nine days and three months. Penicillin cures at this stage in 97% of cases. Six or eight weeks after the first stage, without treatment, a rash develops all over the body apart from the face. This stage is still infectious. The third non-infectious stage appears between three and ten years later. The functioning of any organ in the body can be impaired irreparably.

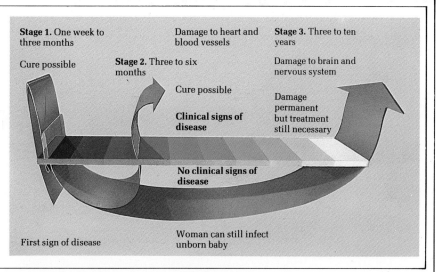

Stage 1. One week to three months

Cure possible

Stage 2. Three to six months

Cure possible

Clinical signs of disease

No clinical signs of disease

First sign of disease

Damage to heart and blood vessels

Stage 3. Three to ten years

Damage to brain and nervous system

Damage permanent but treatment still necessary

Woman can still infect unborn baby

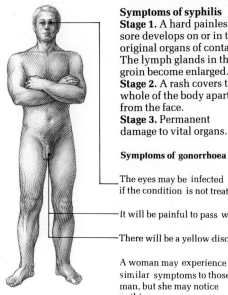

Symptoms of syphilis
Stage 1. A hard painless sore develops on or in the original organs of contact. The lymph glands in the groin become enlarged.
Stage 2. A rash covers the whole of the body apart from the face.
Stage 3. Permanent damage to vital organs.

Symptoms of gonorrhoea

The eyes may be infected if the condition is not treated

It will be painful to pass water.

There will be a yellow discharge

A woman may experience similar symptoms to those of a man, but she may notice nothing.

PRESCRIPTION

Diagnosis
A sample of the discharge will be taken and analysed, or, in the case of a woman who noticed no symptoms, a smear will be taken.

Treatment
A single penicillin injection, or course of injections, is almost always enough to combat a gonorrhoea infection successfully. Abstinence from alcohol and sex for a period of about three months, until a series of tests has proved negative, is a normal requirement. The doctor will probably test the blood for syphilis. If this is present, then appropriate antibiotics have a very high success rate in the early stages. However, the necessary period of testing is about two years.

Enlarged Prostate

Benign enlargement of the prostate gland, an accessory organ of the male reproductive system, is a common complaint among men over fifty. It frequently causes unjustified anxiety amongst its victims, who suspect that such an enlargement must be malignant. This simple, commonplace form of enlargement, however, is not the forerunner of prostatic cancer; only a small proportion of cases prove malignant. Nor has it anything to do with sexual activity.

Physical symptoms

The prostate is part gland and part muscle, surrounding the base of the urethra (urine tube) where it leaves the bladder. Normally, it is about the size of a chestnut, with the point downwards, and consists of three lobes – right, left and median. If the middle lobe enlarges, it projects into the bladder and so it is the most likely element to obstruct the flow of urine. It may act like a valve over the exit from the bladder, so that the more you strain, the more firmly the outlet is blocked. In addition, because the first section of the urethra actually runs through the prostate gland, such compression means that the flow of urine is slow and weak. As a result, the bladder will not be emptied properly.

If your prostate is enlarged, you are likely to have to pass urine more frequently than before, particularly at night. It is also difficult to urinate; you may have to stand and wait for the flow of urine to begin. If your bladder cannot be emptied properly, you may face what is called dribbling incontinence; urine dribbles out of the penis as a kind of overflow. Stagnant urine in the bladder is particularly vulnerable to

RESTRICTING THE FLOW OF URINE

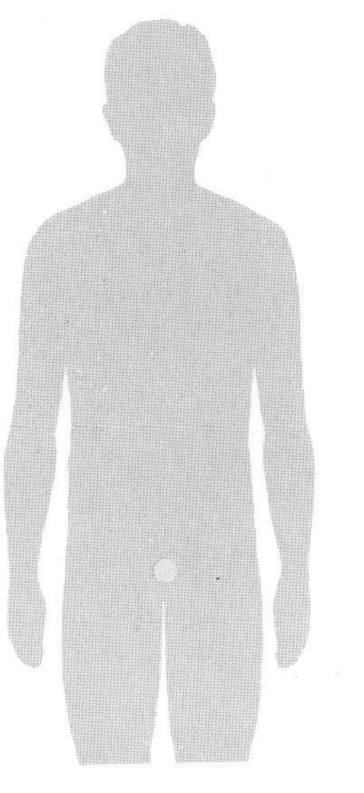

The prostate gland is at the base of the bladder, around the urethra. It secretes some semen fluid and stores unused semen.

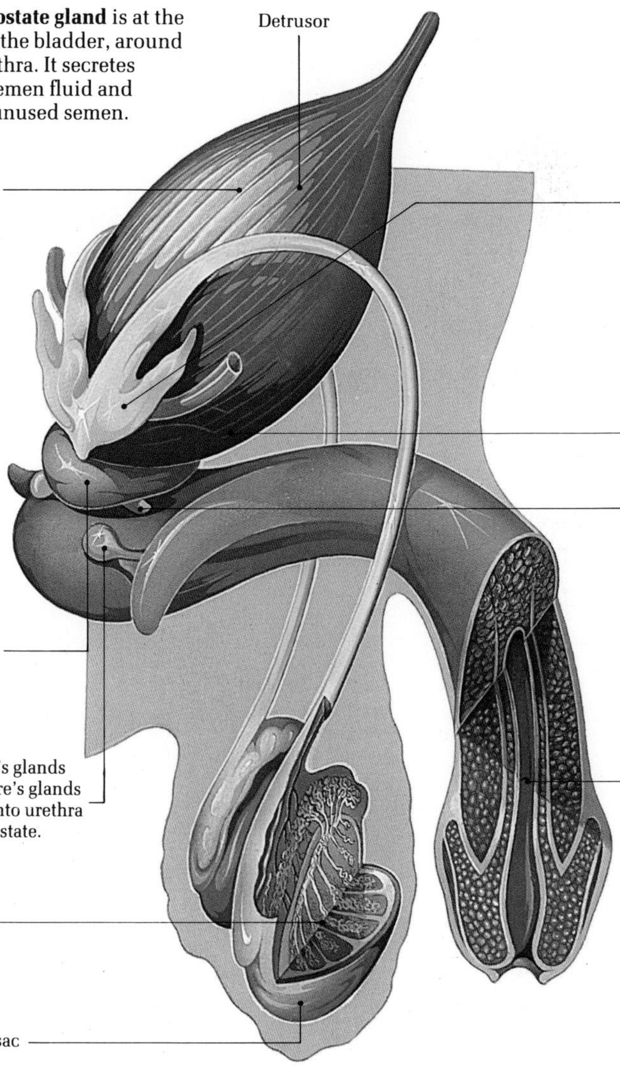

Bladder

Detrusor

Seminal vesicle stores mature sperm

Trigone

Ejaculatory duct

Prostate gland

Cowper's glands and Littre's glands empty into urethra near prostate.

Testis

Urethra

Scrotal sac

The angle at which the ureters enter the bladder prevents any backflow into the kidney. As the bladder fills, the smooth muscle in its wall allows it to stretch. The trigone at the base does not stretch. The internal sphincter maintains continence and is normally contracted. When urine is passed, the sphincter allows it through into the urethra, which is surrounded by the prostate gland. The external sphincter can be used to voluntarily interrupt a urine flow, but if the internal sphincter is damaged after a prostate operation it can take over control.

infection; CYSTITIS, pelvic aching and burning on passing water may result.

Complications can ensue if back pressure from an inadequately emptied bladder damages the kidneys. Urea, the main waste product excreted by them, may mount up in the blood stream, making you ill and mentally confused. With an enlarged prostate, you are also in danger of developing acute retention of urine – no urine can get out of your bladder, which swells up and causes intense pain. This is an emergency, requiring immediate treatment.

Diagnosis and treatment

Rectal examination, done by inserting a gloved finger in the back passage, will enable your doctor to feel the size and state of your prostate. If the bladder is full or over-full, this can be detected by feeling the abdomen and percus-sing it. The doctor does this by putting one finger on the abdomen and tapping it with another to hear if the note is dull, so indicating the presence of fluid. Blood samples, x-rays and other tests give an indication of the state of your kidneys, while a midstream specimen of urine may be examined for evidence of infection. X-rays are also useful in establishing the state of the bladder itself, while cystoscopy may be used to examine its inside.

If there are signs of infection, your doctor will prescribe antibiotics and advise you to drink plenty of bland fluid, such as fruit juice. If you develop acute urine retention, the urine will be drained off through a catheter – a tube passed up the urethra. Occasionally, drainage has to be achieved through the abdomen.

Cases of acute retention, kidney damage, or acute pain require operation.

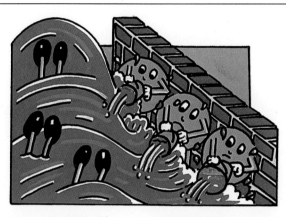

If you suffer from an enlarged prostate it is particularly important to make sure that it is not having an adverse effect on the kidneys. The half-emptied bladder can create a pressure backwards towards the kidneys, returning the waste products which have been expelled.

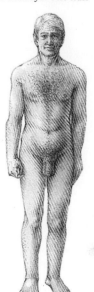

An enlarged prostate will make it necessary for you to pass urine more frequently, basically because each time you do it, you do it inefficiently. The stream is weak, and urine may dribble out. Passing water may be accompanied by a burning sensation. If urea accumulates in your blood stream you will feel ill. If acute retention develops and you cannot pass water, the pain will be intense.

In North America and Northern Europe a third of the men over 50 and half of those over 60 suffer from an enlarged prostate. The combination of long spells sitting down, and a need to frequently delay passing water seems to be particularly conducive to an enlargement of the gland.

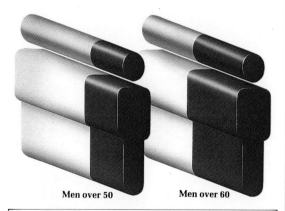

Men over 50   Men over 60

PRESCRIPTION

Diagnosis
It is wise to attend to an enlarged prostate when the symptoms first appear, because the stagnant urine that a patient retains can cause infection which spreads to other parts of the urinary system such as the bladder and kidneys. Your doctor can feel the state of your prostate by inserting a gloved finger into the anus. An over-full bladder can be felt through the abdomen. Blood and urine tests will reveal any infection that has set in.

Treatment
Treatment normally consists of removing the enlarged part of the prostate. If the operation is left too late and the kidneys are already affected, then the number of things that can go wrong is increased. If you have a good idea that your enlarged prostate was caused by some established part of your life-style, such as long-distance driving, then do what you can to avoid this activity.

Gynaecological/Introduction

The female reproductive system functions according to a cycle which, on average, lasts 28 days. The main reproductive organs are the ovaries, which from birth contain the eggs or ova, and the Fallopian tubes, down which the ovum travels into the womb or uterus. The vagina is the passage leading out of the womb and the cervix is the neck of the womb.

During the first half of the menstrual cycle, the lining of the uterus is built up ready to receive the egg, which is released by the ovary around the fourteenth day. If it is fertilized on its way to the womb, it lodges in the womb wall and develops into the foetus. If the egg remains unfertilized, it is expelled from the womb around the twenty-second day. The lining of the womb is also shed at this stage, which lasts about five days and is called the period. At the end of the cycle, the process starts again.

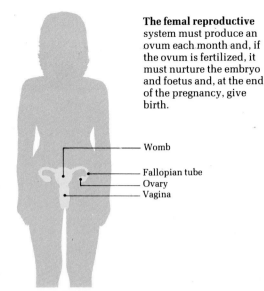

The femal reproductive system must produce an ovum each month and, if the ovum is fertilized, it must nurture the embryo and foetus and, at the end of the pregnancy, give birth.

Womb
Fallopian tube
Ovary
Vagina

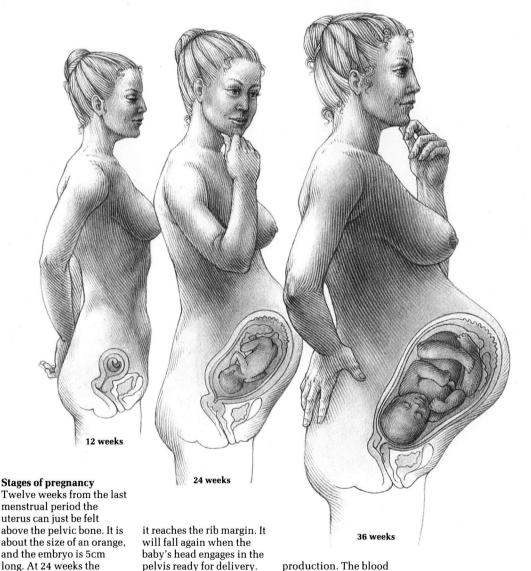

12 weeks

24 weeks

36 weeks

Stages of pregnancy
Twelve weeks from the last menstrual period the uterus can just be felt above the pelvic bone. It is about the size of an orange, and the embryo is 5cm long. At 24 weeks the enlarged uterus reaches to the umbilicus. At 36 weeks it reaches the rib margin. It will fall again when the baby's head engages in the pelvis ready for delivery. The breasts enlarge during this time ready for milk production. The blood volume increases by about 40%.

Fertilization
(1) The ovum is surrounded by a corona of small cells and a membrane called the zona pellucida, which allows one sperm only (2) to penetrate it. (3, 4) The sperm nucleus joins with the ovum nucleus to make a new cell, which contains the genetic inheritance of a new individual. (5) The fertilized egg starts to divide. (6) Each new cell divides again, until (7) there is a ball of cells with a central fluid-filled cavity called a blastocyst. (8) The blastocyst is carried into the uterus, where it sinks into the fleshy tissue.

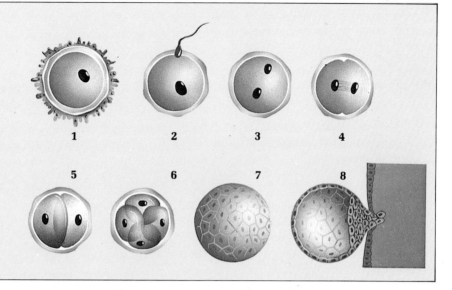

The female reproductive organs

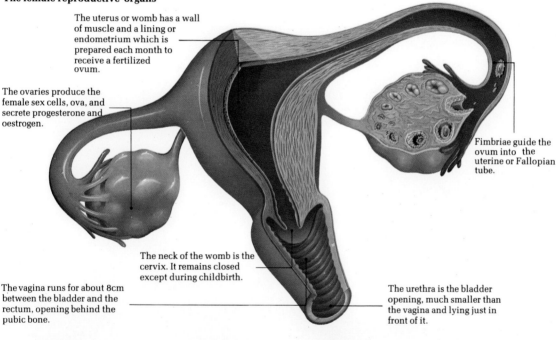

The uterus or womb has a wall of muscle and a lining or endometrium which is prepared each month to receive a fertilized ovum.

The ovaries produce the female sex cells, ova, and secrete progesterone and oestrogen.

Fimbriae guide the ovum into the uterine or Fallopian tube.

The neck of the womb is the cervix. It remains closed except during childbirth.

The vagina runs for about 8cm between the bladder and the rectum, opening behind the pubic bone.

The urethra is the bladder opening, much smaller than the vagina and lying just in front of it.

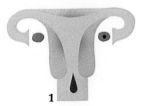 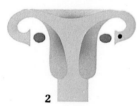 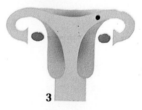 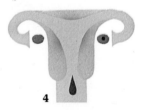

1 **2** **3** **4**

The 28 day menstrual cycle. The menstrual cycle is under the control of the hormones of the ovary and the pituitary gland. **1**. Menstruation occurs. The progesterone level is low. The pituitary gland releases FSH, which stimulates the ovary to produce oestrogen. This helps to build up the lining of the uterus (the endometrium) and stops the flow of FSH. **2**. In mid-cycle the pituitary gland suddenly secretes LH and FSH into the blood. Ovulation occurs. **3**. The empty ovarian follicle or corpus luteum secretes progesterone which along with oestrogen causes the endometrium to prepare for a fertilized egg. If fertilization occurs, the embryo secretes HCG which maintains the production of progesterone. **4**. If fertilization does not occur, progesterone production stops and the lining begins to break up. Menstruation lasts about five days, during which time the low progesterone level allows the pituitary gland to produce FSH again.

Disorders of the Period

The word menstruation comes from the Latin *menses*, meaning month; in fact, more than seventy per cent of women menstruate in the twenty-eight-day cycle, though some take slightly longer and others slightly less. All the activities within this period fall into phases, the most crucial of which is the fertile period.

Physical symptoms

What happens is simple to understand. The ovaries control the period through the hormones they produce. They, in turn, are influenced by the hormones from the pituitary gland, situated in the base of the skull. This lies below, and is attached to, the hypothalamus, the part of the brain concerned with sex. Instructions from the hypothalamus pass to the ovaries via the pituitary hormones.

When a child reaches the age of puberty, her ovaries come to life. Each of these two small glands, lying one on each side low in the abdomen, consists of an outer skin surrounding the cortex, which contains thousands of follicles. These are groups of cells of which one in each forms an egg or ovum. Every month, one follicle matures fully, moves to the ovary's side and bursts, throwing the egg out. This is ovulation. The egg enters and travels down the fallopian tube into the womb. It may or may not become fertilized *en route*.

While the follicle is maturing, the ovaries secrete substantial quantities of the hormones known as oestrogens, reaching peak production at ovulation. After this, the old follicle from which the ovum was discharged reorganizes to form a corpus luteum. This makes another hormone called progesterone, which builds up to a maximum and then falls abruptly when the

WHAT HAPPENS DURING THE PERIOD

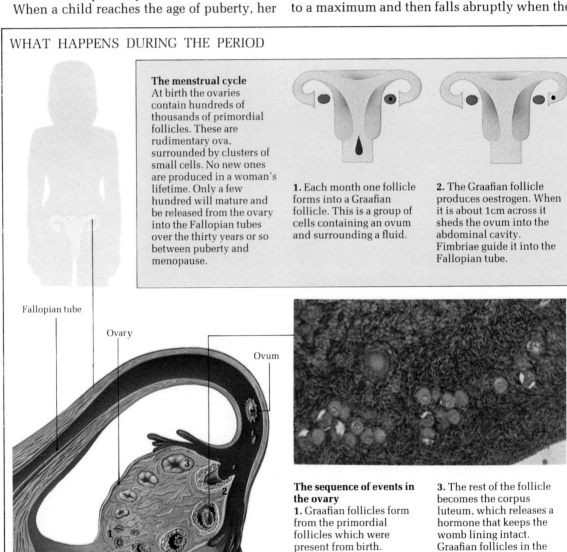

The menstrual cycle
At birth the ovaries contain hundreds of thousands of primordial follicles. These are rudimentary ova, surrounded by clusters of small cells. No new ones are produced in a woman's lifetime. Only a few hundred will mature and be released from the ovary into the Fallopian tubes over the thirty years or so between puberty and menopause.

1. Each month one follicle forms into a Graafian follicle. This is a group of cells containing an ovum and surrounding a fluid.

2. The Graafian follicle produces oestrogen. When it is about 1cm across it sheds the ovum into the abdominal cavity. Fimbriae guide it into the Fallopian tube.

Fallopian tube

Ovary

Ovum

Uterus

The sequence of events in the ovary
1. Graafian follicles form from the primordial follicles which were present from birth.
2. One Graafian follicle per month sends an ovum into the Fallopian tube, where it may or may not be fertilized.

3. The rest of the follicle becomes the corpus luteum, which releases a hormone that keeps the womb lining intact. Graafian follicles in the ovary are photographed above.

corpus luteum degenerates. The period then begins. If you become pregnant, the corpus luteum continues its life, the progesterone level remains high and there is no period.

Period disorders

There are a fair number of disorders that can affect the period. These range from amenorrhoea – having no periods – through to menorrhagia – heavy or prolonged periods, with much blood loss. These are sometimes due to a fault in the womb lining and sometimes to a hormonal disturbance, as in the case of an under-active thyroid. Dysmenorrhoea—painful periods—are the commonest problem.

Primary dysmenorrhoea is marked by cramping pains in the lower abdomen. These usually start just before the menstrual flow begins and continue through the first day of the period. They may be so severe that you feel faint. The disorder is associated with ovulation and starts, as a rule, a year or so after the first period. Fortunately, you usually grow out of it between the ages of twenty-five and thirty. Ordinary analgesics, such as soluble aspirin, are helpful. Secondary dysmenorrhoea occurs when pain with the periods develops after years of painless menstruation. It is caused by some local change, such as inflammation in the pelvis, or a retroverted womb.

Weepiness, irritability or depression may occur in the week or so before a period begins. This is known as premenstrual tension. This is variously attributed to the effect of too little progesterone production or underlying psychological tension. Hormone suppositories or pessaries, pyridoxine (a vitamin) and tranquillizers can all help.

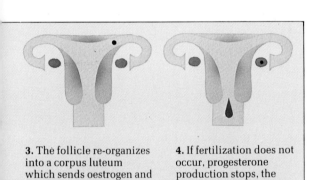

3. The follicle re-organizes into a corpus luteum which sends oestrogen and progesterone into the blood for the next seven to ten days. This keeps the lining in a state of readiness for a fertilized ovum.

4. If fertilization does not occur, progesterone production stops, the lining deteriorates and menstruation occurs.

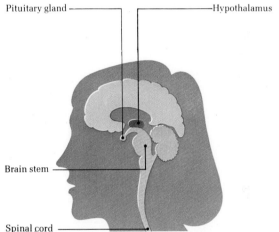

Pituitary gland

Hypothalamus

Brain stem

Spinal cord

The role of the brain
The hypothalamus controls the release of the hormones FSH and LH from the pituitary gland. In males the release of these hormones after puberty is continuous. In women, they are released at intervals, controlling the menstrual cycle by controlling the production of oestrogen and progesterone in the ovaries. FSH stands for Follicle Stimulating Hormone and LH for Luteinizing Hormone. In males these hormones control the production of spermatozoa and testosterone in the testes.

PRESCRIPTION

Diagnosis
Your doctor will want to know about the regularity or otherwise of your periods. He or she may arrange for you to have a cervical smear test. A period disorder can have a wide variety of causes, and the most serious should be eliminated. This test can detect abnormalities at an early stage. For example, cancerous or pre-cancerous cells can be pinpointed many years before any cancer develops. If you keep a record of when your periods start and stop, this information will help your doctor.

Treatment
Restriction of blood flow may be one cause of painful periods, and this can be helped by drugs. Simply lying down may also be beneficial. A hot water bottle rested on the tummy can be a comfort. Premenstrual tension seems to be at least partly caused by a larger than normal accumulation of salt and water. Diuretic drugs increase the rate at which the kidneys pass salt and water through to the bladder and so out of the body. In this way they help to alleviate the symptoms. Alternatively, a woman can simply reduce her intake of salt and water at the appropriate time.

It is not unusual to have some discomfort during the first couple of days of your period. However, if you are at all worried about your periods—if they suddenly become heavier, for example—consult your doctor. An increasingly common remedy for irregular periods is the contraceptive pill.

Fibroids

Fibroids are common, non-malignant tumors of the womb, developing in the uterine muscle tissues either singly or in groups. Frequently, their presence goes unremarked – with no complications or even symptoms – so it is difficult to judge how prevalent they are. It is thought, however, that probably about twenty per cent of women over thirty-five suffer from them. This is borne out by the fact that symptoms due to fibroids usually occur, if at all, towards the end of the child-bearing period, from about the age of thirty-five to forty-five.

Physical symptoms

A fibroid is a solid, round lump which develops in the thick muscular wall of the womb. It may remain the size of a seedling or, if left to grow, become as big as a football. This type of enlargement is especially likely if the fibroid develops in the outer layers of the uterine muscle; this means that there is no pressure from the surrounding muscle tissue to restrict the fibroid's growth. The outside of the fibroid consists of a capsule of fibrous tissue, which makes it easy to remove by operation.

Sometimes there is insufficient blood available to nourish the center of the tumor. Three of the symptoms of fibroids are heavier bleeding during periods, bleeding between periods and anaemia. While this shortage may not lead to problems, on occasion, especially during pregnancy, there may be what is termed 'red degeneration' of the fibroid. This can cause acute pain and tenderness low in the abdomen.

As has already been mentioned, fibroids need not necessarily cause any symptoms at all. Heavy bleeding, usually at the normal period time, may result if a fibroid lies just

THE LOCATION OF FIBROIDS AND THEIR EFFECTS

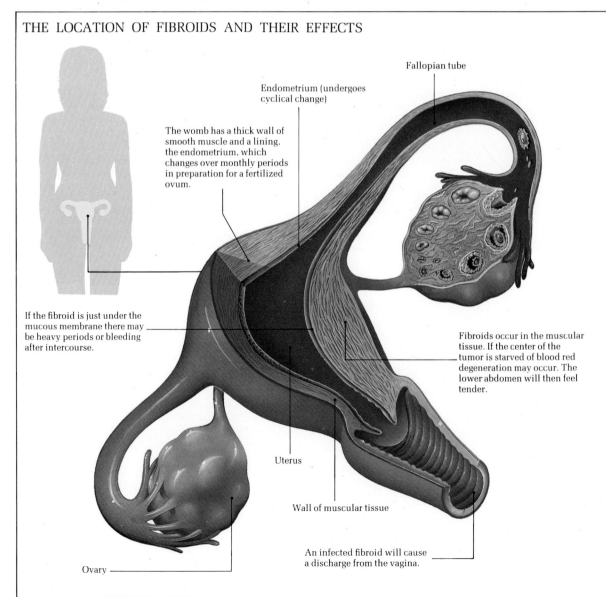

Fallopian tube

Endometrium (undergoes cyclical change)

The womb has a thick wall of smooth muscle and a lining, the endometrium, which changes over monthly periods in preparation for a fertilized ovum.

If the fibroid is just under the mucous membrane there may be heavy periods or bleeding after intercourse.

Fibroids occur in the muscular tissue. If the center of the tumor is starved of blood red degeneration may occur. The lower abdomen will then feel tender.

Uterus

Wall of muscular tissue

An infected fibroid will cause a discharge from the vagina.

Ovary

under the mucous membrane which lines the uterus. Occasionally, bleeding is brought on from a fibroid in this position by sexual intercourse, or a vaginal examination. From time to time, too, bleeding after the menopause is due to fibroids.

Pain is not usual unless there is red degeneration, or a fibroid is pressing on nerves in the pelvis. The discomfort in this second case is felt in the back or thighs. A large fibroid may produce enlargement of the abdomen; an infected one produces a vaginal discharge. Fibroids, too, are often associated with infertility.

Diagnosis and treatment
Diagnosis starts with a general clinical examination, including a vaginal examination, in which the doctor inserts a finger into the vagina and feels through the abdomen with an-

other. Your doctor may also suggest that you have a laparoscopy, in which a fiberoptic instrument is passed into the abdomen to give an internal view.

If you are approaching the menopause and the only problem is heavy periods, it is usually best to wait rather than embark on extensive treatment, as fibroids normally shrink after the change of life. If bleeding is tiresome, it can be controlled by drugs, while iron tablets can cope with any anaemia. Analgesics, such as paracetamol or soluble aspirin, will allay any mild pain and discomfort.

In most cases, however, an operation is the best treatment – either a hysterectomy, removal of the uterus, or a myomectomy, removal of the tumor, if you want to remain capable of reproduction. In all cases, fibroids should be regularly checked.

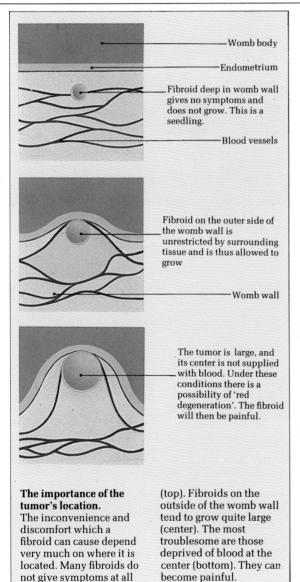

Womb body

Endometrium

Fibroid deep in womb wall gives no symptoms and does not grow. This is a seedling.

Blood vessels

Fibroid on the outer side of the womb wall is unrestricted by surrounding tissue and is thus allowed to grow

Womb wall

The tumor is large, and its center is not supplied with blood. Under these conditions there is a possibility of 'red degeneration'. The fibroid will then be painful.

The importance of the tumor's location.
The inconvenience and discomfort which a fibroid can cause depend very much on where it is located. Many fibroids do not give symptoms at all (top). Fibroids on the outside of the womb wall tend to grow quite large (center). The most troublesome are those deprived of blood at the center (bottom). They can become painful.

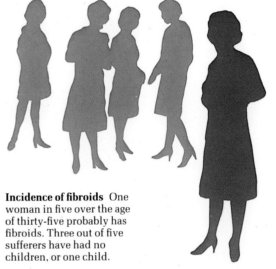

Incidence of fibroids One woman in five over the age of thirty-five probably has fibroids. Three out of five sufferers have had no children, or one child.

PRESCRIPTION

Diagnosis
Your doctor will examine your womb manually. He or she may also examine you using a fiberoptic instrument.

Treatment
The main disadvantages of fibroids are the pain and discomfort they can cause and the large proportions they can assume. For these reasons, it is normally best to have them removed. The operation is reasonably straightforward, but normally involves removal of the womb. This of course means that no more pregnancies are possible, but patients are normally at the end of their childbearing years anyway. There is no connection between fibroids and cancer.

Cancer of the Breast

Breast cancer is caused by an abnormal growth of malignant cells in the breast tissue. If it is not detected and treated, it is an extremely serious disease; breast cancer is a major cause of death in women aged forty and over. It is for this reason that all health authorities and similar organizations urge women to examine their breasts for signs of abnormality every month and to have a regular annual check-up.

Physical symptoms

A cancer is a disorder of growing cells which are not serving any useful purpose to the body. They are like parasitic members of a family, who contribute nothing useful to the family's welfare, interfere with the activities of their relatives and appropriate their nourishment.

Cancers do not necessarily grow quickly; some, like one form of breast cancer, grow so slowly that they cause their victims little damage. Other breast cancers are what are termed 'conditional cancers'. They cannot progress without the aid of certain hormones; in the case of the breast, these may include prolactin or oestrogen, milk producing and sex hormones respectively. This means it has become possible to develop several new methods of dealing with breast cancer along hormonal lines. Altering the hormone environment for the tumor cells does not kill them outright; their activity, however, subsides, the tumor shrinks and the cells become dormant.

Tumor cells may also get into the lymphatic vessels. They are then caught up by the lymphatic glands, often those in the armpit. This serves as a safety device, since these glands retain the unwanted cells for some time. They can then be removed without causing much

HOW BREAST CANCER DEVELOPS

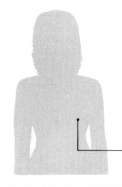

Scanning of the breast tissue. Chemical imaging of hydrogen is used to detect malignant tumors. The image on the right is normal. That on the far right shows the presence of breast cancer.

The breast: a hard lump may indicate breast cancer, but it may also be a sign of non malignant cystic mastitis.

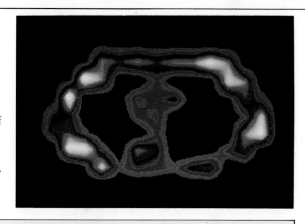

How cancer progresses. Cancer is caused by abnormal cell growth. Cancer cells have somehow been altered so that they behave differently from the normal cells from which they derive. They revert to a primitive function of merely growing and dividing, and are not fitted for any role in the body. The alteration is believed to be caused in some instances by chemicals which are thereby given the name carcinogens. The illustration below shows the way a cancer progresses.

6. Growth may become rapid – Tumor becomes malignant. Cancerous cells may well spread to other parts of the body.

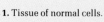

1. Tissue of normal cells.

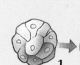

1

2

3

4

5

6

2. Carcinogen causes mutation in cell nuclei.

3,4. Mutations continue to occur in nuclei.

5. Tissue can revert to pre-cancerous state or to slow growth.

damage to the body.

The most obvious symptom of breast cancer is the appearance of a hard, painless lump in the breast tissue; sometimes, the nipple draws in on one side. Other symptoms include tenderness of the nipple, persistent pain under the armpit, areas that feel sore when pressed and discoloration of the skin. It is important to get these checked out by an expert, if only to set your mind at rest. Some women, for instance, become extremely anxious after feeling a hard corner of rib through the breast tissue; more often than not, too, the lump in the breast is often caused by chronic cystic mastitis, a common, non-malignant complaint. Vague symptoms, such as tiredness and loss of weight, are unlikely to be due to breast cancer, unless there are other more obvious signs or indications that malignant cells are present.

Diagnosis and treatment

Your doctor will palpate – feel – your breast thoroughly and have a special form of x-ray, called a mammogram, taken. As a final precaution, he may arrange for you to have a biopsy under anaesthetic. This involves taking a sample for microscopic examination; seventy-five per cent of these prove negative.

If cancer is present, operation is often the answer. Either the entire breast can be removed, plus the lymph glands under the arm – radical mastectomy – or a limited operation, to remove only the unhealthy tissues, is done. This is followed up by radiotherapy. Hormone tablets are particularly useful for older women; conversely, younger women may find anti-hormone tablets a help. Other operations can include the removal of the ovaries, the adrenal glands or the pituitary gland.

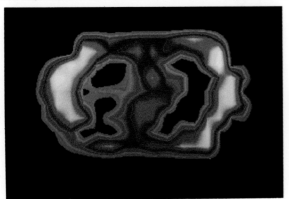

PRESCRIPTION

Diagnosis
Having felt your breasts, your doctor may arrange for a biopsy (sample taking).

Treatment
If the results of the X-ray are positive, then the cancerous tissue will have to be removed. This need not involve the whole of the breast, if the spread of the cancer has been caught in time. Removal by surgery will normally be followed by radiotherapy, to make sure any remaining cancerous cells are destroyed.

Examine your own breasts Using this routine, check your breasts once a month. **1.** Look at your breasts in the mirror with your arms by your side, then with them up in the air. Look for puckering. **2.** Lie down and, with the left arm behind the head examine the left breast with the flat of the right hand fingers. Work from the upper, inner quarter in towards the nipple. **3.** Feel round the nipple, then continue to the lower inner quarter. **4.** Put your arm by your side then working from outside the breast area feel towards the lower outer quarter, the nipple, then the upper outer quarter. **5.** Check the breast tissue across the top of the breast to the armpit. **6.** Feel inside the armpit. For the right breast begin with the upper inner quarter, and your right arm behind your head.

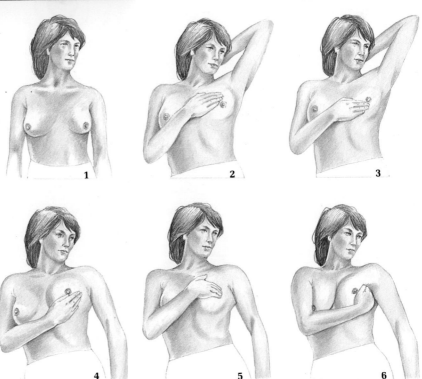

Cancer of the Womb

Cancer of the womb used to be the chief cancer killer amongst women. Now, largely due to modern methods of detection and treatment of the disease, it has fallen to third place. It is divided into two types, depending on whether the cervix, or neck, of the uterus is involved, or the main body of the organ. The cervical type is about two to three times more common than the other. It usually occurs in women over the age of thirty, who have had several pregnancies, several sexual partners and frequent sexual intercourse.

One of the most important factors in the decline of cervical cancer as a threat to life – today, the annual rate is approximately five per 10,000 married women in the Western world – has been the development of the cervical smear, or Pap test. This can detect the precancerous condition several years before the actual development of malignancy. For this reason all women, but most especially those over forty – should have this routine test at least once a year; the potential cure rate is high, provided that the disease is caught in its early stages.

Cancer of the body of the womb arises in the lining of the organ. In contrast to cervical cancer, it is rare for the disease to occur before the menopause; it is also less common in women who have had many pregnancies. Excess weight, DIABETES, and a high or raised blood pressure are conditions often associated with the development of this form of the disease. It is thought that the heavy use of oestrogen (female hormone) therapy for post-menopausal flushes and other such complaints may possibly be a contributory factor, though only if such treatment is excessively prolonged.

WOMB CANCER: LOCATION AND INCIDENCE

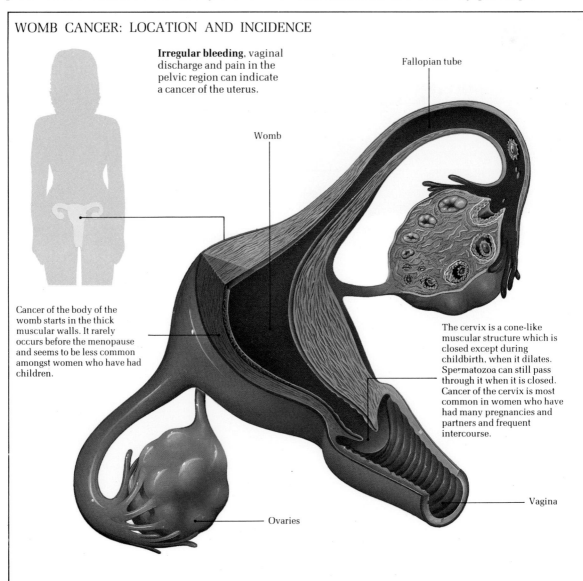

Irregular bleeding, vaginal discharge and pain in the pelvic region can indicate a cancer of the uterus.

Fallopian tube

Womb

Cancer of the body of the womb starts in the thick muscular walls. It rarely occurs before the menopause and seems to be less common amongst women who have had children.

The cervix is a cone-like muscular structure which is closed except during childbirth, when it dilates. Spermatozoa can still pass through it when it is closed. Cancer of the cervix is most common in women who have had many pregnancies and partners and frequent intercourse.

Vagina

Ovaries

Physical symptoms

The main symptoms are usually the same for both types of cancer of the uterus. The most common is irregular bleeding; this can occur either between periods, or, in older women, when you least expect it – after the onset of the menopause. The bleeding is frequently linked to a watery, blood-streaked discharge from the vagina and, usually rather late in the course of the disease, pain in the pelvic region. In cancer of the cervix, bleeding sometimes occurs after sexual intercourse, or after violent exercise. If you fail to take appropriate action in the early stages, you may become anaemic and show symptoms of extreme tiredness.

Diagnosis and treatment

In the case of cervical cancer, precaution and prevention are far better than cure. You should make it a regular routine to have a cervical smear examination. In this, a wooden spatula is rotated against the cervix, via the vagina. The cells obtained are then examined microscopically. About one per cent of married women between twenty-five and sixty have some abnormal cells; fifty per cent of them revert to normal, thirty per cent continue to have atypical cells and some, if untreated, contract cancer after, say, ten years.

Apart from these preventive investigations, your doctor will want to examine you internally under an anaesthetic. Samples from the cervix, the lining of the uterus and the vagina will be taken for examination by a pathologist.

Treatment of uterine cancer is either by hysterectomy (surgical removal of the womb) or by radiotherapy. Hormone and other medical treatment may also be useful.

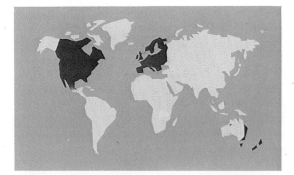

Enlightened sexual attitudes in the West seem to be responsible for an increase in the incidence of abnormal cells in the cervix. An appreciation of the need for early detection should form a part of these attitudes.

Cervical cancer is three times as common as cancer of the body of the womb.

PRESCRIPTION

Diagnosis
The cervical smear or Pap test is a vital tool in the early detection of cervical cancer. It involves scraping off a few cells from the lining and scrutinizing them under a microscope. Other more elaborate investigations may be carried out under anaesthetic.

Treatment
If some of the tested cells are found to be undergoing the changes that typically precede cancer, then the part of the cervix where they occur can be surgically removed, and cancer will be prevented. If the womb itself is the seat of cancer, then it is probable that it will have to be removed. This operation—a hysterectomy—is normally straightforward.

Early detection
Cervical smears are an important means of detecting cancer in its early stages. Right: cells from a patient's cervix are transferred to a slide. Below right: the cells are dispersed for easier testing. Far right: the slide, container and spatula used in testing.

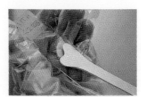

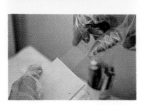

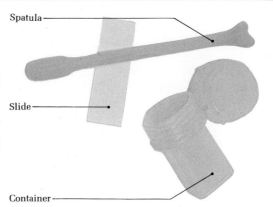

Spatula

Slide

Container

Locomotor/Introduction

Between two fifths and half of the body weight of the average adult is accounted for by muscle. Bodily movements under voluntary control are produced by the action of skeletal muscle, which makes up the largest part of that weight. It is attached directly to bones except where it would interfere with smooth and efficient movement. It is then attached by tendons. Muscles are under the control of the nervous system, and always act in groups. When one contracts, for example, another related but opposing one will relax. Other associated muscles called synergists may also contract, ensuring smooth movement. Contraction is possible because muscle fibers can shorten by up to one third. Two sorts of filament in the walls of the long cells of which the fibers are made slide over each other, and pull the ends of the muscle towards each other.

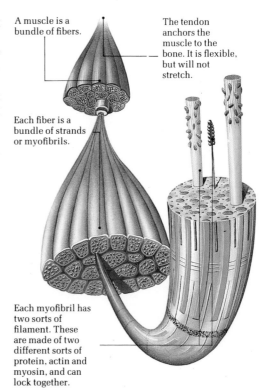

A muscle is a bundle of fibers.

The tendon anchors the muscle to the bone. It is flexible, but will not stretch.

Each fiber is a bundle of strands or myofibrils.

Each myofibril has two sorts of filament. These are made of two different sorts of protein, actin and myosin, and can lock together.

The muscles of the body that are under voluntary control are called the skeletal muscles. They are arranged in opposing pairs. Most have one end attached to a bone that is not moved and the other attached to a bone that is moved. One muscle of a pair will pull this bone, the other will pull it back.

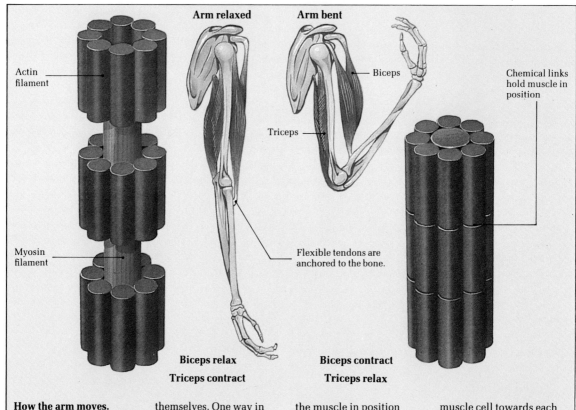

Actin filament

Myosin filament

Arm relaxed

Arm bent

Biceps

Triceps

Chemical links hold muscle in position

Flexible tendons are anchored to the bone.

Biceps relax

Triceps contract

Biceps contract

Triceps relax

How the arm moves. The brain controls the movement of skeletal muscles using information received from the eyes, from the semicircular canals in the ears, and from the muscles themselves. One way in which movements are kept smooth is through the arrangement of opposing muscles. When the arm is bent the biceps contract and the triceps slowly relax. Chemical links hold the muscle in position when contraction is complete. Muscle contraction is brought about through the interaction of the actin and myosin filaments. They draw the ends of the muscle cell towards each other by sliding past one another. The fibers which make up the muscle are thus shortened, and contraction of whole bundles of fibers results in turn in a pull on a bone.

The bones
The bones support the body and give it shape. They protect the internal organs and act as a system of levers, moved by muscles. Red and white blood cells are produced in the red marrow of some bones and reserves of calcium, sodium and phosphorus are stored in them.

The muscles
Muscles act in groups under the control of the nervous system. Skeletal muscle accounts for about half of the weight of an adult. It moves bones by contracting or relaxing. It is attached to the bone directly or by tendons.

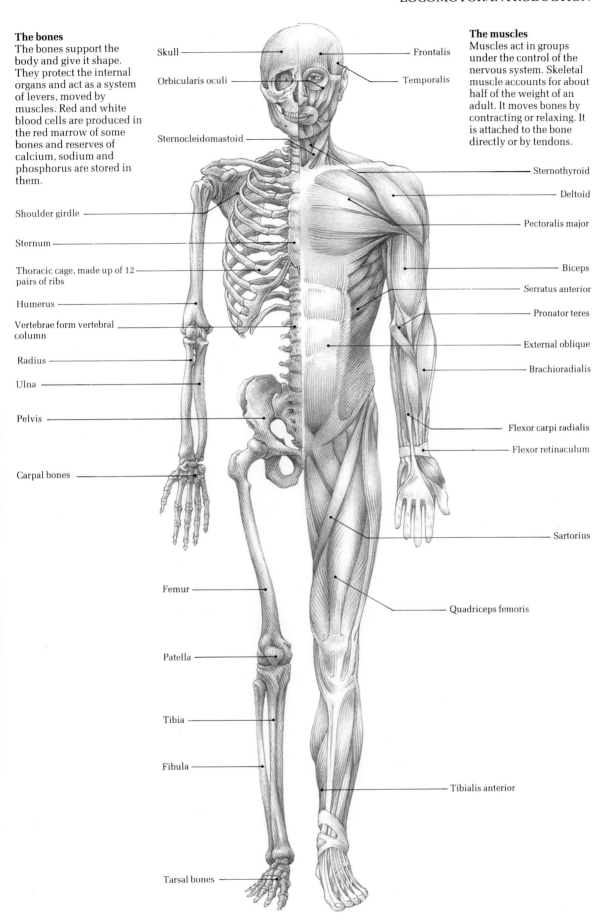

Skull

Orbicularis oculi

Frontalis

Temporalis

Sternocleidomastoid

Sternothyroid

Deltoid

Pectoralis major

Shoulder girdle

Sternum

Thoracic cage, made up of 12 pairs of ribs

Biceps

Serratus anterior

Pronator teres

Humerus

External oblique

Vertebrae form vertebral column

Brachioradialis

Radius

Ulna

Pelvis

Flexor carpi radialis

Flexor retinaculum

Carpal bones

Sartorius

Femur

Quadriceps femoris

Patella

Tibia

Fibula

Tibialis anterior

Tarsal bones

Osteoarthrosis

Osteoarthrosis is a degenerative disease affecting the joints. As a consequence it tends to strike the middle-aged and the elderly almost exclusively. Usually, many joints are affected, including the end joints of the fingers.

The older you are, the more likely you are to contract osteoarthrosis. As the body ages, the joints are more affected by wear and tear, since worn tissue is not repaired and regenerated at the same rate as when you are younger. The disorder can also be secondary to previous injury, a disease such as gout, or hormonal disturbances affecting one or more joints. Obesity is a contributing factor in people with an arthritic tendency, since the extra weight puts more stress on the joints.

Physical symptoms
In osteoarthrosis, the cartilage or gristle – the smooth, slightly elastic sliding surface to the bones of a joint – becomes soft. The parts subjected to most wear are usually those most affected. The surface cracks, fragments and ulcerates. At the same time, outgrowths of bone called osteophytes develop around the joint and may obstruct its movement.

The first indication of osteoarthrosis may be the development of what is known as Heberden's nodes – hard, bony swellings in the last joint of your fingers. They may be painful at first, or merely appear insidiously. Other joints, excluding the wrist joints, may be involved and become painful and stiff after use. Morning stiffness, as associated with RHEUMATOID ARTHRITIS, also occurs in osteoarthrosis, though the stiffness seldom lasts for more than fifteen minutes.

Cervical spondylosis – osteoarthrosis of the

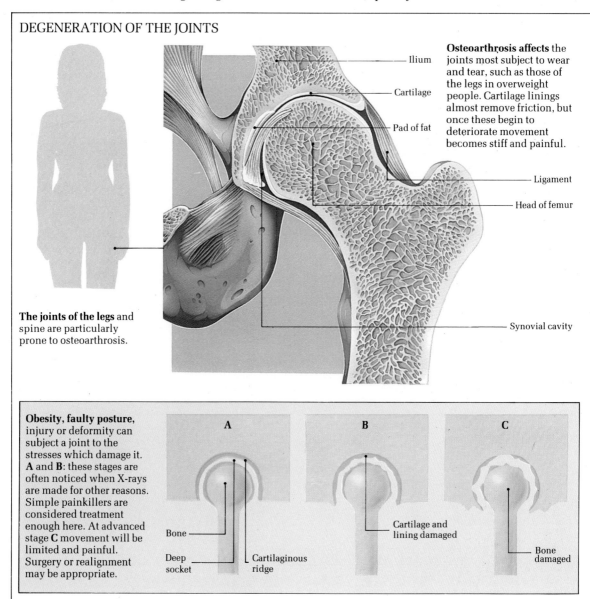

DEGENERATION OF THE JOINTS

Osteoarthrosis affects the joints most subject to wear and tear, such as those of the legs in overweight people. Cartilage linings almost remove friction, but once these begin to deteriorate movement becomes stiff and painful.

Ilium

Cartilage

Pad of fat

Ligament

Head of femur

Synovial cavity

The joints of the legs and spine are particularly prone to osteoarthrosis.

Obesity, faulty posture, injury or deformity can subject a joint to the stresses which damage it. A and B: these stages are often noticed when X-rays are made for other reasons. Simple painkillers are considered treatment enough here. At advanced stage C movement will be limited and painful. Surgery or realignment may be appropriate.

A

B

C

Bone

Deep socket

Cartilaginous ridge

Cartilage and lining damaged

Bone damaged

joints between the vertebrae of the neck – may cause pressure on the nerves of your shoulders, arms and hands. Symptoms include numbness, pins and needles and pain in these areas. Affected joints in general are limited in their range of movement. They also creak or grate as they move.

Diagnosis and treatment

The doctor's first task is to explain to the patient the nature of the disease. This is vital, since many people fear that they have contracted rheumatoid arthritis, which is a much more crippling disease. The main diagnostic tool is x-ray, which shows up narrowing of joint space, osteophytes and loss of cartilage. Drugs may be prescribed, but these can only help to relieve pain; they are not a cure for the disease.

Excessive rest can be as bad as excessive exercise; both should be undertaken in moderation. Swimming is helpful. Sensible measures include reducing your weight, if necessary—especially if the hip or knee joints are involved—and the demands you make on your body. Simple pain killers are useful if you are subject to spontaneous pain in the night. Since pain in osteoarthrosis seems to be influenced by the weather—cold and damp increase pain and stiffness—sufferers should dress warmly. Heat therapy can be soothing.

If one hip joint is affected, the use of a walking stick on the opposite side reduces the load on the joint by three-quarters. A cervical collar can help in cervical spondylosis, or a surgical corset if the lower part of the spine is affected. Physiotherapy may be invaluable to retrain and strengthen the muscles which support your joints.

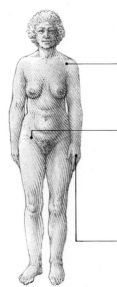

Numbness and pins and needles around the shoulders, arms and hands may indicate osteoarthrosis in the neck joints.

Any affected joint will move less easily. You will sense a grating and may hear a creaking.

Heberden's nodes at the last finger joints may be the first indication of osteoarthrosis.

PRESCRIPTION

Diagnosis
Your doctor will arrange for you to have an X-ray. This will reveal the characteristic closing up of the joint, and the worn cartilage. He or she will want to know how difficult and painful you find movement of joints.

Treatment
The symptoms of osteoarthrosis do not extend beyond the affected joints, and treatment is normally confined to relieving the pain which the complaint gives. Analgesics, keeping warm, supporting joints and applying heat can all help. In advanced cases the joint can be replaced. If the case is not so serious, related muscles will still be either strained or weakened. A walking stick can give help when there is too much strain on one side. Physiotherapy is invaluable in keeping muscles in shape that are in danger of weakening through lack of use. Surgical supports are also useful in specific cases.

Various surgical methods of treating joints affected by osteoarthrosis have been tried, but replacement of the inefficient and painful joint (see X-ray, below left) by a ball and socket joint (right) still gives best results.

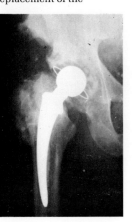

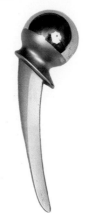

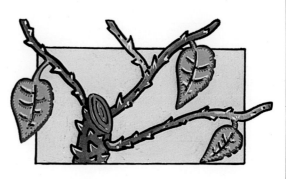

Young leaves have strong but flexible attachments to the parent branch.

Eventually the attachment becomes brittle and loses flexibility.

Rheumatoid Arthritis

Arthritis is a generally-used term to define diseases which give the sufferer painful joints. The definition covers inflammatory disease, or true arthritis, and, in addition, degenerative disorders of the joints, such as osteoarthrosis. These, together with rheumatoid arthritis, are the most troublesome forms of the disease.

Rheumatoid arthritis is a disease of unknown origin. It can begin suddenly, affecting several joints to cause pain and swelling, or gradually, affecting first one joint and then another. The disease affects women three times as much as men; the peak age for its onset is between twenty-five and fifty-five. No age is exempt, however. It can strike in childhood, when it is known as Still's disease, and in the elderly. At sixty-five and over, sixteen per cent of women show signs of the disease. Heredity also plays a part in its development; you stand four times the risk of developing rheumatoid arthritis if you have a close relative with the disease.

Physical symptoms

For some mysterious reason, the problem starts with over-activity of what doctors call the body's immune processes. The effects of this show themselves in the synovial membranes, which form the lining to the joints, the tendon sheaths and bursae. The latter are small water-cushions, which protect prominent joints or bony protuberances. When the synovium is inflamed, it grows thickly and untidily, eroding the gristle that covers the bone end in a joint and even the bone itself. The end result of this may be severe deformity.

The disease normally develops very gradually, with joints on both sides affected symmetrically. Usually, swelling in the joints of the

INFLAMMATION OF THE JOINTS

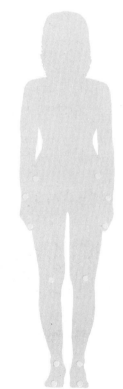

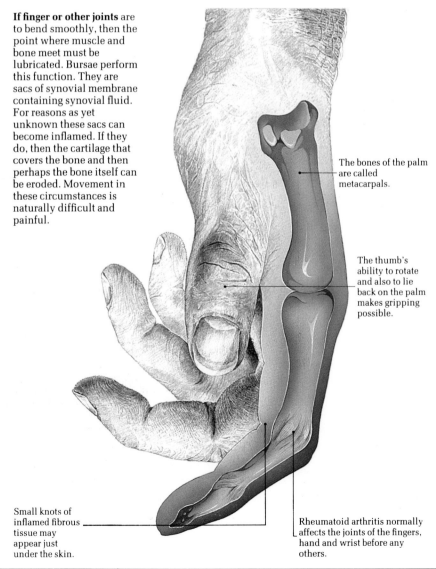

If finger or other joints are to bend smoothly, then the point where muscle and bone meet must be lubricated. Bursae perform this function. They are sacs of synovial membrane containing synovial fluid. For reasons as yet unknown these sacs can become inflamed. If they do, then the cartilage that covers the bone and then perhaps the bone itself can be eroded. Movement in these circumstances is naturally difficult and painful.

Rheumatoid arthritis affects the joints: normally those of the hands and wrists first then, progressively, the feet, the larger ankle joints, the knees and the hips. There may be mild fever and weight loss, pins and needles in the legs and feet, pleurisy and anaemia.

Small knots of inflamed fibrous tissue may appear just under the skin.

The bones of the palm are called metacarpals.

The thumb's ability to rotate and also to lie back on the palm makes gripping possible.

Rheumatoid arthritis normally affects the joints of the fingers, hand and wrist before any others.

hands and wrists is the first symptom to be noticed; the feet and, later, the larger joints in the ankles, knees and hips are then affected. If the disease is active, you will have stiffness and pain in your joints when you wake in the morning, lasting for more than half an hour. Your sleep may be disturbed by pain and you may feel generally below par, with mild fever and loss of weight. After several weeks or months, the joints may return to normal, but such relief is short-lived. Rheumatoid arthritis is a chronic disease. On the other hand, it is common for the inflammation to subside without leaving any aftermath of damage to the joints.

Other parts of your body can be involved. Your nerves may be affected, causing pins and needles in legs and feet. Particularly in men, there is the chance of pleurisy. Anaemia is very common.

Diagnosis and treatment

The main diagnostic tool is x-rays. Swelling of the soft tissues is visible to the naked eye, but the characteristic erosion of the bones near the joints shows up only on radiography.

Because the basic cause of the disease is still unknown, treatment cannot aim at more than control and modification of the effects of the disease. In the early stages, rest and skilled physiotherapy are vital. Pain killers and anti-inflammatory drugs give you some relief. More specific measures include the use of gold salts, given by intramuscular injection in a long course, followed by maintenance injections monthly for two to three years. Other drugs can be useful but, because, they may have toxic effects, all need careful monitoring. Surgery may be helpful, but, at best, can only relieve some of the effects of the disease.

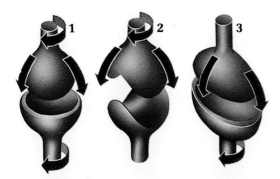

The Synovial Joints
These are known as freely movable joints, although possible movement is in fact limited to various combinations of angular, rotational and gliding movements. (**1**) In a ball and socket joint movement is allowed in all directions. The hip and shoulder joints are examples. (**2**) Ellipsoid joints such as those between finger and palm allow circling and bending but not rotation. (**3**) Saddle joints cannot rotate but angular and circling movements are possible. The ankle joints and the joint of wrist and thumb are saddle joints.

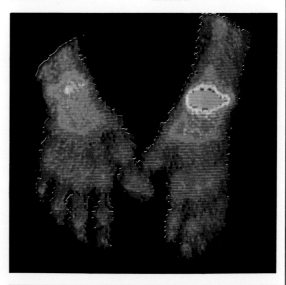

The areas of inflammation of rheumatoid arthritis will show on a thermogram. The red areas are hottest and so most affected.

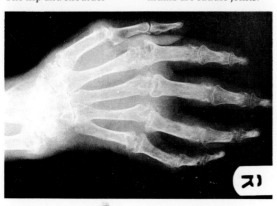

Inflammation around joints causes the muscles to tighten, and this can lead to deforming of the joint. The distortion shown in this X-ray is the result of many years of rheumatoid arthritis.

PRESCRIPTION

Diagnosis
Your doctor will send you for an X-ray. This will reveal the condition of the bones near the joints.

Treatment
In severe cases steroid hormones give massive relief of the arthritic symptoms, but these are not used in less severe cases because the price paid in terms of undesirable side-effects is too high. There is no cure as yet for rheumatoid arthritis, but a good deal can be done to relieve the discomfort and inflammation. Aspirin and other similar drugs are particularly useful. In some cases treatment with gold salts proves effective, but it is not known how these work. Splints are sometimes used to protect affected joints.

Slipped Disc

Slipped disc is the common name for what happens when one of the discs of cartilage that act as cushions between the bones of the backbone slips out of position. It occurs most commonly in the lumbar region – that is, the lower part of the back – mainly as a result of strain caused by lifting.

A slipped disc can occur from adolescence onwards. In a young person, the cause is usually a definite injury or strain; in old age, however, backache is more likely to be due to general degeneration, as the discs dry up and shrink. You are a likely candidate for a lumbar slipped disc if you have had several attacks of acute low back pain over the years, are male and aged about forty. You may precipitate the prolapse by a fall, jarring your spine, or heavy lifting, but there may be no immediate cause you can recall.

Discs in the neck can be affected, too. If this happens, there is likely to be associated degenerative change. You will probably be aged between thirty-five and fifty and of either sex. Though you may have strained your neck through some unaccustomed exertion, it is more likely that there is no apparent reason for the disease to occur. You may well have had a stiff neck on occasions in the past, but without attacks of pain.

Physical symptoms

The backbone consists of a curved, flexible column of twenty-four separate bones – seven in the neck, twelve at chest level and five in the lower back, plus the sacrum and coccyx, or tail bone, at the bottom. Between each of the movable bones, or vertebrae, is a cushion of gristle, or cartilage, called an intervertebral

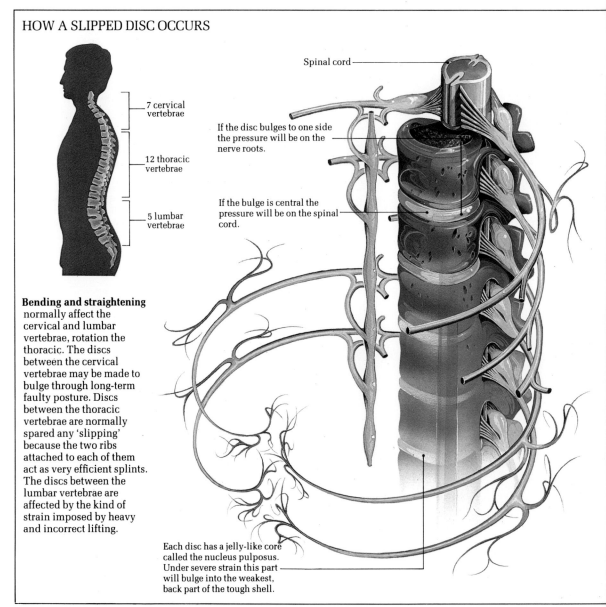

HOW A SLIPPED DISC OCCURS

7 cervical vertebrae

12 thoracic vertebrae

5 lumbar vertebrae

Spinal cord

If the disc bulges to one side the pressure will be on the nerve roots.

If the bulge is central the pressure will be on the spinal cord.

Bending and straightening normally affect the cervical and lumbar vertebrae, rotation the thoracic. The discs between the cervical vertebrae may be made to bulge through long-term faulty posture. Discs between the thoracic vertebrae are normally spared any 'slipping' because the two ribs attached to each of them act as very efficient splints. The discs between the lumbar vertebrae are affected by the kind of strain imposed by heavy and incorrect lifting.

Each disc has a jelly-like core called the nucleus pulposus. Under severe strain this part will bulge into the weakest, back part of the tough shell.

disc. This allows for a small amount of movement in each direction; it also acts as a natural shock absorber.

The ribs impede movement in the chest, or thoracic, part of the spine, while, at the lower end, the bones are fused. This leaves the neck and the weight-bearing lumbar region as the most mobile sections. Because of this, they are the most liable to damage and strain.

If a lumbar disc slips out of place, the usual result – apart from local back pain – is sciatica. Pain is felt in the back, one side of the buttocks and the back or side of the thigh and calf. Either the heel or the top of your foot may be painful, the pain extending into the big toe. You may also get pain in the front of the thigh. You will only be able to lift your leg a small distance because of the pain; if you touch the skin on the foot, the sensation may feel dull or strange.

If a neck disc is involved, you are likely to have severe pain, with tingling and numbness usually affecting either the inner or outer aspect of the arm and hand. You will be unable to move your neck for pain.

Diagnosis and treatment

Examination will exclude such disorders as the virus disease shingles, which affects the nerve roots, DIABETES MELLITUS and rectal problems. During the period of severe pain, rest is essential, combined with generous doses of analgesics. A cervical collar or a corset may be useful during the recovery period, while graduated exercises will strengthen your back and neck muscles and provide a natural, flexible splint. Avoid lifting anything heavy for the foreseeable future. If you have chronic or recurrent sciatica, surgery may be the best answer.

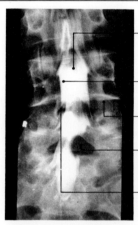

The X-ray above shows how a disc forced out of place presses into the spinal cord. The displaced disc is in the dark area, against the spinal cord.

— Spine

— Dye in the space around the spinal cord.

— The dark 'stripes' are normal discs.

— The black area shows the disc pressing into the spinal cord.

— Dents in the white area show where the nerves leave the spinal cord.

PRESCRIPTION

Diagnosis
Diseases such as shingles and diabetes mellitus sometimes show symptoms similar to those produced by a slipped disc. These will have to be ruled out by appropriate tests.

Treatment
If the pain is acute, it may be necessary to lie on your back for a matter of weeks. If the vertebrae at the neck are affected, then a splint in the form of a surgical collar may make this unnecessary. In less severe cases, the disorder may respond to physiotherapy in the form of teaching on how to improve your posture. Physical manipulation will be administered by a physiotherapist. It is quite feasible, if the disorder persists, to cut out the protruding part of the disc surgically.

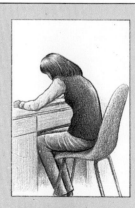
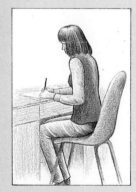
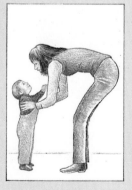
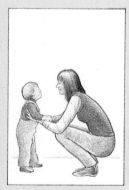

How it happens.
The back can be strained by such activities as slaving over a sink that is too low, or working with a persistently poor posture at a desk (above left). The back should be kept quite straight (right). Incorrect lifting is a common cause of slipped discs in the lumbar region. This is a common industrial accident, but housewives too are at risk. Lifting children, bathing them, and many other household duties have their dangers in this respect. The main rule to remember is that the knees should always be bent (far right) to take the strain that would otherwise impose on the back (center right) and threaten the discs.

Ears/Introduction

The central organ of hearing is the organ of Corti, inside the cochlea of the inner ear. Vibrations are carried to it through the outer and middle ear. The organ acts on these vibrations like a microphone. Any movement in the organ of Corti initiates an electrical current. This is a sort of translation of the original vibration. Notes of different pitches travel varying distances along the organ of Corti, lower notes further than high notes. Each part of the organ has its own nerve fiber to the brain, and in this way the brain can determine the pitch of a sound. Higher notes travel less far down the organ, and so stimulate fewer cells. This accounts for the fact that when hearing is affected by ageing the highest notes are lost first, diminishing sensitivity in the cells cutting out the more delicate responses. The ear also helps to control balance, through the semilunar canals.

Of the organs of the inner ear, the cochlea is concerned with hearing, the semicircular canals detect movement of the head, and the vestibule monitors position. Both the vestibular and the auditory branch of the VIII cranial serve the inner ear.

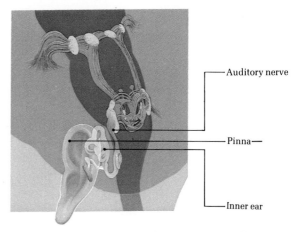

Auditory nerve

Pinna

Inner ear

The ear-drum conveys sound to the three interlocking bones in the air-filled cavity of the middle ear.

Malleus — Incus — Stapes — Utricle — Vestibular and auditory branches of VIII cranial nerve.

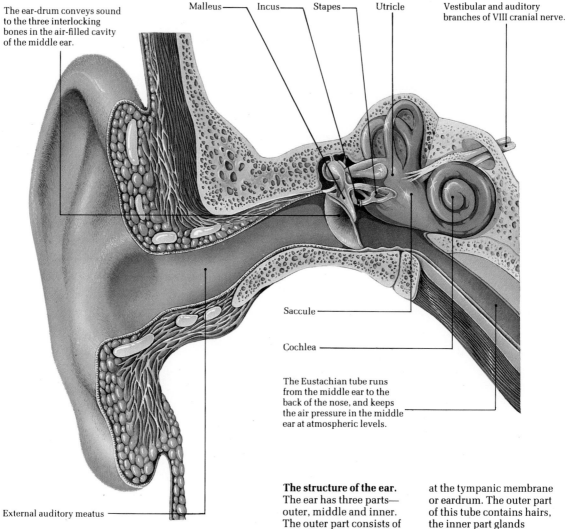

Saccule

Cochlea

The Eustachian tube runs from the middle ear to the back of the nose, and keeps the air pressure in the middle ear at atmospheric levels.

External auditory meatus

The structure of the ear.
The ear has three parts—outer, middle and inner. The outer part consists of the visible pinna, and the external auditory meatus to which it directs sound. This 25mm long tube ends at the tympanic membrane or eardrum. The outer part of this tube contains hairs, the inner part glands which produce wax. The wax drains out dirt and bacteria. Excess should only be removed by a doctor.

The middle ear.

The three bones of the middle ear, the malleus, incus and stapes, are sometimes called the hammer, anvil and stirrup. They are known together as the ossicles. The malleus is attached to the eardrum. It conducts sound by way of the incus to the footplate of the stapes. This is located in the oval window of the inner ear. Vibrations are transmitted from here to the cochlea.

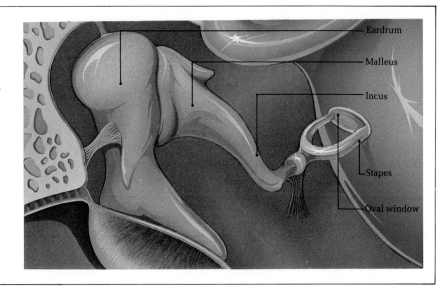

Eardrum

Malleus

Incus

Stapes

Oval window

The inner ear

The cochlea is a coiled tube with a bulbous base. It has three compartments. The upper compartment receives vibrations from the stapes and passes them on to the basilar membrane in the middle compartment. They are then conveyed through the lower compartment to the round window. Because this vibrates in the opposite direction to the oval window's vibration, the fluids in the inner ear can vibrate freely. Loudness discrimination takes place in the middle compartment: the Organ of Corti in the basilar membrane contains hair cells which have varying sensitivities to movement. Nerve impulses caused by the bending of different hairs are interpreted by the brain. Differences of pitch are also detected here. Low-pitched sounds make the whole membrane vibrate. High-pitched sounds make part of the membrane vibrate. The semicircular canals of the inner ear and the ampulla at the base of each detect rotation. Position is also determined here.

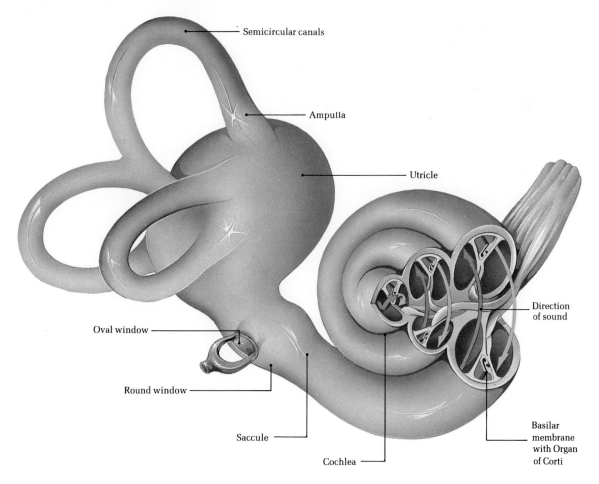

Semicircular canals

Ampulla

Utricle

Direction of sound

Oval window

Round window

Basilar membrane with Organ of Corti

Saccule

Cochlea

Disorders of the Ear

The commonest medical problems that can affect the ear are excess wax in the ear and perforation of the ear drum. In the first case, excessive production of wax, or cerumen, in the ear canal can cause symptoms of deafness or irritation. Perforation of the ear drum means that there is a break in the ear drum, or tympanic membrane. This can be caused by infection in the middle ear (otitis media) – a common complaint in children. Pus builds up behind the drum and eventually bursts through the center, the weakest place. The other cause is injury, which is likelier to occur in children than in adults.

Physical symptoms

The two conditions are fairly common. What actually happens is that wax is produced by the ceruminous glands in the outer ear passage to lubricate the skin of the ear passage, so that it does not dry and crack, and also the surface of the ear drum. This is a thin membrane that stretches across the bottom of the external auditory meatus, or ear passage. The drum is set into vibration by sound waves, which are conveyed by a chain of minute bones in the middle ear to the sensitive inner ear. There, the vibrations are analysed and the signals conveyed to the brain for decoding and interpretation.

If the ear drum has a lump of wax against it, or the ear passage is blocked, this whole system is put out of gear. The result is conductive deafness.

Ear wax is the commonest cause of hearing loss, except for normal deterioration from increasing age. One or both ears may be affected; if infection has set in – often the result of

WAYS IN WHICH HEARING CAN BE IMPEDED

The function of wax. The outer part of the external auditory meatus is covered with protective hairs. The inner part harbours the ceruminous glands which produce wax or cerumen. This has a protective function and helps to get rid of dirt and bacteria. It is important that the ear drum is lightly lubricated by the wax, but if a piece of wax is constantly touching it, or if wax is blocking the ear passage, hearing obviously suffers.

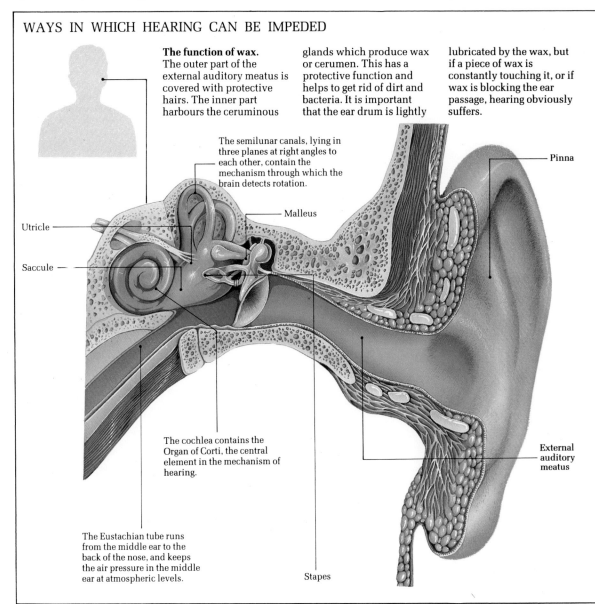

The semilunar canals, lying in three planes at right angles to each other, contain the mechanism through which the brain detects rotation.

Malleus

Pinna

Utricle

Saccule

The cochlea contains the Organ of Corti, the central element in the mechanism of hearing.

External auditory meatus

The Eustachian tube runs from the middle ear to the back of the nose, and keeps the air pressure in the middle ear at atmospheric levels.

Stapes

attempts to hook the wax out – discomfort, irritation and possibly a discharge may occur. Because of the nervous connections of the ear canal, any irritation from the wax itself or infection may set off bouts of coughing or sneezing.

If your ear drum is perforated by injury, you may feel pain. You cannot hear properly and you feel a hollow reverberation in the head. You may be dizzy, nauseated or actually vomit. Blood may appear in the ear canal. If otitis media is the cause, you will already have been experiencing severe, stabbing pain, a feeling of fullness and ringing in the ear, plus a fever as the pressure on the drum builds up.

Diagnosis and treatment

In both cases, physical examination of the ear is made with an auriscope. If otitis media is suspected, the doctor will carry out a blood test. A swab may be taken for bacteriological examination.

Hard lumps of wax can be removed with a special instrument, or syringed out with warm water. Alternatively drops may be prescribed. If cotton wool buds are used, use them only in the outer part of the ear passage; otherwise the chances of infection are high.

Small injuries to the ear drum are usually self-healing. Larger ones may require delicate surgery, sometimes using tissue from a vein to mend the hole. If you have acute pain and the drum is about to burst, the situation can be saved by a minor operation called a myringotomy. A small incision is made in the drum to release the pus and allow rapid healing. If the perforation is established, you will need pain-killers and antibiotics.

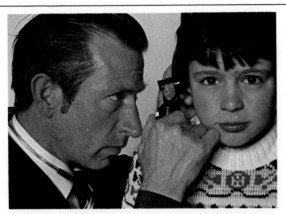

The ear-drum can be inspected with the aid of an auriscope. It will reflect light from the instrument, and so reveal abnormalities.

Where the drum is affected.
The weakest part of the drum is the center, so if the adjacent area becomes infected the central part of the drum will deteriorate first.
If perforation is caused by injury then any part of the drum may receive damage.

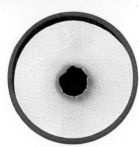

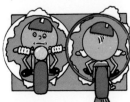

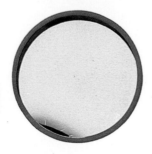

The ear drum is susceptible to damage from the inside through infection—normally the result of a spread along the

Eustachian tube from the nose—or from the outside, through blows or carelessly inserted objects.

PRESCRIPTION

Diagnosis
Otitis media, inflammation of the inner ear, is one possible cause of earache. As this is dangerous, any earache should be given careful medical attention. Your doctor will examine your ear with an auriscope, possibly carry out a blood test, and take a sample of any infecting organism

Treatment
Once the cause of an earache is found, treatment is normally effective. Perforations tend to heal themselves up if they are small enough. Self-administered substances or objects might adversely interfere with this process. If the perforation is large, then surgery should do the trick, Antibiotics may well be prescribed for any infection that has been introduced. Painkillers may be prescribed to deal with what can be most distressing symptoms. If hardened wax needs to be removed, then your doctor may well arrange to have your ears syringed. If your doctor prescribes ear-drops, it is important not to damage the inner part of your ear when giving them. Tilt your head to one side. Squeeze the drops into the center of the outer ear (below left), fold over the visible ear – the pinna – and (below right) allow the drops to run inside the ear.

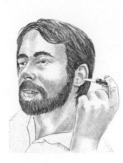

Insert dropper then tilt head to one side before squeezing.

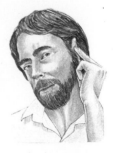

Keep head tilted after removal of dropper so that drops do not run out.

Eyes/Introduction

The arrangement of the different parts of the eye enables a sharp image to be focused on the retina. Light passes through, from front to back: the conjunctiva, a thin lubricated lining; the cornea, a sort of round window; the aqueous humor, a watery fluid; the pupil, a hole in the middle of the iris; the lens; the vitreous humor, a transparent jelly; and finally reaches the retina. Most of the focusing is carried out by the cornea, but its focus is fixed. The lens is flexible, and makes fine adjustments to the focus. There are two sorts of nerve-endings in the retina, rods and cones. Cones are sensitive to color, but need more light than the color-blind rods. Myopia or short sight occurs when the lens is too strong, so that it focuses distant objects somewhere in front of the retina. In long sight or hypermetropia near objects are focused behind the retina.

The structure of the eye.
The eye has three layers. The thick outer sclera surrounds it, except for the transparent window at the front, called the cornea. Behind the cornea is a muscular pigmented screen, the iris. This expands and contracts allowing varying amounts of light through the hole in its center, the pupil. Just behind the iris is a lens, which is secured by ligaments to the ciliary body. This is the front part of the middle or choroid layer. This layer is pigmented and contains blood vessels. As the inner layer, the retina, is almost transparent this middle layer gives the eye's interior a dark brown appearance. The retina is made up of light sensitive cells called rods and cones. Cones are sensitive to red, blue and green, rods to a gradation from grey to white. Light focused by the lens forms an upside-down image on the retina. Nerve fibers from the retina pierce the sclera at the optic disc and form the optic nerve to the brain. The point of entry of the optic nerve is known as the blind spot, as there are no rods or cones at this point.

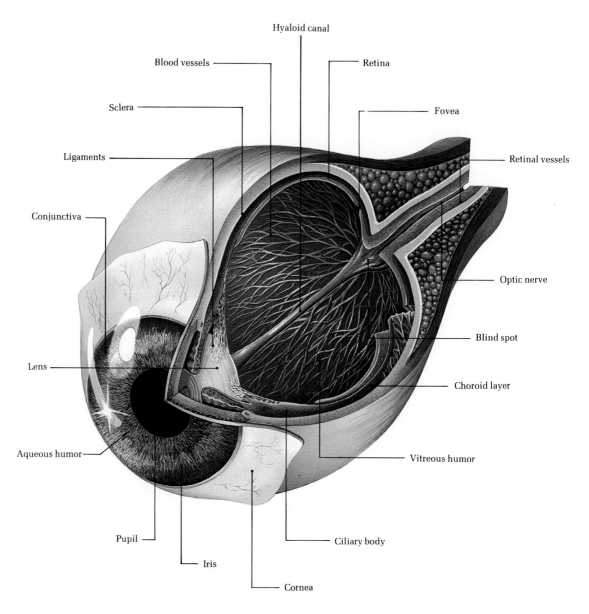

120

How the eye focuses.
Fine adjustments to focus are made by the lens of the eye under the control of the ciliary muscle in the ciliary body. The lens is kept flattened by the suspensory ligaments which pass on the tension of the eyeball. In distant vision (top) the relaxation of the ciliary muscles allows the ligaments to pull the lens into a disc shape. In close vision (bottom) the ciliary muscles constrict so that the ligaments relax and allow the lens to assume the circular shape necessary for focusing.

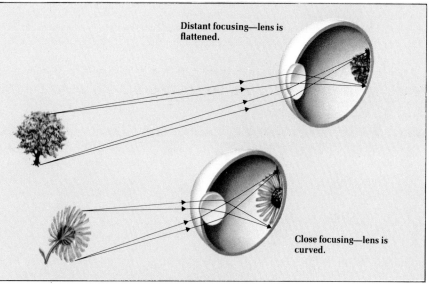

Distant focusing—lens is flattened.

Close focusing—lens is curved.

The visual path.
According to medical convention, the visual field of each eye is divided into the temporal field and the nasal field. The obtrusion of the nose and cheeks makes the temporal field bigger. Light from the nasal field falls on the temporal side of the retina, and light from the temporal field falls on its nasal side. The optic nerves from the two eyes meet at the optic chiasma. Here, the fibers from the nasal sides of the retinas cross over, but those from

the temporal sides do not. The two groups of fibers then pass through opposite sides of the brain to the visual cortex, so that the left visual cortex receives information from the right side of the visual field (that is, the left side of each eye) and the right visual cortex receives information from the left side of the visual field (the right side of each eye). The occipital cortex which surrounds the visual cortex interprets and analyses what has been seen.

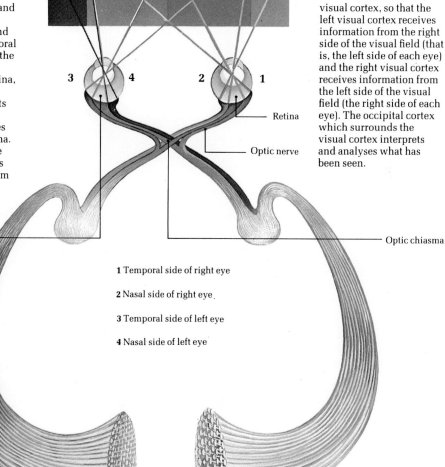

Retina

Optic nerve

Image on retina is clearest at center, where there are most cones.

Optic chiasma

1 Temporal side of right eye

2 Nasal side of right eye

3 Temporal side of left eye

4 Nasal side of left eye

Impulses from right half of visual field.

Impulses from left half of visual field.

121

Cataract

Cataract is an eye disorder, in which the lens of the eye becomes progressively more and more opaque, so blocking the passage of light to the retina and thus making it increasingly difficult to see. The exact cause of the disease is unknown, though it affects most types of mammal in addition to man. The biochemical process involved is now the subject of intensive research and indications are that it involves the activity of specific enzymes.

Cataracts can be caused in several ways, the commonest being through the progressive deterioration of the lens structure due to advancing age. Senile cataracts are the chief cause of blindness amongst the old. This process can be hastened by external factors, such as diseases like DIABETES, infections inside the eye, such as iritis, nutritional deficiencies and, very rarely, poisoning. Other causes are eye injury and, in children, an inherited metabolic disorder called galactosemia. Children can also contract the disease as a result of their mother catching German measles during early pregnancy, in which case they are born with cataracts.

Physical symptoms

If you have normal vision, the light waves from what you see are picked up by your eyes. They pass through the cornea, the window at the front of the eye, and are concentrated by the lens lying just behind the pupil, so that they fall exactly on to the retina. If the lens is out of shape, you get distorted or blurred vision; if it becomes like ground glass – as it does in cataract – you cannot see at all.

You gradually lose your sight, as your vision becomes dim and blurry. There is no pain or discomfort, while it is usual for one eye to be

EFFECTS AND TREATMENT OF CATARACTS

Cataracts affect the lens of the eye. The shape of the lens varies between rounded and disc-like, concentrating rays of light so that they fall on the retina. If a cataract has formed the lens will become opaque, making it impossible for an image to be formed.

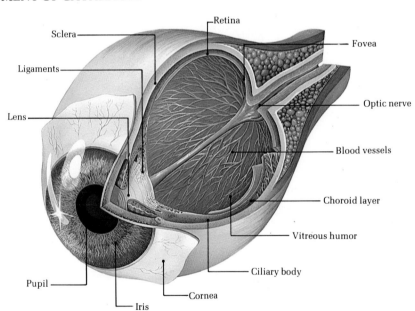

Sclera — Ligaments — Lens — Pupil — Iris — Cornea — Retina — Fovea — Optic nerve — Blood vessels — Choroid layer — Vitreous humor — Ciliary body

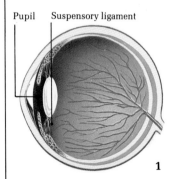

Pupil — Suspensory ligament

1

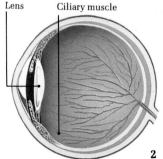

Lens — Ciliary muscle

2

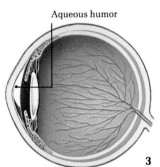

Aqueous humor

3

How the lens is affected. In the normal course of events the lens changes shape through the action of the ciliary muscles and the suspensory ligaments to which they are attached. In focusing on a close object (**1**) relaxed ligaments allow the lens to assume a circular shape. In distant focusing (**2**) the ligaments pull the lens affected into a disc shape. A lens affected by a cataract (**3**) becomes brittle. This means that when the ligaments relax for close focusing it cannot return smoothly to its circular shape.

worse affected than the other at first. A bright light is required for reading and you can only make out objects when you are close up to them. Double vision can occur, you may see spots in front of your eyes and you may be able to see better in twilight than in the full light of day. Eventually, the pupil turns a milky greyish-white.

Diagnosis and treatment

If you are losing your sight, a thorough eye examination is vital. It is important to check that you have not got GLAUCOMA, since speed of treatment is then vital. In cataract, there is plenty of time for diagnosis, as it takes about two years for the disease to develop to the point where the lens becomes totally opaque. During this period, frequent changes of glasses are necessary in order to preserve some vision.

The only treatment for cataract is surgery. The deteriorated lens must be removed, preferably starting with the side first affected while the eye on the other side is still working. The success rate is high; about ninety-five per cent of all cataracts are operable.

There are several techniques open to the surgeon. Either traditional surgical methods can be used; alternatively, the cataract can be broken up and extracted by suction. Another modern technique uses freezing.

After the operation, you will be tested and fitted with special glasses. These are purpose-designed to do the job of the discarded lens. They will compensate for its absence completely and also make up for the change in your vision capabilities that will have resulted from the disease and the operation. The results are almost always excellent.

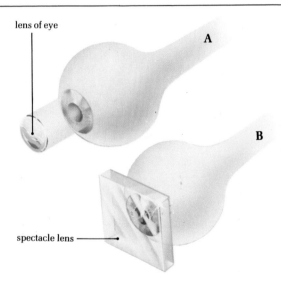

lens of eye

A

B

spectacle lens

Treatment of cataracts.
When an affected lens is removed (**A**) vision returns and only the ability to focus is lost. This is because the front of the eye

acts as a powerful compound lens, the 'lens' itself being involved only in fine adjustments. Spectacles can make up for this loss of accuracy (**B**).

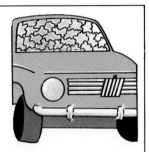

Vision through a lens that has developed a cataract is rather like that through a shattered windscreen. Light and dark can be distinguished, but very little else.

PRESCRIPTION

Diagnosis
A straightforward eye observation should reveal the condition of the lens but your doctor will want to make sure that you are not suffering from glaucoma as well. He may therefore check the pressure in your eyes.

Treatment
Once a cataract is diagnosed, necessary treatment does not really vary. At some point before your vision is lost from the affected eye, the lens must be removed. Sight will then be restored, by the removal of your only real impediment to good vision. The front of the eye will continue to act as a powerful lens, and spectacles will be prescribed to make up for the loss of the removed lens'focusing ability.

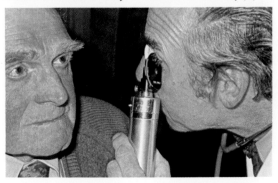

Using an ophthalmoscope.
The eye is the only place where a nerve (the optic)

or blood vessels can be directly observed.
Here the lens is examined.

Conjunctivitis

Conjunctivitis is an inflammation of the conjunctiva, the thin mucous membrane covering the majority of the eye-ball and lining the eyelids. The disease is common amongst children, largely because of their tendency to rub their eyes when they are tired – even though their hands are dirty. This can lead to the virus infection known as 'pink eye'.

There are two types of conjunctivitis – acute and chronic. Acute conjunctivitis can be due to a virus or to bacteria – in which cases it is highly contagious – or to irritant chemicals. It may also be an allergic reaction, as in hay fever. Chronic conjunctivitis is caused by the same things as the acute form of the disorder. It is often found in places associated with air pollution, such as Los Angeles in the USA. Amongst other victims are students and the elderly, whose eyes dry up somewhat through age.

Both forms of conjunctivitis are usually fairly easy to treat, but there is one exception – trachoma. This is a very severe, highly contagious viral conjunctivitis, which is reasonably common in most parts of the underdeveloped world. It is the only form of conjunctivitis likely to lead to blindness.

Physical symptoms
The nature of the conjunctiva varies according to which parts of the eye it is covering; it lines both the upper and lower lids and the visible part of the eye. The palpebral – eyelid – parts are thick and opaque, with a generous blood supply. At the margins of the lids, these run into the skin; they are also continuous with the linings of the tear ducts and the passages from the eyes to the nose. Over the front of the eye, the conjunctiva consists only of epithelial cells

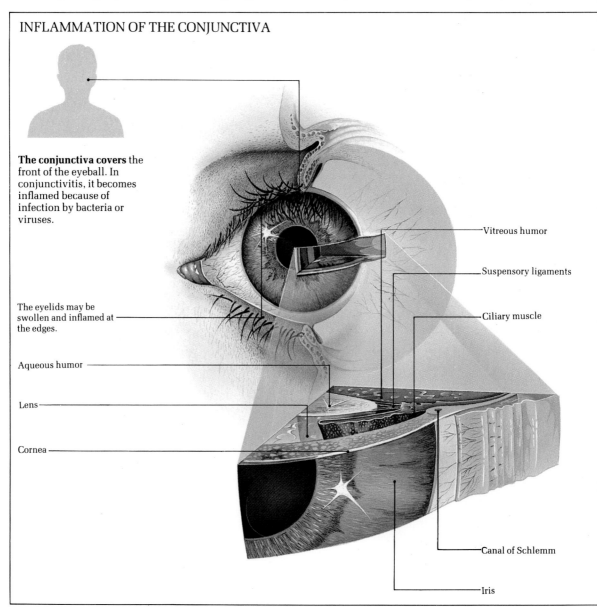

INFLAMMATION OF THE CONJUNCTIVA

The conjunctiva covers the front of the eyeball. In conjunctivitis, it becomes inflamed because of infection by bacteria or viruses.

The eyelids may be swollen and inflamed at the edges.

Aqueous humor

Lens

Cornea

Vitreous humor

Suspensory ligaments

Ciliary muscle

Canal of Schlemm

Iris

– a thin, see-through covering.

When the conjunctiva is inflamed, the eyes are red and watery, with the redness stretching towards the cornea. There may be a purulent discharge. The lids may be swollen, while the eyes feel as though there is grit under the lids as the watery secretions of the inflamed membrane become thicker. Sometimes the edges of the eyelids may become inflamed and red; this is known as blepharitis.

Diagnosis and treatment

Conjunctivitis is fairly easy to diagnose. In mild cases, the complaint responds to routine home treatment through eye irrigation and eye ointment or drops. If only one eye is infected, it is obviously important to prevent the infection spreading to the other eye. This is best done by observing the rules of simple hygiene and using disposable tissues and towels. If you are using drops, take care not to infect one eye with material from the other. You should avoid touching your face and wiping it with towels used by other people.

Cold compresses and dark glasses are comforting. In acute cases, you will probably be given antibiotic eyedrops by your doctor, who will also check that there is no mechanical cause of the infection, such as a trapped eyelash or inbedded particle of dirt. Steroid drops are frequently prescribed for allergic conjunctivitis and bring considerable relief. They will probably contain an anti-fungal agent, such as neomycin.

The outlook is good in conjunctivitis, apart from trachoma. If this is suspected, the doctor will refer you to a specialist for expert treatment of the infection.

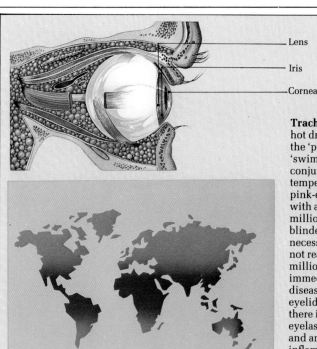

Lens

Iris

Cornea

Trachoma is a disease of hot dry regions, related to the 'pink-eye' or 'swimming bath conjunctivitis' of temperate climates. Like pink-eye, it can be treated with antibiotics, but millions of people are blinded by it because the necessary antibiotics do not reach the hundreds of millions of sufferers. More immediate effects of the disease are threefold: the eyelids become scarred; there is a tendency for the eyelashes to turn inwards; and an opaque inflammatory tissue known as a pannus may obstruct the cornea.

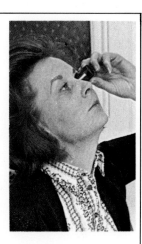

In mild cases of conjunctivitis, disinfection by means of an eye bath can help to ease the inflammation.

A virus, bacteria, or an irritant can lead to inflammation and conjunctivitis. Most forms are infectious or contagious. Pink-eye and trachoma are caused by virus-like parasites which, unlike true viruses, can be treated with antibiotics.

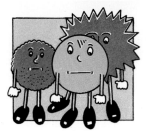

PRESCRIPTION

Diagnosis
A straightforward eye examination should be sufficient for diagnosis.

Treatment
Appropriate treatment depends upon severity. If the inflammation is mild, then mild eye baths should be enough to restore the conjunctiva to health. If the infection is more serious then antibiotics will be necessary. In the case of allergic reactions steroid drops have proved effective. With young children, try to make sure that their hands stay clean and that they do not rub their eyes.

Glaucoma

Glaucoma is an eye disease in which fluid accumulates in the forward part of the eyeball. If the disease is not treated, the resultant pressure builds up to such an extent that the retina and the nerve of sight – the optic nerve – are damaged and blindness is the result. Apart from a rare congenital form, affecting children and teenagers, this disorder is unusual before the age of forty.

There are various types of glaucoma, the commonest being chronic simple glaucoma and acute narrow-angle glaucoma. The exact cause of the disease is not fully understood.

Physical symptoms

To understand how glaucoma strikes, it is necessary to have some knowledge of how the eye works. The eye consists of the eye ball, which is held in its fat-lined socket by liga-ments and muscles. The inside of the back of the eye ball is lined by the retina, which is sensitive to light of different wave lengths, and the information it gathers is transmitted by the optic nerve to the back of the brain. There the input is analysed and interpreted.

The eye also has a transparent front window – the cornea – which is covered by the delicate conjunctiva. The lens lies behind the pupil, which is the hole in the center of the colored part, or iris. The spaces in front of and behind the lens or iris are named the anterior and posterior chambers respectively. They are filled by a transparent salty liquid, called the aqueous humor, derived from the blood from the vessels at the back of the brain.

Normally, this liquid drains away through the veins in the angle between the cornea and the iris at the front; if glaucoma develops

AN EXCESS OF PRESSURE IN THE EYE

Glaucoma is an excess of pressure in the eyeball.

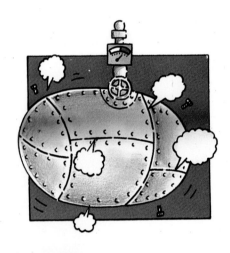

High pressure within the eyeball endangers the optic nerve, and must be treated as soon as it is diagnosed. When the cause is known it is normally found to be attributable to inadequate drainage of the aqueous humor at the junction of the iris and cornea. This can be through a simple tendency for the iris to impede the outlet, to pores which malfunction, or to an inflamed iris.

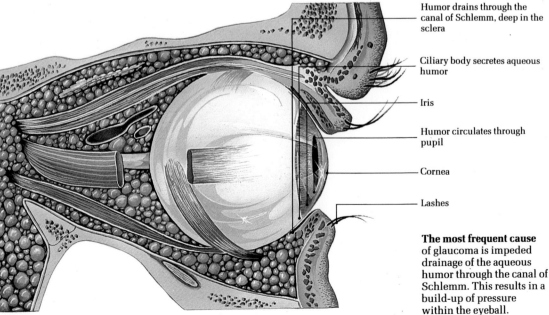

Humor drains through the canal of Schlemm, deep in the sclera

Ciliary body secretes aqueous humor

Iris

Humor circulates through pupil

Cornea

Lashes

The most frequent cause of glaucoma is impeded drainage of the aqueous humor through the canal of Schlemm. This results in a build-up of pressure within the eyeball.

however, this is where the trouble starts. Here, there is inadequate drainage of the aqueous humor and so the pressure rises. This may be due to adhesions between the iris and lens, or because the angle between the cornea and iris has become narrowed.

In chronic simple glaucoma, you may notice nothing unusual until the sight of one or both eyes is impaired. Brow aches and misty vision may be the first rough indications of the disease. You may develop gaps in your field of vision, a curved shape in it, or lose vision around the edges of the field. Rainbow borders, or haloes, may appear around lights and your eyeballs may be hard to the touch.

In acute glaucoma, warning symptoms may include misty vision, colored haloes around lights, pain in the eye, enlargement of the pupils and headaches. There is then a sudden loss of sight; you will be unable to bear light – this is known as photophobia – and you will have a severe throbbing pain in the eye. You may vomit so much that you think you have a stomach upset. The eye is red and hard.

Diagnosis and treatment

If glaucoma is treated early enough, the outlook is good. Glaucoma must always be treated by an eye specialist, who will measure the pressure in your eye simply and painlessly with a tonometer. He or she will also determine whether the angle between cornea and iris is sufficiently open. In chronic simple glaucoma, drops containing pilocarpine are commonly prescribed to promote drainage of the aqueous humour. If these are not effective, an operation may be necessary; in acute glaucoma, this will certainly be the case.

While acute glaucoma is painful, chronic glaucoma is more dangerous, because the symptoms can easily go unnoticed even though the optic nerve is in danger. If your eyes are troubling you, either through pain or disturbed vision, have them examined by a doctor or optician.

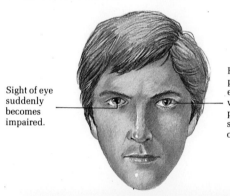

Sight of eye suddenly becomes impaired.

Headaches, pains in the eye or misty vision precede a sudden loss of sight.

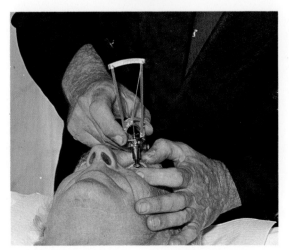

Measuring eye pressure. The tonometer is designed to show whether or not the pressure in the eye is above normal. It does this by measuring the resistance of the eyeball to gentle pressure.

PRESCRIPTION

Diagnosis
The pressure in your eye can be measured simply and painlessly by a trained specialist using a tonometer. He or she will also examine your eyes to find out whether the cause of inadequate drainage is a too narrow angle between cornea and iris, or whether a more likely cause is an an inflamed iris, or a blockage in the canal of Schlemm.

Treatment
This is in the form of drugs or surgery. Some drugs constrict the pupil and so allow easier drainage. Others slow down the production of the aqueous humor that is causing the pressure. Surgery normally involves making an extra hole for the fluid to drain through, but sometimes the angle is simply opened up slightly.

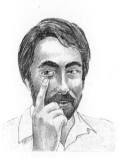 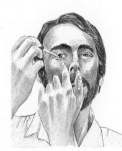

Pilocarpine drops act by constricting the pupil and so decongesting the area around the canal of Schlemm. Excess fluid is thus enabled to drain away. When administering eye-drops, first pull down the lower lid, then allow the drop to fall in the revealed area.

Psychological/Introduction

The dividing line between normal and abnormal behavior is vague. According to one body of opinion a person might be mentally ill, while according to another he may not be. Nevertheless, the more serious disorders are clearly recognizable as disorders. This section explains what form some of the more common of these take. Sometimes the mind deteriorates through a physical cause. The brain may be poisoned by too much alcohol, for example. But in many cases there is no demonstrable physical cause. Neuroses such as anxiety or depression are amongst such illnesses. The neurotic patient does not lose touch with reality, but his normal responses are exaggerated. A psychotic patient loses touch with reality. Sometimes brain damage is known to cause this, but for schizophrenia or manic depression, no physical cause has yet been found.

The brain.
Apart from its role in the maintenance and control of the cells, tissues, organs and systems of the body, the brain is the center of thinking and feeling, and initiates movements by controlling the contraction of the skeletal muscles. The cerebral cortex is the covering of grey matter over the hemispheres. Folds and fissures (gyri and sulci) in the cortex increase its surface area about thirty times. It is densely packed with nerve cells or neurones. Such cells transmit impulses to other cells. They are made up of a cell-body and a number of thread-like projections. These projections are called processes. The branched ones, of which there are several, are dendrites. The unbranched ones – normally one to a cell-body – are conducting fibers or axons. The white matter of the cortex is a mass of these intertwined nerve fibers. These fibers connect the neurones of the cortex with each other and with the brain stem. Their arrangement is immensely complex. The lobes are areas of cortex divided along the lines of major fissures. The areas of concern of the different parts of the cortex are shown below.

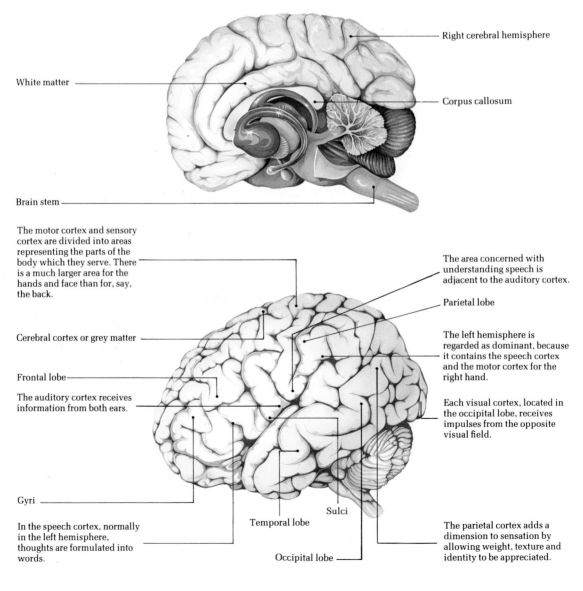

Right cerebral hemisphere

White matter

Corpus callosum

Brain stem

The motor cortex and sensory cortex are divided into areas representing the parts of the body which they serve. There is a much larger area for the hands and face than for, say, the back.

The area concerned with understanding speech is adjacent to the auditory cortex.

Parietal lobe

Cerebral cortex or grey matter

The left hemisphere is regarded as dominant, because it contains the speech cortex and the motor cortex for the right hand.

Frontal lobe

The auditory cortex receives information from both ears.

Each visual cortex, located in the occipital lobe, receives impulses from the opposite visual field.

Gyri

Sulci

Temporal lobe

In the speech cortex, normally in the left hemisphere, thoughts are formulated into words.

The parietal cortex adds a dimension to sensation by allowing weight, texture and identity to be appreciated.

Occipital lobe

Kinds of thinking.
It seems possible to identify two sorts of thinking which proceed in radically different ways. In 'logical' thinking we proceed from one safe step to another until we arrive at a certain conclusion. More 'creative' thinking, on the other hand, makes leaps from related ideas and facts to apparently unrelated ones. Some of these leaps end in failure, but successful ones help us to solve problems not readily amenable to logical solution.

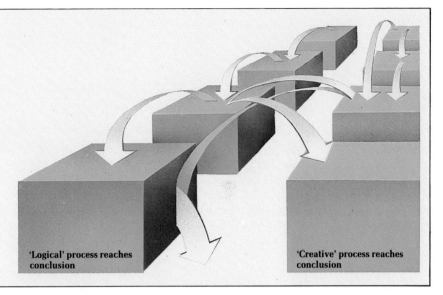

'Logical' process reaches conclusion

'Creative' process reaches conclusion

The two sides of the brain are structurally similar but very different in terms of function. The left side controls speech, reasoning and analytical ability. The right side seems to be responsible more for creative or artistic activity and spatial relationships. The left side is commonly regarded as dominant. Most sensory impulses from the right side of the body reach the left side of the brain and vice versa. The corpus callosum is a thick connecting tract between the two hemispheres. If it is severed the overall effect on a person's efficiency can sometimes be surprisingly small.

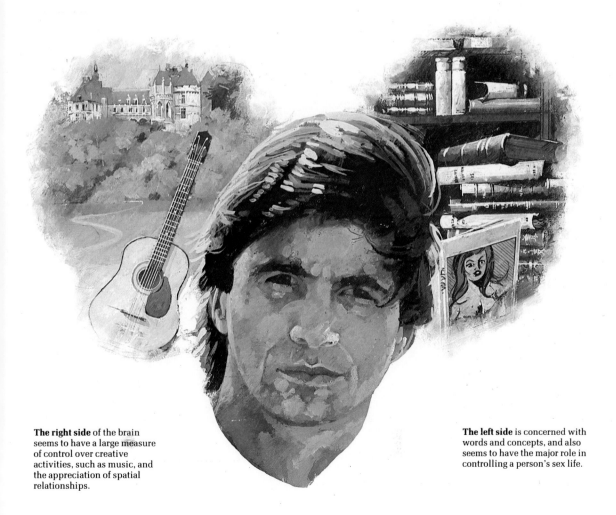

The right side of the brain seems to have a large measure of control over creative activities, such as music, and the appreciation of spatial relationships.

The left side is concerned with words and concepts, and also seems to have the major role in controlling a person's sex life.

Anxiety States and Phobias

Anxiety states and phobias cover a wide range of fearful emotions, which often affect people under different forms of stress. There are several different types, according to the circumstances involved. A general feeling of anxiety, with such physical symptoms as sweating, trembling and palpitations for no apparent reason, is known as free-floating anxiety. Phobia is the same feeling, brought on by something which does not frighten other people to the same extent. The commonest form of this is agoraphobia, fear of open places, while other examples include travel and social phobias. Women are more susceptible to both anxiety states than men.

Physical symptoms

If you are in physical danger, your body will react in ways designed to help you cope with the threat – either by fight or flight. If the danger is extremely intense, you may freeze, all movement and thought being inhibited. The same thing happens now, but with no actual physical cause being present.

Your pupils will widen and the blood drain from your face and muscles. Your mouth will become dry and your heart rate increase – enough for you to become aware of its thumping. Your breathing becomes much faster and you may want to urinate or pass faeces. You may feel nauseated or even vomit. Your legs may tremble and feel weak, enough to make you fear that you may physically collapse.

Diagnosis and treatment

Anxiety is not hard to diagnose in itself; what is important is to check that the condition is not due to a physical disorder. To check this, your

FEAR, FOCUSED AND UNFOCUSED

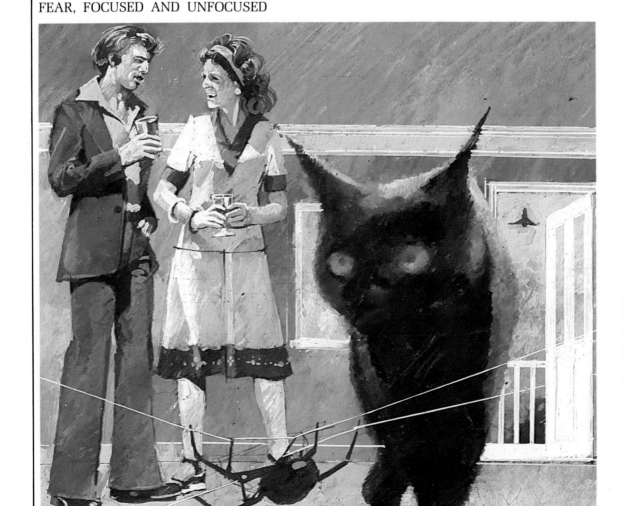

blood may be tested to ensure that your anxiety state is not due to hyperthyroidism, while your gastro-intestinal functions may be examined if your symptoms include diarrhoea or vomiting. You may have an electrocardiogram (ECG), if there is reason to suspect a heart disorder.

Free-floating anxiety, which seems to have no cause, and phobic anxiety, which appears to have a trivial one, both always have a hidden basis, which your mind has suppressed. The best remedy is talking over the problem, usually with a psychiatrist.

There are two effective ways of dealing with the phobias – through behavior therapy and medication. The former chiefly consists of doing whatever you most fear little by little – desensitization – or all at once – maximal exposure. In the first instance, you might deal with agoraphobia by going a few yards down a road with a companion and then alone, increasing the distance every day until you become confident. The second should never be taken without strict medical guidance.

Medication can help by artificially reducing your anxiety; a dose of a suitable drug, for instance, can enable you to fly if you have flight phobia. For a more lasting result, a course of drugs may help to build your courage up by aiding you to increase your store of nervous energy.

For free-floating anxiety, medication is essential. This is because there is no particular situation or object which brings the condition on and which you can practise mastering. Whichever state is involved, it is essential to come to grips with whatever it is that makes you frightened. Otherwise the fear will spread and eventually become uncontrollable.

Anxiety can appear to be vague and undirected, in which case it is termed free-floating, or it can be brought on by a clear external cause. This is phobic anxiety (left). There are some phobias which occur again and again in the case histories. Fear of crowded and busy places is widespread, as is a fear of social gatherings. And animal phobia – snakes, spiders, cats and mice are notorious objects of such fear – affects the lives of many people to a great or lesser degree.

Women are at present far more prone to anxiety than men.

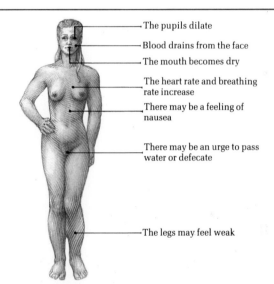

The pupils dilate

Blood drains from the face

The mouth becomes dry

The heart rate and breathing rate increase

There may be a feeling of nausea

There may be an urge to pass water or defecate

The legs may feel weak

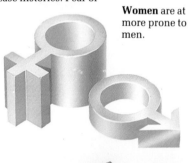

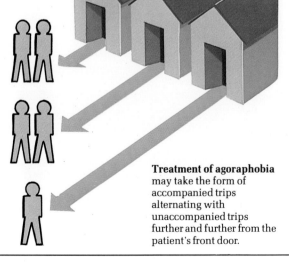

Treatment of agoraphobia may take the form of accompanied trips alternating with unaccompanied trips further and further from the patient's front door.

PRESCRIPTION

Diagnosis
Your doctor will want to rule out a possible physical disorder such as hyperthyroidism as a cause of your anxiety.

Treatment
Once the exact shape that your anxiety takes is as near as possible established, your doctor will have two broad choices: to recommend therapy, or to treat your condition by selecting from a range of available drugs. The therapy will probably take the form of 'desensitizing' you to the cause of the trouble by very gradually making you more and more accustomed to it. In the end, tolerance should be normal.

Alternatively, your doctor may prescribe tranquillizers. If these are mild enough, these will give you relief from the symptoms without causing drowsiness. The muscle tension which accompanies anxiety should also be relieved.

However, drug treatment can never be the whole answer, and the root cause will have to be dealt with at some point, either in psychotherapy or some less structured treatment.

Alcoholism

Alcoholism is a periodic or chronic illness caused by the compulsive drinking of alcoholic beverages. The tell-tale signs of the disease are either the inability to choose whether or not to start drinking or whether or not to stop when you have begun. You are also classed as an alcoholic if you have damaged your physical or mental health by persistent drinking.

Alcoholism is constantly on the increase and is an extremely serious medical problem. Male alcoholics outnumber female ones in the ratio of two or three to one, though alcoholic abuse among women is now increasing more rapidly than among men. Women, too, are more vulnerable to the affects of alcohol, so that the outlook for a female alcoholic is far worse than for her male equivalent.

The person most likely to develop alcoholism is a man or woman with the traditional 'hard head', who thus avoids the debilitating experience of hangovers after drink. Shyness and tension often underly the disease, while reverses of business or personal fortunes often spark it off. It usually takes about ten years for a heavy drinker to become dependent on alcohol, but, with persistent gross excess, five years may be more than long enough. Anything over four pints of beer, four double whiskies (or other forms of spirits), or a bottle of wine a day is enough to induce alcoholic addiction in a man, while between half and three-quarters of this amount can addict a woman.

Physical symptoms

Alcohol has both physical and mental effects on the body, the latter being by far the most noticeable. Physically, alcoholic drinks may make you feel warm in the short term. Mental-

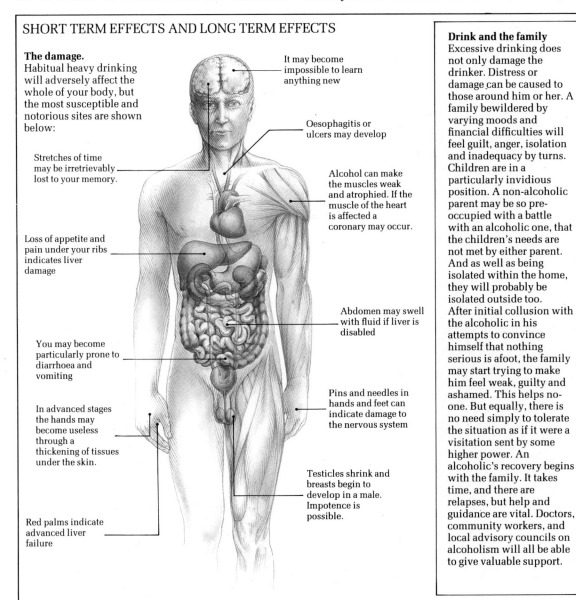

SHORT TERM EFFECTS AND LONG TERM EFFECTS

The damage.
Habitual heavy drinking will adversely affect the whole of your body, but the most susceptible and notorious sites are shown below:

Stretches of time may be irretrievably lost to your memory.

Loss of appetite and pain under your ribs indicates liver damage

You may become particularly prone to diarrhoea and vomiting

In advanced stages the hands may become useless through a thickening of tissues under the skin.

Red palms indicate advanced liver failure

It may become impossible to learn anything new

Oesophagitis or ulcers may develop

Alcohol can make the muscles weak and atrophied. If the muscle of the heart is affected a coronary may occur.

Abdomen may swell with fluid if liver is disabled

Pins and needles in hands and feet can indicate damage to the nervous system

Testicles shrink and breasts begin to develop in a male. Impotence is possible.

Drink and the family
Excessive drinking does not only damage the drinker. Distress or damage can be caused to those around him or her. A family bewildered by varying moods and financial difficulties will feel guilt, anger, isolation and inadequacy by turns. Children are in a particularly invidious position. A non-alcoholic parent may be so pre-occupied with a battle with an alcoholic one, that the children's needs are not met by either parent. And as well as being isolated within the home, they will probably be isolated outside too. After initial collusion with the alcoholic in his attempts to convince himself that nothing serious is afoot, the family may start trying to make him feel weak, guilty and ashamed. This helps no-one. But equally, there is no need simply to tolerate the situation as if it were a visitation sent by some higher power. An alcoholic's recovery begins with the family. It takes time, and there are relapses, but help and guidance are vital. Doctors, community workers, and local advisory councils on alcoholism will all be able to give valuable support.

ly, the pleasant initial affect of alcohol is to lower your inhibitions, so that you can say and do things that would normally make you feel awkward or embarrassed. Your judgement and co-ordination are soon impaired, however, and your reactions are slowed.

If you continue regular hard drinking for long enough, addiction will occur. Not only do you feel a craving for alcohol, but you also experience unpleasant physical symptoms when you are deprived of it. These can include shaking, sweating, diarrhoea, nausea, vomiting and acute anxiety. In extreme cases, you can develop the hallucinatory state known as delirium tremens.

The physical effects of long-term over-indulgence in alcohol can be disastrous. Every organ of your body may be affected by its poisonous influence. If your liver is impaired,

you will lose your appetite and feel pain and tenderness under the right side of your ribs. In the later stages of liver failure, you may notice that the palms of your hands are always red – liver palms, as they are termed. If you are a man, your testicles shrink and your breasts develop like a woman's. You may be impotent. Finally, as your liver ceases to function, your abdomen swells up with fluid.

The effects on your muscles – a condition known as myopathy – are equally serious. They suffer from painful weakness and atrophy. If your heart muscle is damaged – cardiomyopathy – you are liable to coronary attack.

As well as reacting through diarrhoea and vomiting, your digestive system may develop gastric or duodenal ulcers. Then, every drink will make matters worse. Oesophagitis, inflammation of the gullet, can be troublesome. As a

One more for the road.
A double whisky will have a slight effect on your judgement. After two of these you will start to feel warm, cheerful, and not so inhibited. However, your judgement will now be significantly impaired. Four or five doubles will probably make you boisterous and bothersome. You will not be able to speak distinctly and your self-control will suffer obviously. Between six and eight will make it difficult for you to walk. You will probably see double, and your memory will become hazy. Ten may cause collapse and save a drinker from the approaching lethal dose.

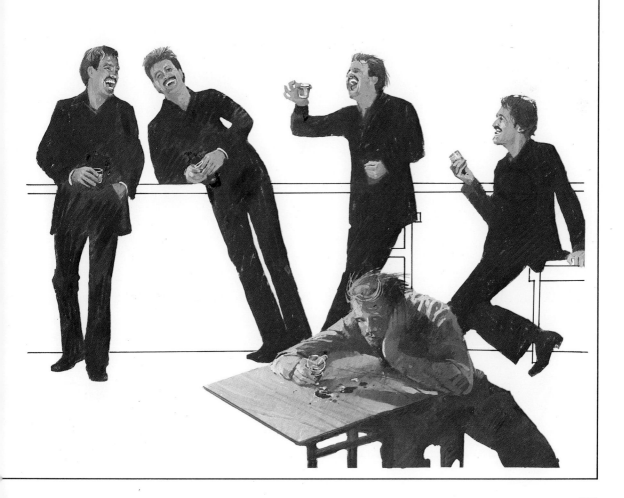

late and extremely serious digestive disaster, you may develop pancreatitis.

If your nervous system is damaged, you may first notice pins and needles plus numbness in your hands and feet. This is called peripheral neuropathy. If your brain is affected, the first sign of alcoholism will be black outs – blank periods in your memory. In due course, this becomes constantly unreliable.

The final stage is that of alcoholic dementia, when, to all intents and purposes, your brain is only capable of keeping the automatic functions of the body operating – breathing, blinking, eating and so on. Some alcoholics develop what is termed Korsakoff's psychosis. In this, you cannot learn anything new. Another consequence may be epileptic fits.

Another characteristic alcoholic condition is termed Dupuytren's contracture. The third and fourth fingers of your hands are pulled down against your palms by a fibrous thickening of the tissues under the skin. The other fingers follow, making your hand or hands useless.

Diagnosis and treatment

Any alcoholic—or anyone in significant danger of becoming one – needs help as a matter of extreme urgency. You cannot cope with the disease or its consequences on your own; it is not worth attempting to do so. Both medical and psychiatric treatment may be needed and, the sooner these are started, the better the chances of an eventual cure.

Physically, the doctor will order blood tests to check how your liver is coping under the strain of drink and also to ascertain the effect that the alcohol is having on your red blood cells. In alcoholism, these often become over-

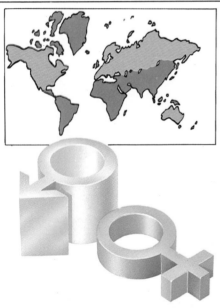

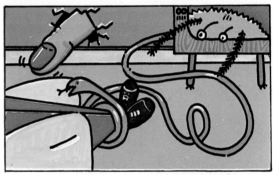

The spread of the illness
The incidence of alcoholism among men is at least twice that among women. It tends to increase along with alcohol consumption which is rising at present in the Western world in general.

Delirium tremens – sights for sore heads The constant craving for alcohol which occupies an addicted person for much of his waking life can, if unsatisfied, be accompanied by hallucinations and highly unpleasant emotions.

The effect on memory.
The way alcohol can wipe out all memory of a drinking bout is well known. But persistent heavy drinking can damage the memory permanently. An acute form of such damage is termed Korsakoff's psychosis. The sufferer may be able to recall distant events – from, say, twenty years previously (**A**), but not recent ones (**B**). This naturally makes

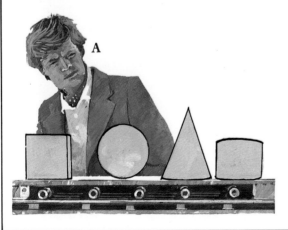

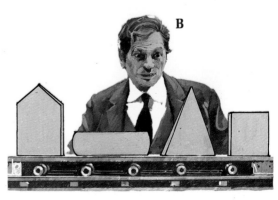

size – a direct poisoning effect. If you have had a fit, he or she, will order an electroencephalogram (EEG) of your brain, to establish whether or not you are truly epileptic. If it is suspected that your heart is affected, an electrocardiogram will be taken.

Though physical treatment is out of your hands, there is much you can do to help yourself under expert medical supervision. The basic problem is how to stop what has become, for you, a dangerous habit.

Firstly, you need to make up your mind to give up drinking alcohol completely for at least several years and, in extreme cases, for the rest of your life. This is a life or death responsibility,which, even with all the help in the world, only you can undertake and carry through. By the end of this time, you will not care whether or not you start drinking again and you would be wiser not to do so.

To make it safer and more comfortable for you for the first crucial week or ten days after you stop drinking, your doctor may prescribe a sedative drug. If there is an underlying mental difficulty, such as tension or depression, you will be prescribed anxiolytic or anti-depressant medicine. In any event, your life will need re-styling; you will need strength of character and all the support you can get from your friends, relatives and doctors to get through the first six months without alcohol. During this period, a technique called antabuse may be used; in this, you are prescribed drugs which have little effect on their own, but produce a violent and alarming reaction if you start to drink again.

The companionship and encouragement of others similarly struggling against alcoholism may be of valuable assistance.

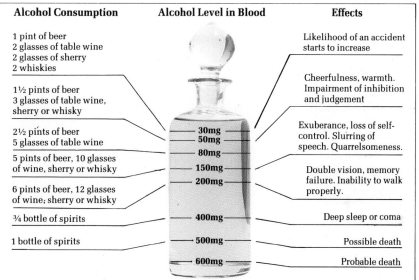

The nearside column shows the volume of different drinks that will contain about the same amount of alcohol. In the center, the alcohol level which such an intake would cause in the blood, in terms of milligrams of alcohol per 100 milliliters of blood, is shown. This figure is approximate, as are the effects on behavior, shown on the right. Different personalities, and different bodies, will vary in their reactions to a given level of alcohol. In all cases, though, alcohol is a depressant, affecting judgement and skills.

Alcohol Consumption

1 pint of beer
2 glasses of table wine
2 glasses of sherry
2 whiskies

1½ pints of beer
3 glasses of table wine, sherry or whisky

2½ pints of beer
5 glasses of table wine

5 pints of beer, 10 glasses of wine, sherry or whisky

6 pints of beer, 12 glasses of wine, sherry or whisky

¾ bottle of spirits

1 bottle of spirits

Alcohol Level in Blood

30mg
50mg
80mg
150mg
200mg
400mg
500mg
600mg

Effects

Likelihood of an accident starts to increase

Cheerfulness, warmth. Impairment of inhibition and judgement

Exuberance, loss of self-control. Slurring of speech. Quarrelsomeness.

Double vision, memory failure. Inability to walk properly.

Deep sleep or coma

Possible death

Probable death

new learning impossible. At (C) he can use memories from time (A) but not from time (B). He may compensate for this disability with elaborate lies. Lack of B vitamins causes the damage.

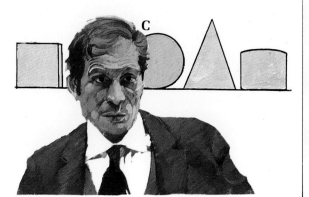

PRESCRIPTION

Diagnosis
It is important to be on the lookout for warning signs that your drinking is getting out of control. If your drinking sprees are frequent, if you drink early in the morning, if you find yourself missing work because of its effects, if you drink in private, if you need a drink to face the world, if others express concern over your welfare, then you will possibly soon need help to combat alcoholism. Remedial action is easier, the earlier it is taken.

Treatment
An alcoholic cannot cure himself but he must decide that he needs help and seek it out. This is the first step of a painful but rewarding process. Your doctor will be able to supply drugs which help you through the difficult early days, and others which assist your will-power by producing distressing symptoms if you drink. The support of your family and friends will be vital. It is a good idea for your family to talk to your doctor.

Anorexia Nervosa

Anorexia nervosa is a neurotic disorder in which the victim – usually female, as twenty women to one man are affected – deliberately reduces weight to the point of emaciation. At the same time, the monthly period stops. The typical, or primary, form of the disease initially affects girls between the ages of eleven and eighteen, who are usually highly intelligent and attractive, with a desire to succeed. The disease often starts when they place themselves under extra strain to fulfil this desire. A secondary form affects older women. This is often sparked off by an unsatisfactory sexual experience, or one for which the woman was emotionally unprepared. In addition, a late form, called anorexia tardive, can occur in women aged forty or more. This usually happens if their influence over husband and children – especially a daughter – is decreasing.

Physical symptoms

Outbreaks of primary anorexia nervosa are normally closely linked to slimming in an attempt to look fashionable. This fits in with a deep-seated, unrecognized, desire to stop growing up. As a consequence of this, the periods stop from the onset of the disease and its victims fanatically pursue an ideal of extreme thinness. At the same time, primary anorexics feel compelled to exercise excessively.

Secondary anorexics are more likely to achieve their loss of weight by eating – sometimes enormously – and then vomiting immediately. Alternatively, they may take ever increasing doses of laxatives. They do not usually take much exercise and often complain of feeling tired. A victim of anorexia tardive goes on hunger strike to gain attention.

In primary anorexia, thoughts of food and

ALWAYS TOO FAT

Profile of anorexia nervosa
Teenage middle class girls are particularly prone to primary anorexia nervosa, where high parental expectation of a child is a frequent contributory factor in bringing on the complaint. Prevalence among this group in Europe, Asia and America has not so far been extended to Africa or to those of African descent.

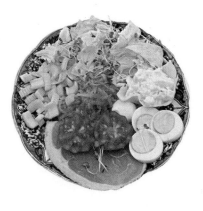
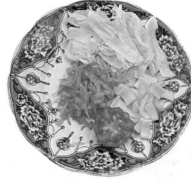

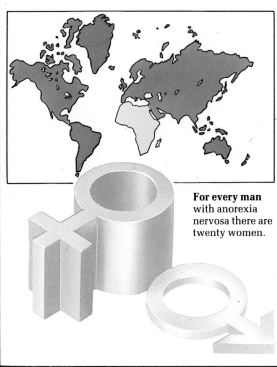

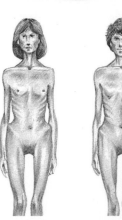

For every man with anorexia nervosa there are twenty women.

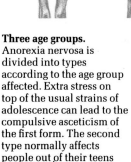

Three age groups.
Anorexia nervosa is divided into types according to the age group affected. Extra stress on top of the usual strains of adolescence can lead to the compulsive asceticism of the first form. The second type normally affects people out of their teens and can follow a bad sexual or emotional experience. Self-control is not so much in evidence here, with frenetic over-eating often followed by vomiting and self-administered laxatives. Anorexia tardive affects women over forty, often when a longstanding and useful role is no longer applicable.

fears of fatness fill your mind. Even though you know mentally you are thinner than your friends, you still feel too fat. It can excite you to find your bones sticking out. You feel deadly cold, your hands and feet being mottled purple. You are afraid of the future and what is expected of you, but you cannot explain your fears – least of all to your parents. In secondary anorexia, obsession with your shape is equally predominant in your thinking. Most of all, you fear the bulge that comes with pregnancy. In anorexia tardive, you are likely always to have been somewhat fussy about what you eat. Now that your family life has lost its savor, it does not seem worth bothering about food.

Diagnosis and treatment

Once physical disease has been ruled out, your weight loss and the stopping of your period is enough to give your doctor the diagnosis. He may order blood tests, particularly if you have been habitually vomiting or taking laxatives, since these may upset your chemical equilibrium. Hormone tests may be needed if your periods are slow to return after your weight is back to normal. The first essential is to restore your weight to its correct level; this process may well need to be started in hospital.

Talking to a therapist is also helpful in all forms of anorexia. You need to explore your relationship with your family and others, your inner feelings and your fears. As your weight gradually increases, you will become more sensible and mature in your thinking.

The outlook for you is good. Most victims of primary anorexia, for instance, grow up to have highly successful careers, to marry and become good mothers.

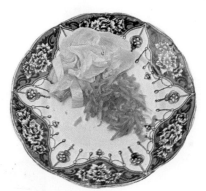 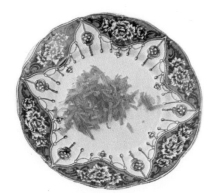

Diminishing diet.
In primary anorexia nervosa you feel too fat even though the objective perspective of which are still capable tells you that you are lighter than anyone else. Over a period of time (left), you cut out all the ingredients of your diet which could contribute to an increase in weight. Your protruding bones and constantly cold hands and feet do not distress you or impel you to eat more.

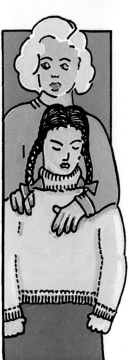

A dread of the future underlies primary anorexia nervosa, along with a keen concommitant desire for success. The conflict is temporarily resolved by something akin to a physical choice to remain a child. This brings about a hiatus in sexual development, or even a regression. Periods which have already started as part of the normal physical development towards adulthood are interrupted, and so, temporarily, is the progress towards motherhood and fully fledged relationships with the opposite sex which they imply.

PRESCRIPTION

Diagnosis
Once you have told your doctor about the cessation of your period, your weight loss, and your diet, the diagnosis should be quite straightforward. However, it is just possible that other illnesses are giving these symptoms, so he or she will want to rule these out.

Treatment
Your resistance to disease will be very low if, as is possible, you have become markedly undernourished. So the first priority, in the interests of your general health, is to put your weight back on. This may not be possible without sorting out the anxiety about puberty, or growing older, which is at the root of this problem. This is an area where psychotherapy has proved extremely successful. It is particularly important because attempts at support from the family are unlikely to work. An emotional tangle rooted in family conflicts is far too likely to have contributed to the disorder in the first place.

Depression

Depression is a psychiatric illness, in which your vitality is reduced and your emotional state is low. The chief feeling in acute depression is that life is simply not worth living; it can strike at any age, though there are two peaks – one between twenty and thirty and the other from fifty upwards – and women are three times as often affected as men.

Physical symptoms

Depression is caused by a shortage of the chemicals within the body which are essential to the smooth running of the nervous system. The whole system operates on various chemicals, which are manufactured by your brain cells during your sleep. Normally, you have enough of these for routine requirements, plus a reserve for contingencies and emergencies – like a bank account, in which there is some capital to back up your income. In depression, you are short of these supplies. There may be two reasons for this. You can be overwhelmed because of a heavy emotional drain – a bereavement, a marriage full of conflict, or a physical illness, for instance. This form of the disease is called reactive depression. Alternatively, the shortage of chemicals may be due to constitutional deficiencies. You usually run on a low reserve and a slight exaggeration of the normal fluctuation in the chemical supply is enough to push you into depressive illness. This type of depression is termed endogenous depression.

Such obvious disasters as the death or loss of a parent when you were a child can make you more vulnerable to a depressive illness later. If you are anxious or unhappy, your sleep is likely to be impaired; this also makes depression more of a risk.

WHAT DEPRESSION IS AND WHAT IT DOES

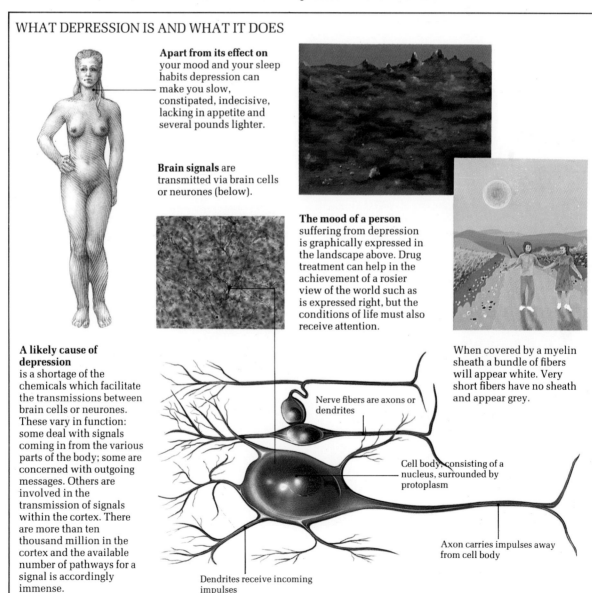

Apart from its effect on your mood and your sleep habits depression can make you slow, constipated, indecisive, lacking in appetite and several pounds lighter.

Brain signals are transmitted via brain cells or neurones (below).

The mood of a person suffering from depression is graphically expressed in the landscape above. Drug treatment can help in the achievement of a rosier view of the world such as is expressed right, but the conditions of life must also receive attention.

A likely cause of depression is a shortage of the chemicals which facilitate the transmissions between brain cells or neurones. These vary in function: some deal with signals coming in from the various parts of the body; some are concerned with outgoing messages. Others are involved in the transmission of signals within the cortex. There are more than ten thousand million in the cortex and the available number of pathways for a signal is accordingly immense.

When covered by a myelin sheath a bundle of fibers will appear white. Very short fibers have no sheath and appear grey.

Nerve fibers are axons or dendrites

Cell body, consisting of a nucleus, surrounded by protoplasm

Axon carries impulses away from cell body

Dendrites receive incoming impulses

Depressive illness will affect you differently, depending on whether it is endogenous or reactive. In reactive depression, you are more likely to be under forty. You feel unhappy and unable to cope with your day-to-day life. You cannot sleep easily and feel exhausted when you wake. You feel worse as the day wears on and you are inclined to blame other people for your state of mind. You may have lost four or five pounds in weight.

If you are suffering from endogenous depression, you will slow down both mentally and physically. You will be constipated, lacking in appetite and may lose a stone or more in weight over a month. Though you can get off to sleep, you wake in the early morning and cannot get back to sleep again. The world around you seems unbearable, especially in the mornings, and you feel that this is your own fault. You cannot make a decision, read, or do anything efficiently.

Diagnosis and treatment

In most cases, there is no difficulty in diagnosing depression. Your doctor may order blood tests, to check that you are not slowing down because of a disorder such as HYPOTHYROIDISM, or that the depression is not secondary to a physical illness.

Depression is like being in a locked room without a key. Medical help is the only answer. The chief forms of treatment are various forms of anti-depressive drug; most anti-depressants take a week or more to produce any beneficial effects. In extremely severe depression, the most effective form of treatment is electroconvulsive therapy (ECT).

After recovery, review your life style.

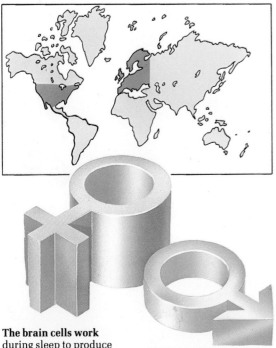

The brain cells work during sleep to produce those chemicals which we need to deal effectively with the vicissitudes of life. These chemicals may be chronically low, and periodically insufficient for dealing with these ups and downs efficiently.

Women are more prone to depression than men, particularly those who live in Western Europe or the USA. Among these women, those most at risk are in the twenty to thirty age group, or over fifty.

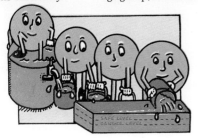

PRESCRIPTION

Diagnosis
Your doctor may try to ascertain whether your depression is 'reactive'—that is, an extreme reaction to circumstances that would depress anyone, but not normally to such a great extent; or endogenous—that is, without any easily discernible cause and seeming to arise from a persisting condition within the patient.

Treatment
A clinically depressed person cannot be talked out of his or her depression, and it is often necessary to use drugs, at least in the first instance, so that he can achieve a mood that is in any way receptive. The risk of suicide is not negligible, so this can reinforce the arguments in favor of drug treatment. If the drugs used need supervision, the patient may be admitted to hospital.

Chemical disturbances in the nervous system, quite beyond the control of the patient, may well be associated with many cases. Drugs have been devised which combat these deficiencies and so relieve the symptoms. Whether or not these disturbances are ever the simple cause of depression is not known.

Psychotherapy can also play an important part in restoring a patient's self-esteem and initiative, making him or her feel more able to deal with the sorts of daily demands that present themselves to all of us in varying degrees. Sometimes, particularly in emergency cases, electroconvulsive therapy can have surprisingly beneficial results.

Schizophrenia

Schizophrenia is a major psychiatric illness. In it, there is no obvious damage to the brain, but thinking, behavior and emotions are all disordered. Complete recovery cannot be counted upon, though, with proper treatment, there is a high cure rate.

Physical symptoms

No one knows precisely what underlies the development of a schizophrenic illness. An hereditary element is involved; this probably concerns the chemistry of the brain, while stress may be the trigger to the symptoms. Mothers have often been blamed for schizophrenic illness in their children, but it is more likely that anxiety and over-protectiveness develop in response to a child's abnormal behavior, rather than causing it.

In schizophrenia, the victim's perceptions are distorted. This involves his or her perception of sound, sight, other people and sensations from the body. While intelligence remains intact, a schizophrenic may have the unshakeable belief that, for instance, a foreign power is plotting to destroy him, that his thoughts are being transmitted to others, or that his every mood is under observation by an enemy. Such false beliefs are termed delusions. If he sees, hears or feels anything that is invisible outside his brain, these experiences are called hallucinations.

If you are developing schizophrenia, your main emotion is likely to be perplexity. Something is happening to you, or around you, which you cannot understand. You may hear voices talking when there is no one present – these often sound hostile. You may feel certain that you are threatened by danger. You may

DISTORTED PERCEPTIONS

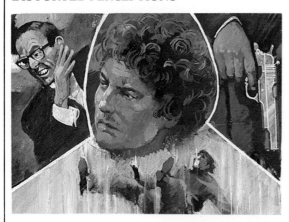

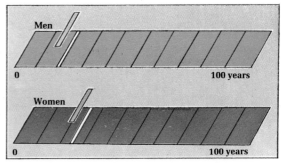

One person in a hundred develops schizophrenia, the ages of greatest risk being late adolescence in men and the mid-twenties in women.

Hallucinatory or paranoid experiences are typical schizophrenic symptoms. Paranoia is characterized by intense anxiety over imagined persecution or by highly inflated ideas of one's own importance. Hallucinations are sensations without any physical origin.

The Maze.
The term schizophrenia means separation of thought from reality. Whereas most people select heavily from their experiences a schizophrenic will bestow equal validity on everything that impinges on his mind. The notion of common sense has no force. The painting on the right, 'The Maze', may give some idea of such a state.

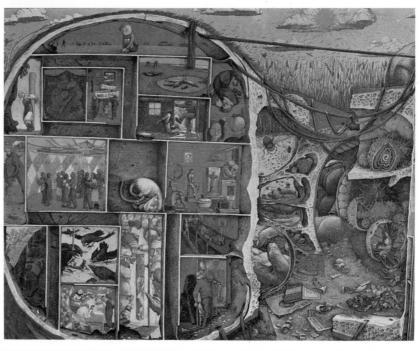

become angry or upset if others do not enter into your feelings. Eventually, you may look inwards so much that you lose contact with reality and seem completely indifferent to whatever is going on around you. Since you are totally wrapped up in yourself, your speech may become garbled or meaningless; so, too, do your answers to any questions you may be asked.

Diagnosis and treatment

Treatment by a psychiatrist is vital in schizophrenia. Because such illnesses are more subtle to diagnose than physical ones, the best way for your doctor to find out what is wrong is to keep you under observation in a hospital for a week or two. Thyroid tests may be carried out, together with a check on your blood chemistry and a test to see if you are short of vitamins –

B12 in particular. An electroencephalogram may be taken to rule out a brain disorder called temporal lobe epilepsy.

Medical treatment involves the use of drugs, psychotherapy and rarely electroconvulsive therapy. The first step is usually to prescribe a strong tranquillizer to calm the disturbed mental state of the patient. The tranquillizer normally takes the form of tablets at first, but later these are frequently replaced by injections every few weeks. If your body reacts to the tranquillizer – the symptons of this are muscle stiffness and a fine trembling – a drug will be prescribed to counteract this.

If you have had a schizophrenic illness, it is important to continue the course of treatment for as long as the doctor prescribes. It usually requires a minimum of two years' treatment after recovery from a first attack.

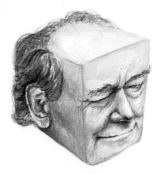

The hallucinatory experiences of a person suffering from schizophrenia extend to his perceptions of his own body – for example, the feeling that his head is square.

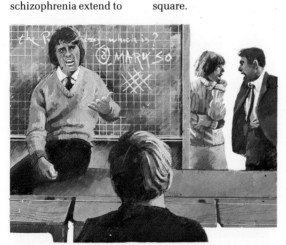

Because families share the same environment it is hard to distinguish hereditary from environmental factors when looking for the causes of schizophrenia. Changes in brain chemistry are associated with the disease, but may not cause it.

PRESCRIPTION

Diagnosis
The term schizophrenia covers a variety of conditions rather than a single one, but in general your doctor will diagnose schizophrenia from such symptoms as hearing voices, other hallucinations and delusional beliefs.

Treatment
It will probably be necessary to carry out some of the treatment in hospital, but this period should be as short as possible. Living with other people and carrying out a normal job are therapeutic rather than the reverse, and a schizophrenic is unlikely to represent a danger to those around him or her. The tranquillizer chlorpromazine is the most useful drug against schizophrenia as it enables a patient to start living a normal life so much more quickly. Therapeutic activity (below) is a crucial follow up to this drug treatment. Complete recovery is a long process.

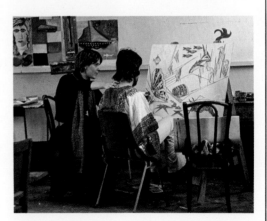

Once the symptoms of schizophrenia have been brought under control, occupational therapy (above) is an important aspect of the ensuing healing process.

Psychosomatic Illnesses

Psychosomatic disorders can affect men, women and children of any age. Such illnesses are physical disorders, which can be caused or kept active by psychological factors to a substantial extent. There are many such diseases; examples include bronchial asthma, peptic ulcer, ulcerative colitis, anorexia nervosa and migraine. Though such illnesses are obviously not imaginary, the trigger or stimulus to development of symptoms may be mental rather than physical.

Physical symptoms

Everyone's body is affected by emotional ups and downs. If you are scared, for example, your heart beats faster, so raising your blood pressure, while you tremble and sweat. Similarly, the digestive processes inside your stomach may be upset by stress. The first sign is indigestion, which, in the event of repeated incidents, may develop into ulceration. Asthmatic attacks, especially early on in the disease, can often be precipitated by emotional arousal; even the anticipation of pleasant events is enough to set off an attack.

Three things affect which part of the body becomes disordered. It can depend on your basic constitution, whether there has been any previous injury or disease in a particular organ, or sometimes whether a key relative has had a particular disease. In the last case, your attention may become focused on it. You are more likely to develop psychosomatic illness if you are the type of person who bottles up your worries, resentments and problems in general. If there is an inadequate outlet for your feelings in words or actions, emotion is liable to be displayed in physical symptoms.

THE MENTAL TRIGGER

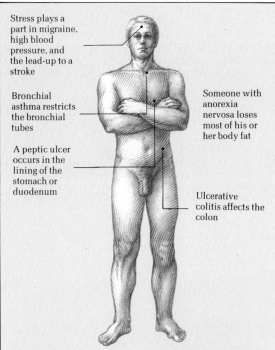

Stress plays a part in migraine, high blood pressure, and the lead-up to a stroke

Bronchial asthma restricts the bronchial tubes

A peptic ulcer occurs in the lining of the stomach or duodenum

Someone with anorexia nervosa loses most of his or her body fat

Ulcerative colitis affects the colon

The suddenness of the occurrence of a psychosomatic illness such as a coronary attack is somewhat misleading. The body normally needs to have been subjected to long stretches of unremitting tension, either through worry or persistent over-exertion, before its organs are incapacitated. It is the daily routine, and the habits learned over long periods of time, which are damaging. However, sudden crises may be instrumental in setting up the habits in the first place. The stresses of modern urban life, often combining physical overcrowding or degradation with psychological isolation make investigation of our repressed and unresolved emotions that much more difficult.

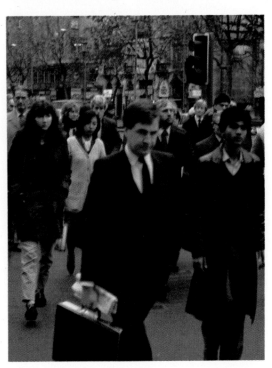

A patient's state of mind can almost always be said to have some bearing on the illness from which he is suffering, but the degree to which the state of mind is responsible varies widely. Those illnesses where it is of paramount importance are called psychosomatic, and include bronchial asthma, peptic ulcers, ulcerative colitis, anorexia nervosa, migraine, strokes and high blood pressure. The physical element in the cause of these complaints is abetted in varying degrees by an emotional element. The balance between these two elements can vary from person to person. In the case of bronchial asthma, for example, the agent most responsible for the narrowing of the air passages may be the allergy or the emotional state.

If you develop a psychosomatic illness such as a gastric or duodenal ulcer you will be far more concerned with the physical symptoms rather than any underlying mental cause. While you are doubled up with pain, or unable to sleep, all you will care about is to be freed from your physical distress. When the immediate problem has subsided, however, you may be able to work out what it was in your life that put such a strain on you initially and so learn how to cope with it.

Diagnosis and treatment

Your doctor will first of all concentrate on the physical aspects of whatever psychosomatic disorder is affecting you. Obviously, the first concern will be your physical well-being and it is only after this has been established that the underlying mental state can be treated.

When the symptoms are under control, you must review the way you live your life. Try to search out any areas of conflict or anxiety in your relationships or in your work. See what needs to be altered, but, most of all, try to make an adjustment in the way that you cope with fears, upsets or other difficulties. Some people give vent to their emotions and diffuse them by free expression of their feelings; others, who often appear self-contained and stoical, try to contain their feelings without fuss or complaint. Try to be like the former rather than the latter. The ostrich syndrome – denying that problems exist – is asking for trouble.

Practise bringing your feelings into the open, where they will do less harm to you. An open fire may be dangerous and damaging, but it is better where everyone can see it, like a bonfire, than shut away from view inside your body.

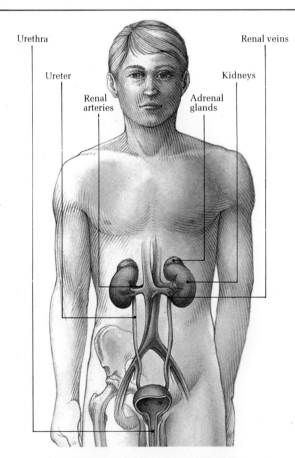

Urethra

Ureter

Renal arteries

Renal veins

Kidneys

Adrenal glands

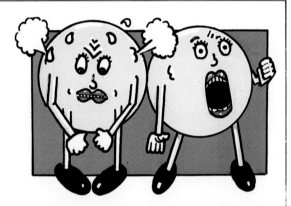

You are most likely to develop a psychosomatic illness if you keep your worries and resentments corked up. It is important to remember that emotion expresses itself somehow.

The body under stress
Physical injury, prolonged exposure, and all sorts of diseases are forms of stress. If the body is having to cope with one chronic aggravation, then it will have fewer resources to maintain its equilibrium if it is troubled by additional ones. Of all its organs, the adrenal glands are affected most by stress. Situated against the kidneys, they are made up of a medulla, which releases adrenaline and noradrenaline, and a cortex which produces hormones called steroids. Some steroids maintain the equilibrium of the body chemistry.

PRESCRIPTION

Diagnosis
The symptoms of certain illnesses are notoriously prone to exaggeration by psychological or emotional factors. If your doctor diagnoses one of these, he or she will naturally treat the disorder which has shown itself, but may also want to find out which particular anxiety is triggering or aggravating your illness.

Treatment
It may be beneficial simply to talk over any problems which you are finding particularly oppressive with your doctor. It is very easy to feel isolated by some anxiety, and the very act of sharing it, and finding out that, first, you are not alone in your predicament and, second, that someone is willing to approach your problems in a constructive manner, will make a positive impression on your state of mind. If your doctor thinks you need more specialist treatment, he or she may recommend psychotherapy appropriate to your case.

General/Introduction

This section of the book will deal with a range of diseases much more loosely related to each other than those assembled together in previous sections. What most of them have in common is some sort of breakdown or malfunction in one or more of the glands of the body. However, not all glands are of the same type. It is most helpful here to talk of three different sorts. The primary definition of a gland is that it is an organ that produces substances then releases them to act elsewhere in the body. One kind releases them into a duct, another directly into the blood stream. The glands in the third group treated here – lymph glands, are not really glands at all in this primary sense. They filter the lymph which the lymph vessels carry away from the tissue spaces, and so prevent the spread of infection.

The biologically useful substances produced by glands are distributed in two main ways. Glands such as salivary glands, sweat glands and gastric glands pass their secretions down a duct to the 'target' area. These are 'exocrine' glands. Others, such as the thyroid, have no duct. They pass their secretions, called hormones, directly into the blood stream. These are 'endocrine' glands. Their effect is not confined to one area. It is partly through these hormones that body functions are co-ordinated. No gland acts independently of others.

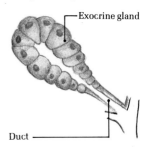

The thyroid gland produces the hormone thyroxine. This controls the rate that glucose is burned in the body.

The parathyroid gland produces parathormone, which regulates the amount of calcium in the blood.

The two adrenal or suprarenal glands each consist of a medulla and a cortex. These two parts are completely separate in function. The medulla produces adrenaline and noradrenaline, which prepare the body for physical effort. The cortex produces cortisol and aldosterone, which are vital in maintaining the balance of body chemistry in the face of stress of all kinds. It also produces sex hormones like those produced in the testes and ovaries.

The pancreas has both endocrine and exocrine functions. It releases pancreatic juice down the pancreatic duct into the duodenum. This neutralizes the acid. coming into the intestine from the stomach and contains digestive enzymes. It also produces insulin and glucagon. The former enables sugar to be taken up from the blood, the latter promotes its release into the blood.

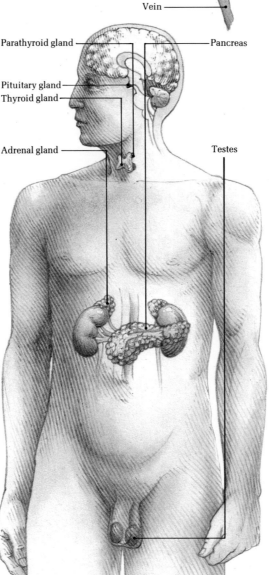

The pituitary gland is suspended from the hypothalamus of the brain, and the nervous system directly affects its functioning. Hormones released by this gland affect the release of many other hormones from other glands. In turn, hormones which these other glands release affect the release of related ones from the pituitary. This is how the right balance of hormones in the blood is maintained. For example, the pituitary releases a hormone TSH that stimulates the thyroid into producing more thyroxine if the blood thyroxine level is low. An excess of thyroxine will suppress the release of this hormone. It should be remembered that there is no one 'correct' level: this varies with the circumstances of a person, his state of mind, and so on. The nervous system provides the hypothalamus with information on these factors, so that the right level for a particular moment can be determined.

The testes and ovaries, apart from producing sperm or ova, produce the male and female sex hormones.

144

The saliva secreted by the salivary glands contains enzymes which start to break down food. There are three pairs of glands. The parotid extends from the front of the ear to the jaw angle. Its duct opens inside the cheek. The submandibular is under the back teeth, the sublingual in the mouth floor.

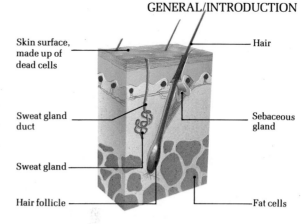

Parotid gland

Sublingual gland

Submandibular gland

Skin surface, made up of dead cells

Hair

Sweat gland duct

Sebaceous gland

Sweat gland

Hair follicle

Fat cells

Sweat and sebaceous glands.
Sweat, a solution of salt in water, helps the body to lose heat by evaporating and so cooling the skin surface. In a very humid atmosphere water cannot evaporate. When it is very hot 10 liters of water can pass through the sweat glands in one day. Sebaceous glands produce sebum, a greasy substance.

The lymphatic system drains tissue fluid and filters off bacteria and other foreign bodies from it. It also produces white blood cells, and antibodies which attack infection. Both these functions, the production of cells and antibodies and the prevention of the spread of bacteria are carried out by lymph glands, or lymph nodes. Only the tissue of the central nervous system has no lymph vessels.

Lymphatic vessels are made up of lymphatic capillaries. These capillaries are larger than blood capillaries.

Lymph nodes or glands lie along the course of lymph vessels. They are between 1 mm and 10 mm in diameter. The largest groupings are in the groin, neck, armpits, abdomen, and between the lungs.

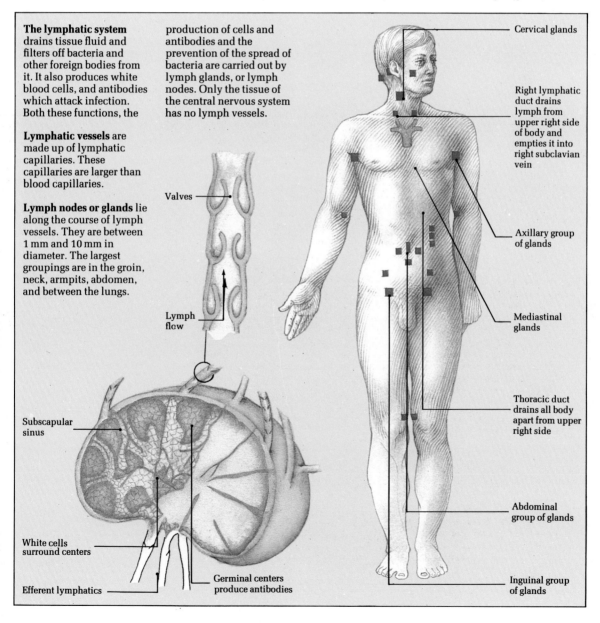

Valves

Lymph flow

Subscapular sinus

White cells surround centers

Efferent lymphatics

Germinal centers produce antibodies

Cervical glands

Right lymphatic duct drains lymph from upper right side of body and empties it into right subclavian vein

Axillary group of glands

Mediastinal glands

Thoracic duct drains all body apart from upper right side

Abdominal group of glands

Inguinal group of glands

Diabetes

Diabetes mellitus, commonly known as diabetes, occurs when the body is unable to utilize the sugar it absorbs as a source of energy. It is not a single entity; it includes several metabolic disorders, all associated with an unduly large amount of sugar in the blood stream and urine.

The body normally controls this level through the action of a hormone called insulin, which it produces in the pancreas. Insulin plays a vital part in the conversion of the sugar the body takes in into a form it can use. In diabetes, however, either one of two things can interfere with this process; either there is too little insulin available, or, for some reason, the insulin that is produced is ineffective.

Diabetes is a common ailment – for every diagnosed case, there is an undiagnosed one. In the UK alone, there are more than 300,000 known cases, while in the USA the total is as high as 3.5 million. The likelihood of developing the disease increases with age – it is particularly common among overweight people over fifty – but it can strike at any time. 'Juvenile onset' is a severe, acute illness, which develops in thin, young adults and children; 'maturity onset' is, by contrast, often mild and tends to run in families.

The exact cause of the disease is unknown, but there can be several contributory factors. Whilst an emotional shock cannot actually cause the ailment, it can make mild diabetes worse, or reveal a latent disorder. Injury, or disease, of the pancreas, the gland which makes insulin, may lead to the disease; occasionally, diabetes can be caused by MUMPS, pancreatitis, alcoholic damage, or cancer of the pancreas, though it is likelier to occur with thyroid disorders or rheumatoid arthritis.

THE ACTION OF INSULIN

One function of the pancreas is in digestion. It secretes pancreatic juice into a duct which enters the duodenum at the same point as the bile duct. The juice is alkaline, neutralising acid from the stomach. It also contains enzymes which break down substances from the food so that the intestine can absorb them. However, the pancreas also regulates the use of sugar by the body. Its 'islets of Langerhans' produce two hormones, insulin and glucagon. Not part of the pancreatic juice, these are released directly into the blood stream. Insulin enables the tissues to take sugar from the blood and store it or burn it up. Glucagon stimulates the liver and other tissues to release sugar into the blood.

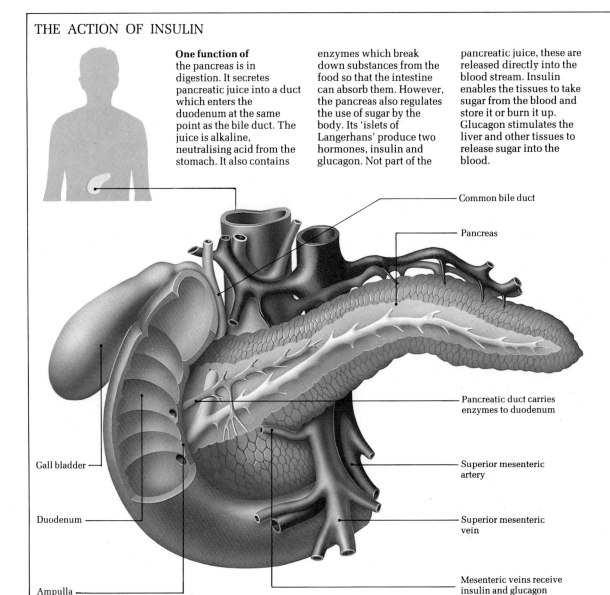

Common bile duct

Pancreas

Pancreatic duct carries enzymes to duodenum

Superior mesenteric artery

Superior mesenteric vein

Mesenteric veins receive insulin and glucagon

Gall bladder

Duodenum

Ampulla

Physical symptoms

Diabetes occurs when the body is provided with insufficient insulin for effective use of glucose, the main fuel for all its activities and essential for the working of the brain. In diabetes mellitus, the body behaves as if it is starved of sugar and the sugar level in the blood rises accordingly. What is happening is that lack of insulin means that glucose cannot enter cells so that the cells are starved despite plenty of glucose in the blood. So fat and protein are changed into glucose by the cells to make up for the glucose they can't get. Only the liver, brain and red cells can absorb glucose without insulin.

Classic symptoms of diabetes vary according to age. In younger victims, these can range from the frequent passing of large amounts of urine, as the body tried to dispose of the excess sugar in the blood, to thirst, lack of energy, dizziness and acute weight loss, despite, on occasion, a huge appetite. In middle-aged and elderly diabetics, a range of so-called secondary symptoms may be more prominent. There is a tendency to skin infections, boils, numbness in the feet, night cramp, impaired vision, angina and high blood pressure. If you are young, the first indication of the disease may be diabetic coma; in this, you feel ill for some hours and then begin to vomit and become mentally confused. Finally, you lose consciousness.

Complications in the case of acute diabetes can be twofold. The first occurs if the body breaks down excess amounts of fat and protein as a replacement for the missing sugar. If this happens, harmful poisons – ketones – are produced. This can lead to a condition called diabetic ketoacidosis, which may result in

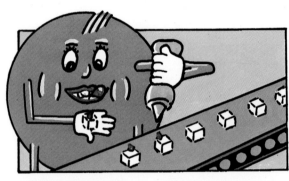

Sugar is an extremely concentrated form of carbohydrate and for this reason is best avoided by anyone with diabetes. However, it is wise for someone injecting his own insulin to carry some sugar, in case he has injected too much, or not eaten enough carbohydrate. Sugar reaches the blood very quickly and so the blood glucose level can be prevented from reaching a level where consciousness might be lost.

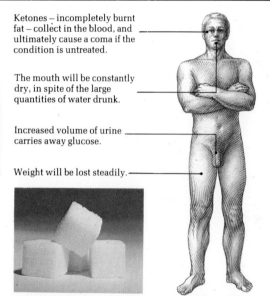

Ketones – incompletely burnt fat – collect in the blood, and ultimately cause a coma if the condition is untreated.

The mouth will be constantly dry, in spite of the large quantities of water drunk.

Increased volume of urine carries away glucose.

Weight will be lost steadily.

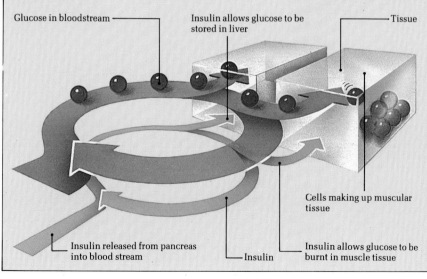

Glucose in bloodstream

Insulin allows glucose to be stored in liver

Tissue

Cells making up muscular tissue

Insulin released from pancreas into blood stream

Insulin

Insulin allows glucose to be burnt in muscle tissue

How insulin works. It is not yet known precisely how insulin works, but it is crucial in the process of providing energy for the body. In normal circumstances the liver releases glucose into the blood. The cells of the body then take it up and burn it. In a way not yet fully understood, insulin enables glucose to pass into the cells, and also allows the liver to store it. Without insulin, glucose would simply build up in the blood and pass out in the urine.

diabetic coma. The second complication is of long-term side effects, such as heart disease, STROKE and kidney damage.

Diagnosis and treatment
Diagnosis is usually made by testing the urine for glucose and also for ketones. The doctor will also test your blood to see if its sugar level is abnormally high. If it is constantly and irregularly raised, no further tests are needed.

Treatment of the disease varies, depending on whether insulin is completely absent from the body, or whether the existing insulin needs stimulating in some way to do its job effectively. In the first case, insulin is given by injection. The process is a simple one – the injections being easy to self-administer; the patient also monitors the diabetic process by testing his or her own urine. In the second case, oral med-

icines are frequently prescribed. These come in two groups – the sulphonylureas.

If you are overweight and a sufferer from mild diabetes, the best option open to you is often to control what doctors term the diabetic tendency by careful diet. Reducing body weight to the correct level means that the diabetes normally remains quiescent. Extra care about cleanliness helps to avoid the possibility of complicating infection.

One possible complication is hypoglycaemia, a condition produced by the administration of excess insulin, which, in turn, means that there is too little sugar in the blood. The remedy is to chew two or three lumps of sugar if you feel the symptoms coming on. These include a feeling of hunger, sweating and tingling sensation around the mouth. Sugar will quickly raise the blood glucose level.

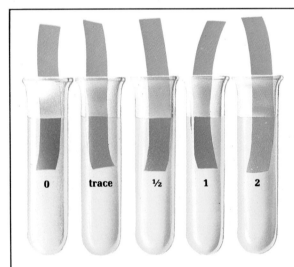

Testing for glucose
If you have diabetes it is important to keep a daily check on the level of glucose in your urine. The level should read negative or, to insure against hypoglaecaemia, a trace.

PRESCRIPTION

Diagnosis
A test for glucose in the urine is one of the important indicators of diabetes. A blood test to determine the level of sugar and ketones will confirm the diagnosis. Your doctor will also want to know whether you have been drinking an inordinate amount of fluid, and whether you have lost weight.

Treatment
Treatment depends on the form of diabetes present. Juvenile diabetes—unlikely to be contracted after the age of thirty—must be treated by daily insulin injections. These are made not into the veins but into the subcutaneous layer just below the skin. The blood capillaries then take up the insulin so that it can be carried around the body. Whether a patient has one or two injections a day, they should be administered before a meal. Late onset diabetes can, in mild cases, be controlled simply by careful diet. In other cases oral drugs are needed.

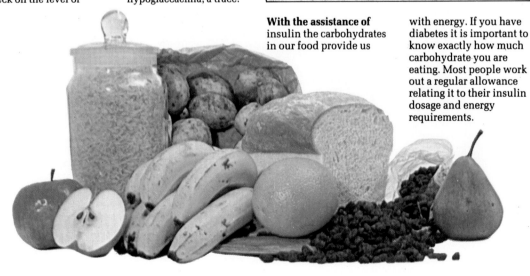

With the assistance of insulin the carbohydrates in our food provide us with energy. If you have diabetes it is important to know exactly how much carbohydrate you are eating. Most people work out a regular allowance relating it to their insulin dosage and energy requirements.

Goitre

A goitre is an enlargement of the thyroid gland, producing a swelling on the front and side of the neck. There are two types – toxic (see HYPERTHYROIDISM) and simple goitre. A simple goitre is usually smooth and uniform in appearance at first, but, as years go by, it may become bumpy and nobbly. The disease is common in areas where the soil is deficient in iodine. It may also occur sporadically in those whose diet is deficient in iodine, or for no obvious reason.

Women are five times more subject to goitres than men. Goitre may reveal itself at puberty, during pregnancy, or at a time during the period when the body is making extra demands on the thyroid gland. Stimulated to produce more thyroxine, it will respond by growing in size. Certain medicines may cause a goitre, by interfering with the thyroid's functioning.

Physical symptoms

The thyroid gland is shaped like a butterfly. It lies in the front of the neck, near the larynx, or voice box. It produces two hormones which control the rate at which the body uses its fuel; if you are short of thyroid hormones, you are likely to feel cold, rather fat and sluggish, whereas excess production makes you hot, thin, sweating and over-anxious. If there is a shortage of hormones, the gland enlarges to enable it to work harder with the consequent production of a simple goitre; the end result, however, is not the production of an increased amount of hormones, but the correct amount.

All you are likely to notice at first is a disfiguring smooth, symmetrical enlargement in the front of your neck. Sometimes, when the goitre gets bigger, it may make it uncomfortable for you to breathe or it may make you cough,

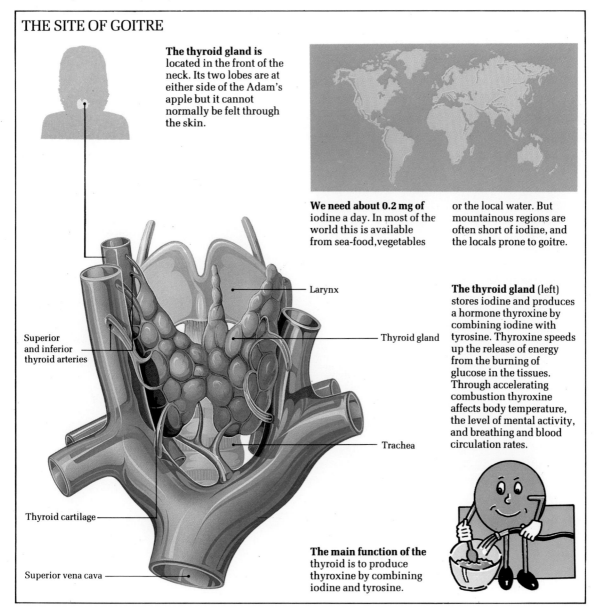

THE SITE OF GOITRE

The thyroid gland is located in the front of the neck. Its two lobes are at either side of the Adam's apple but it cannot normally be felt through the skin.

We need about 0.2 mg of iodine a day. In most of the world this is available from sea-food, vegetables or the local water. But mountainous regions are often short of iodine, and the locals prone to goitre.

Superior and inferior thyroid arteries

Larynx

Thyroid gland

Trachea

Thyroid cartilage

Superior vena cava

The thyroid gland (left) stores iodine and produces a hormone thyroxine by combining iodine with tyrosine. Thyroxine speeds up the release of energy from the burning of glucose in the tissues. Through accelerating combustion thyroxine affects body temperature, the level of mental activity, and breathing and blood circulation rates.

The main function of the thyroid is to produce thyroxine by combining iodine and tyrosine.

because of its proximity to the larynx. This last symptom may only be noticeable when you are lying in bed.

Diagnosis and treatment

The first step your doctor will take is to have blood tests carried out. These are to check that your thyroid is producing the normal amount of hormones, even if it is enlarged. If it is, this excludes the possibilities of HYPERTHYROIDISM or HYPOTHYROIDISM. To distinguish a simple goitre from an auto-immune disorder of the gland – that is, when the body decides to reject one of its own constituents in the mistaken belief that it is a harmful invader – a blood test for anti-thyroid antibodies must be made.

Obviously, if you live in an area where goitre is common, the first step to take is to make sure you eat iodized salt with your food. This has been strikingly effective in reducing the number of goitre cases in places as far removed as Switzerland and North America. The recommendation of the World Health Organization is one part in 100,000. If a medicine – lithium, say – is involved, it should be stopped, if possible. If you are an adolescent or in the twenties, the best treatment for an established goitre is usually a small dose of thyroxine given daily for several years. This helps the thyroid by doing some of its work for it, so that it no longer needs to enlarge.

If you are older than this and the gland is causing you discomfort, the treatment may fail. In this case, surgery to remove most of the gland may be necessary. Thyroxine should be given after the operation to help the small remnant of the gland to do its job. No long-term ill-effects are likely.

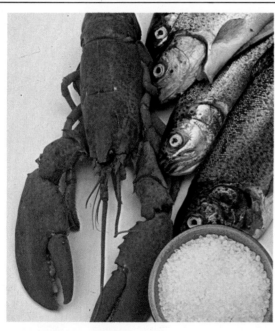

The reason for the enlargement of the thyroid gland is that in the absence of iodine the gland is constantly stimulated into producing more thyroxine. It responds by growing to a vast size.

You may be more prone to coughing than usual.

Enlarged gland will give the neck a thick appearance.

You may find it more difficult to breathe.

If you are short of thyroxine you will probably feel cold and rather overweight and sluggish.

Fish and sea-food are the richest sources of iodine in the diet. But in most non-mountainous regions the local water and vegetables will contain plenty for everyday needs. It is usual to make good deficiencies by adding iodised salt to the diet.

Women are five times more prone to goitre than men.

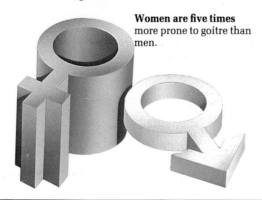

PRESCRIPTION

Diagnosis
It is necessary to test your blood to see whether your enlarged thyroid is producing the right amount of thyroxine. Once hyperthyroidism or hypothyroidism is ruled out, it will be necessary to check your intake of iodine

Treatment
Apart from the adding of iodised salt to your food, there are two main ways of treating a goitre. For young people, daily doses of thyroxine stop the thyroid from growing any bigger. For older people, it may be necessary to remove a large part of the enlarged gland. Thyroxine will then be given in appropriate amounts, and the patients should be spared further symptoms.

Hyperthyroidism

Hyperthyroidism is an abnormal condition resulting from excess production of the thyroid hormones. The characteristic sign of the disease is a GOITRE on the neck. Graves' Disease, affecting the whole gland, is the commonest type; in a few cases, however, only a small part of the gland is over-working – this is known as toxic nodular goitre. This usually appears in people over the age of fifty.

In common with toxic nodular goitre, the exact cause of Graves' Disease is unknown, though statistics show that women are more prone to it than men, particularly during the reproductive years. It often runs in families and, although there is no firm evidence to this effect, it seems likely that the disease is frequently precipitated by some great emotional shock or trauma, acting on someone who has inherited a tendency to the disorder.

Physical symptoms

The thyroid hormones control the body's metabolic rate – that is, how fast the body operates and uses its fuel. An excess of thyroid hormone in your blood means that you burn up your food supply at a high rate, so that, even if you eat heartily, you do not put on weight. You use more oxygen than usual, so your breathing rate increases as do the demands on your lungs. Your heart beats faster, too; you look and feel warm, but not feverish.

A goitre – a visible swelling of the enlarged thyroid gland in the neck – is likely to appear. Your eyes may seem to stand out, giving you a startled expression, and they may feel sore and gritty. If this protrusion of the eyes – called exophthalmos – is severe, you may see double when you look in certain directions. You will feel tired, conscious of your heart beat and

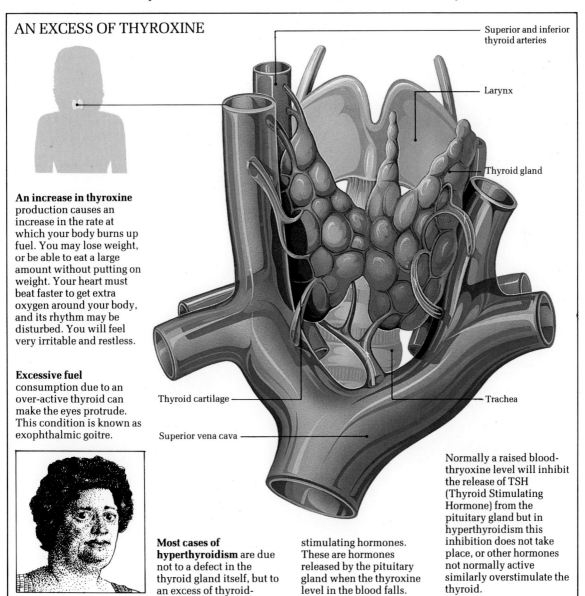

AN EXCESS OF THYROXINE

Superior and inferior thyroid arteries

Larynx

Thyroid gland

An increase in thyroxine production causes an increase in the rate at which your body burns up fuel. You may lose weight, or be able to eat a large amount without putting on weight. Your heart must beat faster to get extra oxygen around your body, and its rhythm may be disturbed. You will feel very irritable and restless.

Excessive fuel consumption due to an over-active thyroid can make the eyes protrude. This condition is known as exophthalmic goitre.

Thyroid cartilage

Superior vena cava

Trachea

Most cases of hyperthyroidism are due not to a defect in the thyroid gland itself, but to an excess of thyroid-stimulating hormones. These are hormones released by the pituitary gland when the thyroxine level in the blood falls.

Normally a raised blood-thryoxine level will inhibit the release of TSH (Thyroid Stimulating Hormone) from the pituitary gland but in hyperthyroidism this inhibition does not take place, or other hormones not normally active similarly overstimulate the thyroid.

muscularly weak. Your hands may tremble rapidly. Because of your raised metabolism, you will sweat freely all over. If you are a woman, your periods will probably become scanty. Despite a big appetite, you may lose weight. Diarrhoea may develop. Your increased breathing rate may lead to shortness of breath. Your ankles may swell and you will feel anxious and restless. Breathing problems, palpitations and swollen ankles are also signs of toxic goitre or hyperthyroidism.

Diagnosis and treatment
The signs and symptoms of hyperthyroidism are usually enough to alert your doctor, but diagnosis will be confirmed by laboratory tests. In toxic goitre, you may need to have a special x-ray called a scintiscan.

You may be treated by medicines or opera-tion. The main indications for surgery are a large goitre, the failure of medical treatment or social factors. Any side effects of medical treatment – especially sore throat – should be reported to your doctor immediately. Usually, treatment lasts from eighteen to twenty-four months, though sometimes you have to continue it indefinitely. One important point is that babies should not be breast-fed if the mother is taking anti-thyroid drugs, as the drugs will pass into the mother's milk, and so be conveyed to her child.

An alternative form of treatment for patients over forty is radio-iodine in the form of a drink. Usually, one dose of this is enough. Thyroxine may have to be prescribed after this to compensate for the decrease in hormone level. The treatment also leads to possible gene mutations, so it is best after the menopause.

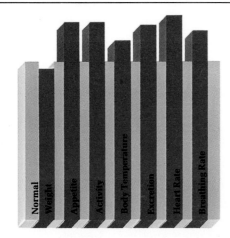

When the thyroid gland is overactive then many bodily functions are accelerated.

PRESCRIPTION

Diagnosis
Your description of your symptoms will be highly suggestive of toxic goitre, but final confirmation may depend on laboratory tests.

Treatment
Complete rest relieves the symptoms, but this obviously cannot be continued indefinitely. Ultimately, part of the thyroid may have to be removed, so decreasing the thyroxine produced. This operation must be preceded by damping down the thyroid activity by means of iodine, or drugs which act in a similar manner. Unlike iodine, these drugs sometimes cure the patient completely, but normally surgery is still necessary.

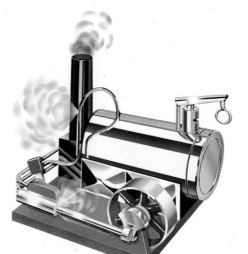

When the body over-produces thyroxine, it is rather like a steam engine with a leak. A large portion of the increased energy it generates is dissipated.

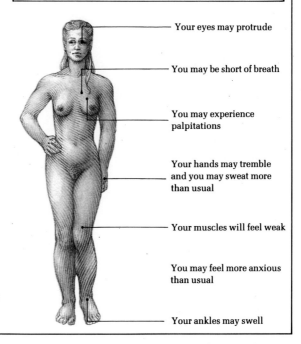

Your eyes may protrude

You may be short of breath

You may experience palpitations

Your hands may tremble and you may sweat more than usual

Your muscles will feel weak

You may feel more anxious than usual

Your ankles may swell

Hypothyroidism

Hypothyroidism occurs when the thyroid gland is under-active. The result is a deficiency in the production of the essential thyroid hormone, thyroxine. Lack of this secretion means that the body's mental and physical activity slows down to well below the normal level.

The condition can arise in new-born babies, the disease developing before birth. Unless treatment is given, the child will not develop properly, either physically or mentally. Among adults, the disease is termed myxoedema. It is more common in women than men, the peak period of risk being between the ages of thirty and fifty. Particular danger comes around the time of the menopause.

Causes of hypothyroidism vary. You may have had a GOITRE at some stage, or live in an area where there is a lack of iodine in the soil and water. But, far more often, the thyroid cells simply shrivel up; alternatively, what is termed an auto-immunity reaction occurs, in which the body turns its own defences against some of its own cells. In the thyroid's case, this is called Hashimoto's thyroiditis. There are also two further possibilities. If you have been taking excess amounts of a cough medicine containing iodine, say, the effect may be to poison the thyroid gland and interfere with its working. Treatment for over-active thyroid can also result in under-activity, which must also be countered.

Physical symptoms

The job of the thyroid gland is to manufacture, store and distribute the two thyroid hormones, for which iodine is an essential ingredient. This is normally obtained from sea-water fish, vegetables, meat, milk and water. The impor-

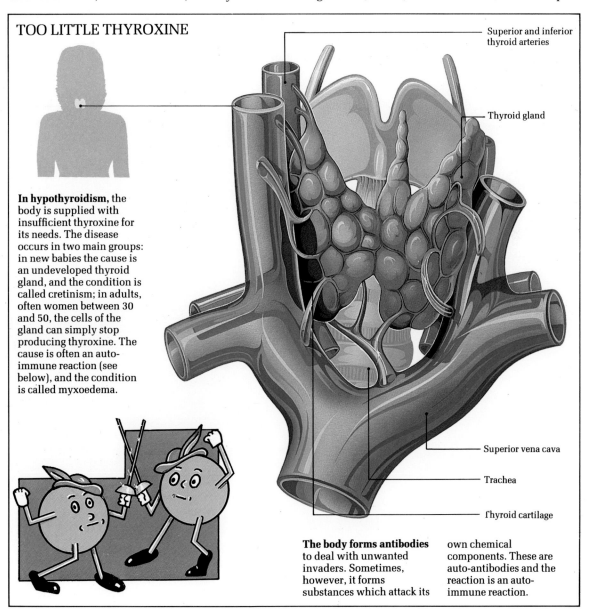

TOO LITTLE THYROXINE

Superior and inferior thyroid arteries

Thyroid gland

In hypothyroidism, the body is supplied with insufficient thyroxine for its needs. The disease occurs in two main groups: in new babies the cause is an undeveloped thyroid gland, and the condition is called cretinism; in adults, often women between 30 and 50, the cells of the gland can simply stop producing thyroxine. The cause is often an auto-immune reaction (see below), and the condition is called myxoedema.

Superior vena cava

Trachea

Thyroid cartilage

The body forms antibodies to deal with unwanted invaders. Sometimes, however, it forms substances which attack its own chemical components. These are auto-antibodies and the reaction is an auto-immune reaction.

tance of the thyroid hormones cannot be understated; they influence growth, sexual maturing and mental development, as well as the amount of cholesterol in the blood.

When you are short of thyroid hormones, your pulse rate slows and your blood cholesterol level rises, leading to silting of the arteries. Your heart muscles may eventually be damaged because of this. The changes come on insidiously, but you will find yourself becoming increasingly cold, weak, stiff and lethargic. Your thinking is slowed down; so, too, is your intestinal action, with the result that you are constipated. Your skin will be dry and you will have a puffy appearance, due to the development of abnormal tissue beneath the skin of the face, arms and legs. Your hair thins. Your voice sounds croaky and you may become deaf. Weight increases and periods falter or cease.

Although the effects of hypothyroidism are complex and far-reaching, the treatment for the disease is simple and extremely effective. It usually consists of taking thyroxine tablets by mouth once or twice a day, plus some thyroid extract if necessary.

Diagnosis and treatment
Your doctor will strike your achilles tendon with a hammer to see it react; the characteristic jerk is slowed down in hypothyroidism. A blood sample will also be taken. This will be checked to assess both the level of the thyroid hormones and of thyroid-stimulating hormone, the production of which is automatically increased in the case of deficiency. He or she may also measure the amount of cholesterol in your blood and have an electrocardiogram (ECG) taken to check your heart.

Cretinism
A baby with a congenital thyroid deficiency will be normal at birth, having had access to its mother's thyroxine, but will not be able to develop properly without the hormone.

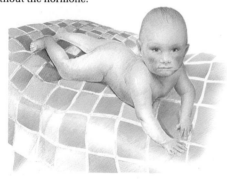

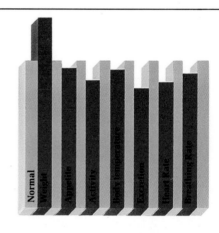

If the thyroid is under- active then bodily functions such as breathing rate and heart beat are below normal. Weight may rise.

Abnormal tissue develops on limbs and face

Pulse rate will be slow

You will be constipated

The main symptoms of myxoedema are loss of appetite and energy, low temperature, dry, puffy skin, slow thought reactions, croaky voice and weight increase.

PRESCRIPTION

Diagnosis
Your doctor will check the various functions that may have been adversely affected by a lack of thyroxine. These include your heartbeat and your reflex reactions.

Treatment
Treatment of hypothyroidism is simple and straightforward. Thyroxine is given, in tablet form, in quantities that make up for the deficiency in the gland's output.

Mumps

Mumps is an acute, contagious illness, usually caused by the infection of one or both of the parotid glands, which are the largest of the salivary glands, lying in front of the ear on each side of the face. The other three pairs of salivary glands can be affected, but in ninety per cent of cases it is the parotid glands that are involved. The characteristic sign of such infection is inflammation and swelling.

Mumps occurs all over the world and is endemic – that is, always present – in any large community. Localized outbreaks – epidemics – are most likely in the spring, but the disease can be contracted at any time of the year. You can get it at any age, though it is commonest in childhood.

Mumps is caused by a virus. In most cases, it is passed from person to person by the droplets from the victim's coughs, sneezes and breath, though, on occasion, the attack may be so mild that the carrier may not realize that he or she is spreading the disease. To all intents and purposes, one attack confers life-long immunity from re-infection; very young babies, especially those which are breast-fed, are also usually protected by an immunity carried over from their mothers.

Physical symptoms

The mumps virus enters the body through the linings of the nose and mouth. From there, it passes into the blood stream, which transports it to the gland and nerve tissue, for which it has a particular predilection. There is a 'silent' incubation period, during which you feel your normal self; this usually lasts between eighteen and twenty-one days, though it can be as little as fourteen days or as long as thirty.

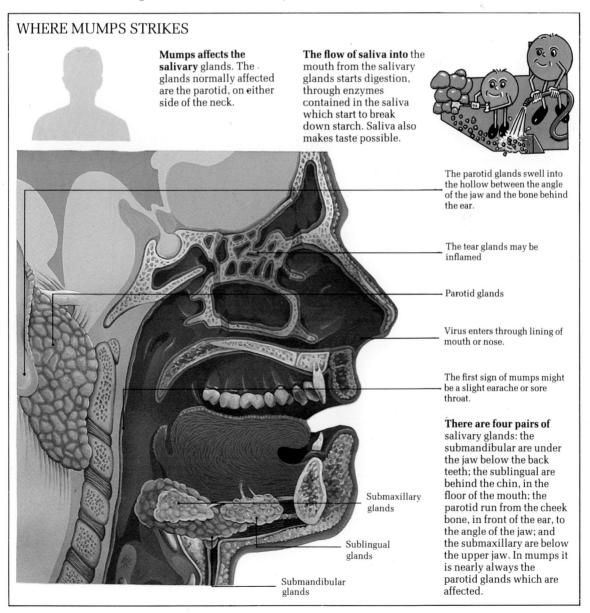

WHERE MUMPS STRIKES

Mumps affects the salivary glands. The glands normally affected are the parotid, on either side of the neck.

The flow of saliva into the mouth from the salivary glands starts digestion, through enzymes contained in the saliva which start to break down starch. Saliva also makes taste possible.

The parotid glands swell into the hollow between the angle of the jaw and the bone behind the ear.

The tear glands may be inflamed

Parotid glands

Virus enters through lining of mouth or nose.

The first sign of mumps might be a slight earache or sore throat.

There are four pairs of salivary glands: the submandibular are under the jaw below the back teeth; the sublingual are behind the chin, in the floor of the mouth; the parotid run from the cheek bone, in front of the ear, to the angle of the jaw; and the submaxillary are below the upper jaw. In mumps it is nearly always the parotid glands which are affected.

Submaxillary glands

Sublingual glands

Submandibular glands

At the end of this, the numbers of the virus suddenly increase and the affected tissues – glandular or nervous – become inflamed. They also swell, due to the presence of fluid and an influx of white blood cells, particularly small lymphocytes. The ducts within the glands become blocked with white cells – some having died in the battle with the virus – and their broken-down remnants. Temperature rises to 38.3° to 38.9° C (101° to 102° F), though, in contrast to fever, the rate at which the heart beats does not increase.

The first symptoms are so mild that they may well pass unnoticed. These are likely to be slight earache or sore throat, a shivery feeling, and perhaps fever. A day or so later, one side of the face suddenly becomes swollen and painful; the parotid gland involved swells increasingly for two or three days. The hollow between the jaw angle and the knob of bone – the mastoid process – just behind your ear disappears. Your ear lobe is pushed upward and forward, compared to the other one.

After a few days, the swelling on one side subsides, but, meanwhile, the other parotid has begun to go through the same process. The other salivary glands and, occasionally, the tear glands at the inner corners of the upper eyelids, become inflamed. The swollen glands are tense and painful; when you see – or even think of – food, they ache more because of increased pressure from the production of saliva. The lymph glands in the neck may become swollen and slightly tender. It will be difficult and painful to open your mouth.

The disease, in itself, is not serious, but complications can result. If you are a male of fourteen or over, you stand a twenty-five per

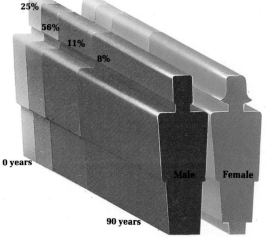

The progress of mumps

Between two and four weeks after infection the affected glands start to become inflamed.

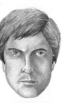

One parotid gland will swell more and more over two or three days. One ear lobe is pushed higher than the other.

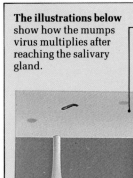

As the swelling in one gland subsides, it begins in the gland on the other side of the neck.

Who it strikes
25% of cases of mumps occur in children between 1 and 4 years. 56% of cases occur in children between 4 and 9 years. 11% of cases occur between the ages of 10 and 14. 8% of cases occur between the ages of 14 and 90.

The illustrations below show how the mumps virus multiplies after reaching the salivary gland.

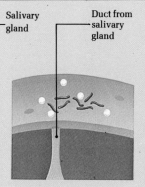

Salivary gland

Duct from salivary gland

Virus

White blood cells

Swelling subsides

The infection reaches the gland from the blood stream and lies almost dormant for about three weeks.

It suddenly starts to multiply. The surrounding tissue becomes inflamed and swelling begins.

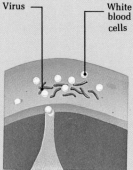

The white blood cells, some of them dead, block the duct and increase the swelling. The disease is at its height.

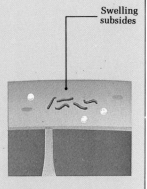

Swelling in the first gland will subside, but the same process will be well on the way in the other gland.

cent chance of developing orchitis, inflammation of one or both testicles. One or two weeks after the first facial inflammation, you may have acute pain in one testicle, or in the abdomen. The testicle becomes swollen and your temperature shoots up. You may vomit. Usually, only one testicle is affected.

In women, the ovaries may be involved, producing pain in the pelvic region and fever. This is more unusual and not nearly as painful as orchitis. The breasts may, even more rarely, be affected. Pregnancy presents no problems, as mumps does not cause any damage to the foetus. Inflammation of the pancreas, will give you sudden, sharp pains near the stomach, with associated vomiting, for about three days. Other glands sometimes involved are the thyroid gland in the neck and Batholin's gland in the female genital area. Meningitis is the com-

monest complication affecting the nervous tissue. You develop a severe headache, vomiting and stiff neck, all of which quickly subside.

Diagnosis and treatment
Mumps is usually easy to diagnose and there is no specific treatment. It is infectious for two or three days before the swelling appears until seven days after the last gland begins to swell. Take reasonable precautions to avoid spreading the disease, but quarantine is not necessary.

You should rest in bed from the time of diagnosis until all the glands have subsided. This lessens the risk of any complication, especially in adult men when it is particularly important not to get up until after the twelfth day from onset. This considerably lessens the chance of orchitis. Take plenty of fluids, mouth washes and analgesics.

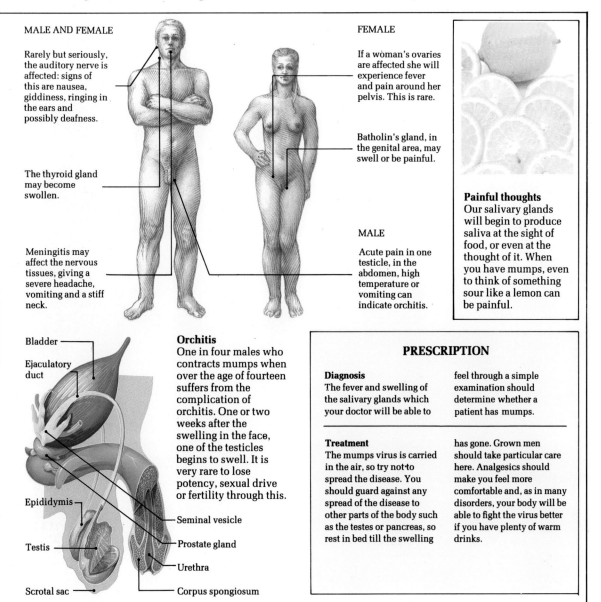

MALE AND FEMALE

Rarely but seriously, the auditory nerve is affected: signs of this are nausea, giddiness, ringing in the ears and possibly deafness.

The thyroid gland may become swollen.

Meningitis may affect the nervous tissues, giving a severe headache, vomiting and a stiff neck.

FEMALE

If a woman's ovaries are affected she will experience fever and pain around her pelvis. This is rare.

Batholin's gland, in the genital area, may swell or be painful.

MALE

Acute pain in one testicle, in the abdomen, high temperature or vomiting can indicate orchitis.

Painful thoughts
Our salivary glands will begin to produce saliva at the sight of food, or even at the thought of it. When you have mumps, even to think of something sour like a lemon can be painful.

Bladder

Ejaculatory duct

Epididymis

Testis

Scrotal sac

Seminal vesicle

Prostate gland

Urethra

Corpus spongiosum

Orchitis
One in four males who contracts mumps when over the age of fourteen suffers from the complication of orchitis. One or two weeks after the swelling in the face, one of the testicles begins to swell. It is very rare to lose potency, sexual drive or fertility through this.

PRESCRIPTION

Diagnosis
The fever and swelling of the salivary glands which your doctor will be able to feel through a simple examination should determine whether a patient has mumps.

Treatment
The mumps virus is carried in the air, so try not to spread the disease. You should guard against any spread of the disease to other parts of the body such as the testes or pancreas, so rest in bed till the swelling has gone. Grown men should take particular care here. Analgesics should make you feel more comfortable and, as in many disorders, your body will be able to fight the virus better if you have plenty of warm drinks.

Glandular Fever

Glandular fever is an acute, infectious illness, most commonly affecting children and young adults of either sex. Some eighty-five per cent of sufferers are aged between fifteen and thirty and it is rare for the disease to occur after forty. Its prevalence is world-wide and all races are affected.

Since the symptoms of glandular fever range from the barely noticeable to severe illness, it is often a difficult disease for doctors to diagnose. The main features are sore throat, swollen lymphatic glands and fever. The disease occurs sporadically and in epidemics, particularly in early spring.

Physical symptoms
Though it is certain that glandular fever is mildly infectious, little is known about how it is transmitted from person to person. It is often

termed 'the kissing disease' and there is some evidence to show that it is indeed sometimes passed on by kissing. Doctors believe that a virus called the Epstein-Barr virus (EBV), which is similar to the viruses that cause cold sores on the lips and SHINGLES, is almost certainly responsible for the disease, but the exact cause has still to be isolated.

The normal incubation period is from five to fifteen days after the initial contact; however, if you have been exposed to infection from someone who has the illness, it may be as long as seven weeks before it develops.

The onset of the disease is marked by a few days during which you feel generally out of sorts. You lose your appetite and have a slight fever – up to 38° C (100° F) – at night. Two to three days later, your glands begin to swell up; the major symptom is a painful swelling of the

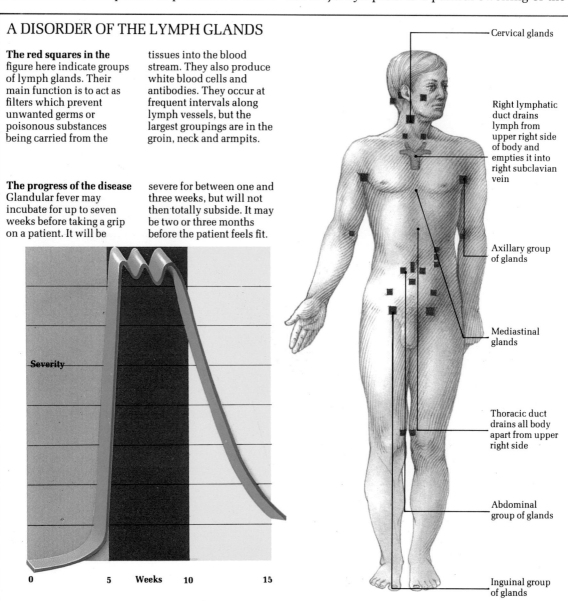

A DISORDER OF THE LYMPH GLANDS

The red squares in the figure here indicate groups of lymph glands. Their main function is to act as filters which prevent unwanted germs or poisonous substances being carried from the tissues into the blood stream. They also produce white blood cells and antibodies. They occur at frequent intervals along lymph vessels, but the largest groupings are in the groin, neck and armpits.

The progress of the disease Glandular fever may incubate for up to seven weeks before taking a grip on a patient. It will be severe for between one and three weeks, but will not then totally subside. It may be two or three months before the patient feels fit.

Severity

0   5   **Weeks**   10   15

Cervical glands

Right lymphatic duct drains lymph from upper right side of body and empties it into right subclavian vein

Axillary group of glands

Mediastinal glands

Thoracic duct drains all body apart from upper right side

Abdominal group of glands

Inguinal group of glands

lymph nodes just under the lower jaw, though the glands in the armpits and the groin may also be involved. Acute sore throat can be accompanied by severe headache.

At this stage, you are likely to have an extremely high temperature. Your skin and the whites of your eyes may look yellowish and jaundiced; in general, the eyes are likely to be sore and red. A rash may develop on your trunk and arms, particularly if you have been pre-scribed an antibiotic for the initial sore throat.

This severe stage usually lasts for one to three weeks; however, it sometimes takes two or three months to completely recover, as the associated symptoms of weakness and general debilitation can last much longer than the actual disease. The consolation is that there is no such thing as chronic glandular fever and it is exceedingly rare to have a second attack.

Diagnosis and treatment

Blood tests will indicate to your doctor whether or not you have glandular fever, as the ailment produces certain characteristic changes in the state of the blood. Chief amongst these is the presence of atypical lymphocytes (a type of white blood cell), while a special serum test will be positive.

There is no specific medicine for glandular fever. It is usually wise to avoid antibiotics because of the likelihood of inducing a rash. Bed rest, plus a light diet with plenty of sweetened fruit juices, are the main forms of treatment. Avoid fat, particularly if you are jaundiced. Soluble aspirin may be helpful if your temperature is high and you have a headache. Tepid sponging will cool you. You will remain infectious for seven days after the fever subsides.

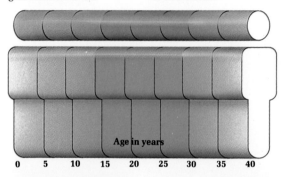

The age group affected. 85% of the people who get glandular fever are between 15 and 30. It is rare for anyone over forty to be affected.

Age in years

0   5   10   15   20   25   30   35   40

PRESCRIPTION

Diagnosis
Your doctor will check the parts of your body—your neck, under your arms, your groin—where the lymph glands are most heavily clustered, and so where any swelling will be most apparent. A blood test will be arranged for you and this will clinch the diagnosis.

Treatment
The disease must be allowed to run its course, as neither cause nor cure has yet been discovered. You will need no encouragement to rest. Diet should be light, but with plenty of liquids. When the fever is at its height, you will sweat profusely, and need frequent changes of bed-wear. Take special care for three months.

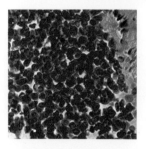

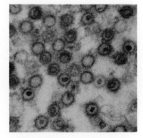

The virus responsible for glandular fever – the Epstein Barr virus – is attacked by abnormal white cells. These are shown (above right) next to normal cells (above left). Detection of these cells in the blood can be used to diagnose glandular fever.

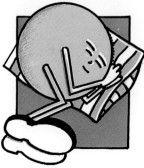

The Epstein Barr virus can lie dormant for up to seven weeks before it begins to multiply and attack the lymph glands.

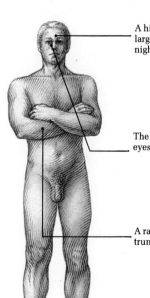

A high fever may set in, with a large amount of sweating at night.

The skin and the whites of the eyes may be jaundiced.

A rash may spread over the trunk and arms.

The lymph glands of the neck, armpits and groin swell most obviously in glandular fever.

Acne

Acne is a disorder of the sebaceous (oil) glands and ducts which produce a substance called sebum to lubricate the skin and hair. In acne, too much sebum is produced and consequently the ducts through which it is conveyed to the surface become blocked. The fatty sebum then accumulates to produce blackheads, pimples and whiteheads.

Almost all adolescents suffer from acne. It is usually more severe in boys, but starts and subsides earlier in girls. The peak period is around fourteen for the latter and sixteen for the former in normal acne; however, the severe forms of the disease normally occur a year or two later. Usually, acne clears before you are twenty, but in some rare cases it continues into the forties. In girls it is often worse just before their menstrual period. The distress that acne can cause should not be underestimated.

Physical symptoms

As you grow up, your skin changes. The very fine, downy hairs on the face and trunk disappear, while, on the other hand, strong beard hairs may grow. Each hair has a sebaceous gland associated with it, with the sebum it produces draining out along the hair follicle duct. Acne occurs when there is imperfect synchronization in the process; the hairs and their ducts may atrophy, while the associated sebaceous ducts either remain active or even increase production. The material cannot escape and remains trapped in the duct. When the sebum is blocked like this an organism called *Corynebacterium acnes* develops and it is this which leads to the subsequent inflammation. Additional factors which block the ducts to the skin are extra lipid production – a feature of adolescence – and also overgrowth of the

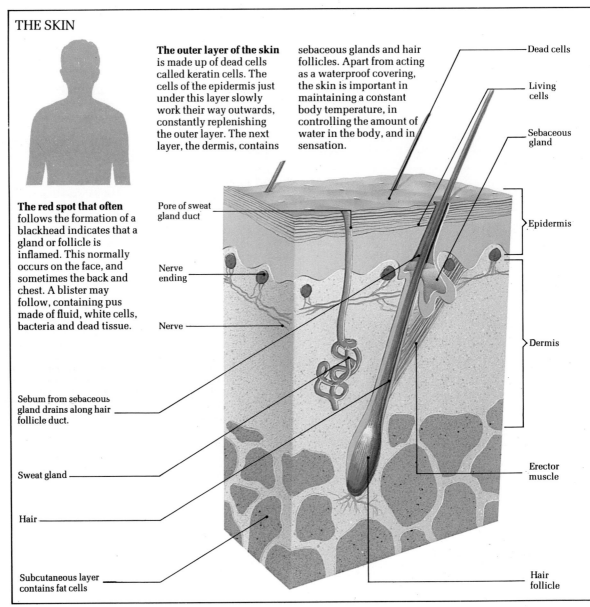

THE SKIN

The outer layer of the skin is made up of dead cells called keratin cells. The cells of the epidermis just under this layer slowly work their way outwards, constantly replenishing the outer layer. The next layer, the dermis, contains sebaceous glands and hair follicles. Apart from acting as a waterproof covering, the skin is important in maintaining a constant body temperature, in controlling the amount of water in the body, and in sensation.

The red spot that often follows the formation of a blackhead indicates that a gland or follicle is inflamed. This normally occurs on the face, and sometimes the back and chest. A blister may follow, containing pus made of fluid, white cells, bacteria and dead tissue.

Pore of sweat gland duct

Nerve ending

Nerve

Sebum from sebaceous gland drains along hair follicle duct.

Sweat gland

Hair

Subcutaneous layer contains fat cells

Dead cells

Living cells

Sebaceous gland

Epidermis

Dermis

Erector muscle

Hair follicle

stiff, top layer of the skin.

Blackheads, whiteheads, red spots and scars may all appear, usually on your face at first. They may spread to your upper chest – back and front – upper arms and bottom. They do not itch. Blackheads are inactive hair follicles, plugged with sebum but not infected. Raised red spots – papules – indicate inflammation in a blocked-up sebaceous duct; pustules, or whiteheads, are the same thing one stage further on, when infection has developed. Cystic acne consists of swellings in the skin, which leave noticeable large scars.

Diagnosis and treatment

While adolescence is sufficient cause for acne, your doctor will want to know if you are taking any medicines which could produce or exacerbate the disorder. Examples include cortico-steroids, iodides, androgens (male hormones), drugs used for epilepsy and phenothiazines. Exposure at work to certain chemicals, oils and petroleum may also result in an acne eruption.

The acne bacillus can be controlled, if not killed, by tetracycline taken four times a day. This must be taken on an empty stomach, at least thirty minutes before a meal. Occasionally, another antibiotic is required. Ultra-violet light, from the sun or a sun lamp, is the second most useful approach. Lotions or soaps which make the skin flake slightly help; you will also derive some satisfaction from taking an active part in treating your skin. Cleanliness is obviously vital. Anti-antrogen medicines are usually too drastic a method to be contemplated unless acne makes your life a complete misery on a psychological level. Squeezing spots is almost always counter-productive.

The formation of a spot. Sebum has the function of maintaining the suppleness of the skin. It reaches the surface by draining along the ducts of the hair follicles. Sometimes the hairs atrophy but the glands continue to produce sebum. A blockage is then likely.

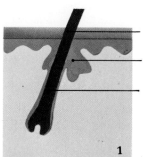

— Hair follicle duct

— Sebaceous gland

— Hair follicle

1. The sebaceous gland produces sebum which drains along the hair follicle duct.

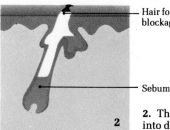

— Hair follicle dies, leaving blockage

— Sebum

2. The hair follicle falls into disuse but sebum continues to be produced.

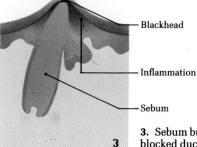

— Blackhead

— Inflammation

— Sebum

3. Sebum builds up in the blocked duct, and a blackhead forms.

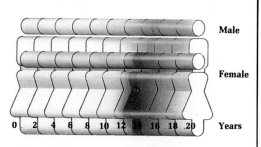

Male

Female

| 0 | 2 | 4 | 6 | 8 | 10 | 12 | 14 | 16 | 18 | 20 | Years |

In adolescence the sebaceous glands are unusually active, so blockages in hair follicle ducts tend to be more frequent in these years.

PRESCRIPTION

Diagnosis
The characteristic appearance of the blackheads and the age of the patient are normally sufficient for a diagnosis

Treatment
When an adolescent has stopped growing and reached maturity, the hormonal imbalance which seems to be behind the occurrence of acne will probably right itself, and the acne disappear. However, it is not really satisfactory to wait until this time as acne can cause considerable emotional stress at this especially sensitive time of life. Sunlight definitely helps acne, and ultraviolet light, used carefully and in moderation can sometimes be beneficial. Squeezing spots increases the risk of scars, but it is possible for a specialist to remove blackheads if this proves necessary. Some lotions go some way towards combating the condition.

Anaemia

Anaemia is a term used to describe a number of blood disorders in which the concentration of haemoglobin in the blood is abnormally lowered. You are considered to be anaemic if your haemoglobin, measured in grams per decilitrs, is below thirteen in an adult male, twelve in an adult female, the same in a child aged between six and fourteen and eleven for infants aged between six months and six years.

Anyone of any age can develop anaemia and the possible causes are numerous. Factors that can cause the disease include a diet deficient in iron, folate, vitamin B12 and/or protein; loss of blood, most commonly from heavy periods; chronic illness of many kinds, from hypothyroidism to cancer; and congenital blood disorders, such as thalassaemia. Women are more prone to anaemia than men, the poor and the elderly being particularly at risk.

Physical symptoms

If your diet is lacking in iron, if there are extra demands upon you from, say, pregnancy, or if you suffer long-term mild blood loss, the type of anaemia you may develop is called microcytic. In this the red blood cells are too small. Another type of anaemia is called macrocytic and in this the cells are oversize. This may be the result of vitamin B12 and folate deficiency; liver and lettuce provide these substances respectively. It is more likely, however, that you have not absorbed the vitamin B12 from your food. This happens quite frequently as an after-effect of a stomach operation.

You may notice that you are pale. The appearance of your skin is not a reliable indicator of the state of your blood, however; a more reliable check is to examine the inside of your lower eyelid or your nail beds. If your

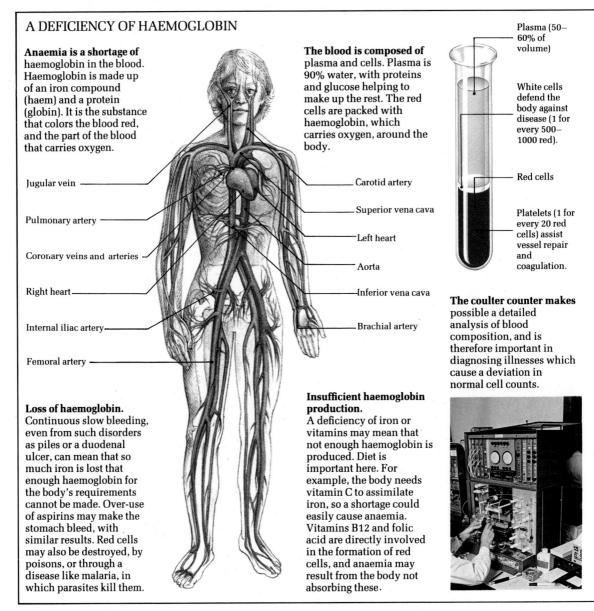

A DEFICIENCY OF HAEMOGLOBIN

Anaemia is a shortage of haemoglobin in the blood. Haemoglobin is made up of an iron compound (haem) and a protein (globin). It is the substance that colors the blood red, and the part of the blood that carries oxygen.

Jugular vein

Pulmonary artery

Coronary veins and arteries

Right heart

Internal iliac artery

Femoral artery

The blood is composed of plasma and cells. Plasma is 90% water, with proteins and glucose helping to make up the rest. The red cells are packed with haemoglobin, which carries oxygen, around the body.

Carotid artery

Superior vena cava

Left heart

Aorta

Inferior vena cava

Brachial artery

Plasma (50–60% of volume)

White cells defend the body against disease (1 for every 500–1000 red).

Red cells

Platelets (1 for every 20 red cells) assist vessel repair and coagulation.

The coulter counter makes possible a detailed analysis of blood composition, and is therefore important in diagnosing illnesses which cause a deviation in normal cell counts.

Loss of haemoglobin. Continuous slow bleeding, even from such disorders as piles or a duodenal ulcer, can mean that so much iron is lost that enough haemoglobin for the body's requirements cannot be made. Over-use of aspirins may make the stomach bleed, with similar results. Red cells may also be destroyed, by poisons, or through a disease like malaria, in which parasites kill them.

Insufficient haemoglobin production. A deficiency of iron or vitamins may mean that not enough haemoglobin is produced. Diet is important here. For example, the body needs vitamin C to assimilate iron, so a shortage could easily cause anaemia. Vitamins B12 and folic acid are directly involved in the formation of red cells, and anaemia may result from the body not absorbing these.

blood is low in haemoglobin, it will have poor oxygen-carrying power; the blood will therefore have to pass round the body more quickly in order to supply the tissues adequately. To achieve this, your heart must beat faster and more strongly. If an adult's haemoglobin has fallen below seven grams per decaliter, palpitations are likely to be noticed, while any exertion will make you tired and breathless. If the anaemia gets worse, your heart may not be equal to the strain; indications of this are swollen ankles and shortness of breath even when you are not exerting yourself.

You will also be subject to mental fatigue, loss of sexual drive, irritability, headache, dizziness and fainting. You may feel nauseated and vomit. Your bowels may be either too loose or constipated. In women, periods may either become heavy or stop completely.

Diagnosis and treatment

Your doctor will check your general health, especially as another disease may underlie the anaemia. The haemoglobin level of your blood will be measured and the red cells, white cells and platelets counted. An increase in white cells may indicate infection. A sample may be taken of your bone marrow to obtain information about the state of blood cell production. In microcytic anaemia, the iron level must be established; in macrocytic anaemia, the folate and B12 levels. Tests may look for bleeding.

Treatment depends on the type and cause of the anaemia. In severe, acute blood loss, transfusion is life-saving. Iron deficiency requires iron tablets or, rarely, iron injections. Deficiencies of folate or B12 are dealt with through tablets and injections respectively. Your doctor will recommend a suitable diet.

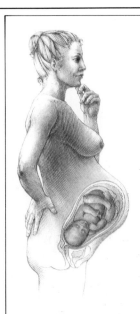

Pregnancy and anaemia
Pregnancy makes two major demands on a woman's chemical resources which put production of red blood cells under strain. Firstly, she has to provide iron for the baby from her own reserves. Ceasing menstruation offsets this to some extent, but not completely. Secondly, folic acid, essential to the process of red cell formation and found in fresh vegetables, may be in short supply.

Irritability, headaches, dizziness and faintness are all likely.

A little exertion may make you tired and breathless.

The heart may beat faster.

The inside of the eyelids or the nail beds may be pale.

Sexual drive will be diminished.

The ankles may swell, even when you are at rest.

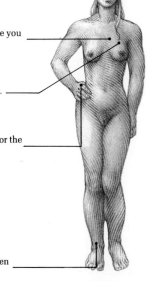

The red blood cells shown here are the parts of the blood which contain haemoglobin. This combines with oxygen so that the tissues can receive constant supplies.

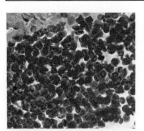

The magnification on the left shows the blood of an anaemic patient. His body will suffer from lack of oxygen, through lack of haemoglobin to carry it.

PRESCRIPTION

Diagnosis
Your doctor will want to find out whether your anaemia is caused by blood loss or iron or vitamin deficiency.

Treatment
If aspirin abuse has caused bleeding into your stomach the main remedy is clearly to refrain from taking aspirins. Other sorts of bleeding—from an ulcer, for example, will have to be dealt with in the appropriate manner. If the bleeding is serious, a transfusion may be necessary. If you are pregnant, your clinic should in any case be giving you iron tablets for you to take daily. Diet is important: meat, eggs and cereals are rich in iron, and the vitamin C of fresh fruit and vegetables is needed for its absorption. If you are short of folic acid, then your diet may be responsible. Eat more fresh vegetables, and take the tablets prescribed.

You and Your Health

This book tells you how the systems of your body work, what can go wrong with them and how modern medical techniques set about solving the problem. Medicine advances all the time, and many diseases that were once most serious are cured routinely; there is now hope in many cases of the long-term progressive afflictions that once made a normal life impossible. But even modern medicine does not completely understand how every disease works or how to treat every illness, and it is generally acknowledged that the most effective form of medicine is preventitive. If you can understand how your body works you stand a better chance of maintaining it sensibly and so avoiding many diseases; by following a few simple rules and using 'common sense' you will be in a good position to prevent the onset of disease and your body will be better equipped to resist any infection that you do contract. These rules relate to five main areas – diet, exercise, abuse of the body, stress factors and safeguards against disease.

Diet

The diet common in the Western world is a major cause of disease. The problem is that Western man's diet has undergone a revolution over the last 200 years; a digestive system that evolved to cope with a high bulk of food, consisting mainly of vegetable fibers with occasional meat and a small amount of sugar now has to process a smaller bulk of food that is generally low in fiber but high in animal fats and sugar – more than 45 pounds of sugar are eaten by each person in the West every year.

As a result of this highly refined diet, Western man is prone to tooth decay, *diverticular disease* and *piles*; in association with other factors the low bulk, low fiber, high sugar and high animal fat diet may cause *hypertension*, *heart* disease and *strokes*. All of these problems are seen much less often in those who eat food that has the opposite characteristics, for example the majority of Africans. For social and cultural reasons it is obviously difficult to live on a high bulk, high fiber, low animal fat and sugar diet in the Western world – the habits of generations are difficult to break, and consumer pressures predispose children towards 'junk foods', sweets and candies from an early age. But it is sensible to try and moderate your intake of highly refined foods. You should avoid sugar and excessive amounts of animal fat; try and eat more vegetables, cereals and pulses (the less these are cooked the more the fiber retains its original structure); make up bulk in your diet with bran and roughage, perhaps from wholemeal bread. This is the basis of a healthy diet, because this is the diet for which man's digestive system was designed.

Your diet must also be 'balanced' - that is, it must contain *protein, carbohydrates, fats, vitamins*, minerals, trace elements and roughage in sufficient quantities to sustain life. Proteins are essential for the growth of new tissues and the repair of damaged tissue – it is especially important for children, pregnant or lactating women and convalescents; eggs, meat and fish are the best sources, but protein is also found in bread and some vegetables. Carbohydrates, such as starch, and fats are either broken down in the body to provide energy or stored; water and mineral salts are used in the *metabolic* processes, or chemistry, of the body, while vitamins are essential for growth and health; roughage helps the process called *peristalsis* by which food is transported through the intestines and eventually excreted. A balanced diet contains a sensible, but not excessive amount of all these substances.

A lack of one or more of the various vitamins may well cause disease. All the vitamins should be found in the quantities that the body needs in the diet, but there is no harm in taking a regular proprietary multivitamin pill to make up any shortfall – as may be seen in children who traditionally never like the foods that are good for them. The large quantities of vitamin supplement pills that some people take daily are normally unnecessary – in fact in excess they may be dangerous, for no systematic research has been done into the effects of regular high doses of vitamins. Vitamin A, for example, is poisonous in very large doses: the early Arctic explorers ate the livers of polar bears and arctic foxes with fatal results – they contain a massive concentration of the vitamin. Vitamin C, however, is simply excreted when more is eaten than the body requires, so you can eat as much fresh fruit and vegetables as you wish – but remember that Vitamin C is denatured by cooking, and so all vegetables should be cooked as lightly as possible.

A sensible, balanced diet is good for you, but too much of it is not. Unfortunately, food substances that are not burnt up as energy are stored in the body as fat; if you consistently eat more food than the body requires to perform its functions you will become fat. A large number of people in the Western world are *obese* (i.e. 20% over the normal body weight for their height and build) and obesity can lead to a number of problems, including heart disease and circulatory problems. Contrary to popular opinion, obesity is almost always the result of over-eating, for whatever cause, and there is only one effective way to lose weight – to diet. The best way to start off a diet is to work out roughly the number of calories (expressed as kilocalories, kcals or Cals) of energy that you burn up each day, then estimate the number of calories that you take in as food. The average daily requirement for a sedentary man is 2700 Cals, and for a woman 2100 Cals. This requirement is increased if an individual's work is physical and decreased by inactivity and age. You can soon reach the 2000 calorie mark: a cheese sandwich is 400 Cals, a pint of milk is 300 Cals, and a spoonful of sugar 23 Cals. There are a number of publications available that give fuller details. You will probably be surprised to see how many more calories you eat than you use. To lose weight you need to reduce your calorific intake to somewhere around 1200 Cals a day, but you should always consult your doctor to see what rate of weight-loss would be best for you. There is really no easy way to diet and the only safe aid is strong personal motivation. The so-called 'slimming pills' usually contain amphetamines; they can have dangerous side-effects and are often addictive, so much so that a doctor will normally only prescribe them in exceptional circumstances. Once you have reached your target weight, try and keep a check on your calorific intake, because an excess of only 50 Cals a day over a long period will make you fat again.

Exercise

A controlled programme of exercise will help your diet. It is very difficult to lose weight through exercise alone, but the human body does need regular exercise to keep it in good working order. A lack of physical activity increases the likelihood of *coronary artery disease* and reduces the efficiency of the muscles of the chest, thus decreasing the amount of *oxygen* that can enter the body. Regular exercise improves both these factors; indeed a controlled exercise programme is often prescribed for those suffering from coronary artery disease. Apart from the physical benefits of strenuous activity, you will actually feel better.

If you have not taken exercise for a long time, you should never overdo things at first – otherwise you may have the heart attack that you have been trying to avoid. Take things slowly: start off with light, undemanding exercise and gradually work up to strenuous activity over a period of months. It may be sensible to consult your doctor about your plans, especially if you are being treated for any condition. Jogging has recently become popular, and even fashionable, and it is a very practical form of exercise. If you find it impossible to jog, or embarrassing, you may prefer swimming, cycling, yoga, isometric exercises, activities at your local gymnasium or even physical jerks in the privacy of your own bedroom. Whatever type of exercise you take it will be good for you, and a preventitive measure against disease.

Abuses of the Body

There is not much point in eating a sensible, balanced diet, keeping your weight in check and taking regular exercise if you abuse your body. The most common abuses are the use of tobacco and the excessive use of alcohol. Both are socially acceptable, though tobacco is becoming less so, and both are made to appear respectable and even desirable by consumer pressure such as advertising and cultural pressure that makes their use seem 'tough' or sophisticated. In fact there is nothing clever about the use of tobacco or about alcohol consumption: they are both *toxic* substances that are in many ways almost as dangerous as heroin, and kill more people each year than that drug.

Tobacco, especially in the form of cigarettes, kills. It causes *lung cancer, bronchitis, emphysema, atherosclerosis* and *coronary artery disease*, as well as contributing significantly to the seriousness of many other conditions. Some people fall back on the argument that nobody has actually proved that cigarettes cause cancer. This is true, but only in a very limited statistical sense. A 'causal' link has not been proven, mainly because it is impossible to show conclusively that those who are likely to smoke are not also predisposed towards cancer – but this argument is an evasion. It is hard to find a single scientist or doctor who does not believe that tobacco kills, one way or another, and at the very least takes years off your life. If you smoke, stop – otherwise you cannot seriously want to stay healthy and live out your natural life-span.

Alcohol is a slightly different problem. In moderation alcohol is a pleasant and sociable relaxant; in fact small quantities may help to stop or slow down the formation of arterial obstructions in *atherosclerosis*. Alcohol becomes a problem when too much of it is taken too regularly. It then becomes addictive, and the addiction, called *alcoholism*, can develop insidiously to destroy an addict physically, mentally and socially. The most important stage in the treatment of alcoholism is the recognition on the part of the heavy, problem drinker that he or she is an alcoholic; after that admission the various forms of therapy used can become effective. If you are a heavy drinker you should ask yourself when you last went without a drink for a day; whether you often feel a strong urge to have a drink; whether you drink as a solution to your problems; and whether your work or home-life is suffering because of your drinking habits. If the answers to these questions worry you, you should cut down your drinking immediately or stop it altogether, and see a doctor.

Tobacco and alcohol are the main substances with which we abuse our bodies, but there are others. Drugs such as heroin, opium and cocaine are taken for pleasure by some, but they are all highly addictive and highly dangerous; heroin in particular normally leads to death. Recent research shows that marijuana, a drug that has become illicitly popular over the last decade, is not nearly as harmless as its proponents would have us believe; it seems to be more *carcinogenic* than tobacco, causes brain damage and leads to *personality disorders*, such as a lack of motivation. Many people who would be horrified to think of themselves as drug addicts are in fact addicted to drugs such as amphetamine stimulants, barbiturate depressants and tranquilizers – withdrawal from these drugs can often be as traumatic as from the 'hard' drugs. Others, quite unnecessarily, purge themselves with laxatives every day, with potentially ruinous effects on their digestive system. There are many different ways in which you can abuse your body, and it is wise to examine your life-style to find out how you can eliminate these abuses and so make your life healthier.

Stress

The pace of life in the overcrowded, demanding 20th century inevitably produces stress, which in turn can cause psychological problems and physical disease. *Hypertension* and the formation of *peptic ulcers* can both be associated with stress, while the psychological problems it causes may range from *depression* and anxiety to *neurosis* – sometimes these psychological problems may manifest themselves as aches and pains in the *psychosomatic diseases*. Stress itself may have a number of causes; some people, especially when they have been promoted above their ability, experience stress as a result of the pressures and expectations of their jobs. Others find that problematic family or social relationships become too much for them, and commonly stress is associated with sexual difficulties and insecurities.

The best way to treat stress is to remove its cause. Your doctor may well, through counselling, be able to sort out your family, social and sexual difficulties, often by making you understand the root of your problem and helping you to work out a way of adjusting to it. A doctor, however, cannot find you a new job; you are ultimately the only person who can solve the problem of job-related stress. The answer may be to change your job or to reconsider the way in which you earn your living – after all there is no point in achieving success at work at the expense of your health.

Safeguards Against Disease

No matter how diligently you look after yourself there is always the possibility of disease. The chances of contracting an illness can, however, be considerably reduced if you use common sense and take advantage of all the available safeguards against disease. The most obvious safeguards are those that confer a degree of *immunity* against specific diseases – *vaccinations*, or *immunizations*. Vaccinations are routinely performed during childhood, but some of them, for example *tetanus*, need 'boosters' every so often in adult life; different vaccinations may be necessary if you are travelling abroad or if you are particularly at risk from a specific disease. It is always sensible to ask your doctor whether your programme of vaccinations is up to date.

There may be specific illnesses, called *occupational diseases*, that are associated with your type of job. You should never be complacent about wearing any protective clothing that is provided and observing safety regulations precisely, because occupational diseases and industrial accidents affect thousands of people each year. Around the home hygiene is very important, especially when there are children in the house, and it is sensible to teach children the habits and routines of hygiene at an early age. Disease can often be contracted from food that has indirectly been contaminated by *faeces*, while in the kitchen an awareness of the shelf-life of foods and careful hygiene is most important. Most people know that flies carry germs, but it is also important to be careful with your pets. Children can catch *worms* from dog faeces, while adults can catch a disease called *psittacosis* from caged birds that may be fatal if untreated. Of course it is important for both you and your children to keep well away from anyone suffering from an infectious disease – unless of course you decide that it would be sensible for your child to catch *German measles*, for example, and so 'get it over with'.

If you follow the simple rules relating to diet, exercise, abuses of the body, stress and safeguards against disease that have been described above, you will reduce, but not unfortunately eliminate, the chances of illness. You will, however, most probably feel a great deal better for their observance. If you do think that you have contracted a disease, or you have psychological or physical problems, self-help and preventitive medicine must be temporarily forgotten. It is time for professional medicine to take over, and you should see a doctor.

Glossary of medical terms and symptoms

Numbers in italics after headings in this
glossary indicate page references in the
Guide to Ailments

THE PURPOSE OF THIS SECTION of the book is to cut through some of the mystique surrounding medicine by explaining the meaning and implications of the medical words and symptoms that can be so confusing. You will often find that a word that means something quite specific in everyday life means something very different when used in a medical context. Medicine has a language all of its own, and to learn how your body works and what goes wrong with it you will need a phrase book.

This glossary does not set out to be complete – 500 pages of text would still not cover every medical term and its usage – but for further information you are referred where appropriate to the Guide to Ailments that is the core of the book. Similarly, only the main causes for any particular symptom are listed.

As you will have seen in the previous section, You and Your Doctor, no one symptom indicates a specific disease. A doctor reaches a diagnosis by relating every symptom to a whole range of other factors and observations. For this reason you should never attempt self-diagnosis. You will rarely be right, and more often dangerously wrong.

If any symptom is causing severe pain you should see a doctor immediately; if a minor problem is persistent you should also see a doctor as soon as possible. Most important of all, always see a doctor when you are worried about your condition or in doubt about it.

A QUICK GUIDE TO MEDICAL TERMS

A large number of medical terms are derived from Latin and Greek. If you know the meaning of the Latin and Greek components, it will become easy to interpret many medical terms that at first sight seem complex. A selection is listed below. The position of the hyphen shows whether the component is placed at the beginning or the end of the term. In the United States the 'a' has been dropped from 'aemia' and 'haem'.

a-, an-: a lack of, an absence of
ab-: away from
ad-: towards, near to
-aemia: of the blood
andr-: of the male sex
anti-: against, opposing
-arch-, -arche-: first
arthr-: of a joint
audio-: of hearing, or sound
aut-, auto-: self
bi-: two
brady-: slowness
-cele: a swelling
-centesis: perforation
chron-: time
-cide: destroyer
contra-: against, opposite
cryo-: cold
-cyte: a cell
de-: removal, or loss
derm-: of the skin
dipl-: double
dys-: difficulty, abnormality
ec-, ect-: outside, external
-ectomy: surgical removal
em-, en-: inside, internal
end-: inner, within
enter-: of the intestine
epi-: upon, over
erythr-: red
ex-, exo-: outside of, outer
extra-: outside, beyond
fibr-: of fibrous tissue
-genic: producing
-gram: record, trace
-graph: a device that records
haem-: of the blood

hepat-: of the liver
hetero-: dissimilar
homeo-: alike
hydr-: of water, or fluid
hyp-, hypo-: deficiency in, lack of
hyper-: excess of
-iasis: a disease state
inter-: between
intra-: inside
-itis: inflammation
laparo-: of the abdomen or loins
leuc-, leuk-: white
-lysis: breaking up
macro-: large
mal-: disorder, abnormality
-mania: compulsion, obsession
mast-: of the breast
megal-: abnormally large
-megaly: abnormal enlargement
mes-: middle
met-, meta-: a) change, e.g. metabolism; b) distant, e.g. metastasis
micro-: small
myo-, my-: of the muscles
myelo-: of the spine
nephr-: of the kidneys
neur-: of the nerves
-oma: a tumor
-osis: a disease state
ost-: of bone
-otomy: a surgical examination
pan-: all
para-: a) near, e.g. paramedian; b) like, e.g. paratyphoid; c) abnormal, e.g. paraesthesia
path-: of disease

-pathy: disease
-penia: deficiency
peri-: near, around
-philia: craving, love for
phleb-: of the veins
-plasia: formation
-plegia: paralysis
pneo-: of respiration
-poiesis: formation
poly-: many
pre-: a) before, e.g. prenatal; b) in front of, e.g. prevertebral
pro-: before, in front of
proct-: of the anus and rectum
rhin-: of the nose
-stasis: standing still
sub-: below
tox-: poisonous
trans-: through, across
-trophy: growth, development
vas-: a vessel

ABDOMINAL PAIN 52,92

The abdomen houses a number of important organs, so abdominal pain can have many different causes and characteristics. It is generally divided into:

Colicky pain – a sharp, severe spasmodic pain that comes and goes. It is usually caused by the gut twisting and contracting, and when followed by *diarrhoea* may be due to *enteritis*.

Indigestion pain – typically comes on after food and is felt high up in the abdomen. It may be accompanied by *heartburn* or *waterbrash*.

Renal and *gallstone* colic – probably the most severe pain ever felt in the abdomen. It is agonizing in intensity. It is a colicky pain that comes on intermittently. Renal colic may be accompanied by *haematuria*, or blood in the urine.

Appendicitis – usually causes abdominal pain. At first this is felt around the navel and is accompanied by fever and vomiting. It then moves to the lower right.

Urinary tract infections and *cystitis* may be felt as pain above the pubic bone at the front of the *pelvis*, along with a characteristic pain on passing urine.

In children *tonsillitis* and ear infections may manifest themselves as abdominal pain.

Severe lower abdominal pain and tenderness may also be caused by *salpingitis*, an inflammation of the *Fallopian tubes*.

ABDOMINAL SWELLING 43,50

A swelling in the abdomen may be general or confined to one area; it is sometimes difficult to tell the difference if the person is fat, or the swelling is very large.

A general enlargement, associated with a bloated feeling, may be due to swallowed air. It can be aggravated by *constipation*. Another common cause is *obesity*, which, surprisingly enough, often goes unrecognized. When the enlargement is accompanied by pain and illness it can be caused by an obstruction of the *intestine*, or by *ascites* – the accumulation of fluid in the *peritoneal cavity* that indicates *cirrhosis* of the liver, chronic

peritonitis, *kidney disease* or *heart failure*.

A localized swelling in the upper right of the abdomen may be due to an enlarged *liver* – indicating alcoholic disease, *heart failure* or *cancer* secondaries, or be due to a swollen *gall bladder*. In the lower region of the abdomen, localized swelling may be caused by *gas* in in the intestines, *fibroid* or other cancer secondaries – or be due to a *cyst*. A full *bladder*, probably in a man of middle age or more with *prostate* trouble also produces a lower abdominal swelling. In women the earlier stages of pregnancy cause a local swelling. Sometimes a loop of intestine bulges through the abdominal wall, and is called a *hernia*, though this is much more common in men. Swollen *kidneys* from *polycystic disease* or *hydronephrosis* can also be felt in thin people.

ABORTION 146

Spontaneous abortion, or miscarriage, is the undesired expulsion of the *foetus* from the body, normally before the 28th week of pregnancy. After 28 weeks the foetus is considered a separate entity from the mother for legal purposes and the miscarriage is called a *still birth*. It may be caused by drugs, severe illness, *diabetes*, physical or emotional *shock* or by a fault in the foetus. Occasionally the abortion can be caused by a physical problem such as a weak neck of the *womb*, which can be treated surgically in subsequent pregnancies. Once the foetus is dead abortion is inevitable, but may sometimes be incomplete when part of the *placenta* is retained in the womb.

Induced abortion carries little risk during the early part of pregnancy, though complications become more likely after the 12th week.

ABSCESS

A local accumulation of *pus* in the body can create an abscess that is treated by the surgical removal of pus or with *antibiotics*. An abscess can be formed in almost any body tissue, but two of the most common types are a skin abscess, or *boil*, and a tooth abscess.

ACIDOSIS 146

A disturbance of the acid-base balance of the body in which the acidity of the body's fluids and tissues is

increased. Acidosis is characterized by sickness, drowsiness and an increase in the rate of breathing; acetone can sometimes be smelt on the breath. The condition is caused by *metabolic diseases*, *kidney failure*, *diabetes mellitus*, or an increase in the amount of *carbon dioxide* retained in the body.

ACID REGURGITATION 45

The rising into the mouth of sour, burning fluid, often associated with *heartburn*. Acid regurgitation may occur in association with *dyspepsia*, pregnancy, *abdominal swelling* or a *peptic ulcer*. In itself it is of no significance.

ACNE 160

Acne vulgaris, or adolescent spots, can cause enormous distress to the sufferer. During adolescence *hormonal* changes in the blood stimulate the production of a skin lubricant called sebum. This can get trapped by the growth of the top layer of skin to form a sebum plug called a comedone or blackhead. The skin becomes inflamed as a reaction to the presence of this plug and the result is a mixture of blackheads and red and purplish spots of all sizes, which can cover the face, neck, back and chest. The condition, which affects boys and girls equally, usually clears up on its own, but some improvement can be obtained by frequent washing and the use of proprietary preparations.

Acne rosacea is a skin disease of the face. It starts with a flushing of the cheeks and nose after meals, hot drinks or alcohol. Gradually the flush can become permanent, with a visible *dilation* of the blood vessels and an enlargement of the nose and cheeks. It is sometimes seen during the *menopause* and with those who have a fondness for hot drinks or alcohol. Though ugly, the condition is not dangerous.

ACROMEGALY

A disease in which overproduction of growth *hormone* by the *pituitary gland* leads to an increase in the size of the hands, face and feet. It is treated by *x-ray* therapy or by surgery.

ACUPUNCTURE

A centuries-old method of treatment and *anaesthesia* in the Far East, acupuncture is now being seriously investigated by Western doctors.

Needles are placed in selected positions beneath the skin and then either rotated or used to apply a weak electric current. It is not certain how the method works, but it can be used to relieve symptoms in the hands of a practised operator. In China acupuncture has become accepted as an alternative to conventional anaesthetics during major surgery.

ACUTE

In medicine, acute does not simply mean severe. It refers to a sharp, severe pain or condition which has a rapid onset and a short course – see chronic.

ADDISON'S DISEASE

A condition caused by inadequate hormone production on the part of the adrenal glands which is characterized by a dark pigmentation of the skin, weakness, lethargy and low blood pressure. At one time this disease was fatal, but it can now be cured by the replacement of the under-produced hormones.

ADENOIDS

Otherwise called pharyngeal tonsils, the adenoids are a mass of lymphatic tissue situated at the back of the nose. Most commonly during childhood or early adolescence, infections of the throat may cause inflammation of the adenoids and make it difficult to breathe through the nose. The tissue is often removed surgically at the same time as the tonsils, in a simple operation called an adenoidectomy.

ADENOMA

A tumor of the epithelium, or lining, of a gland or glandular tissue. Normally it is benign, but can turn into a malignant tumor called an adenocarcinoma which requires surgical treatment or X-ray therapy.

ADIPOSE TISSUE

Fibrous tissue that is packed with common fat. It forms a thick layer under the skin, which tends to be more pronounced in women than in men. Adipose tissue not only acts as an insulating agent but also as an energy store. Too much of it may be a danger to health – see obesity.

ADRENAL GLANDS

The triangular adrenal glands sit like caps on the tops of the right and left kidneys. Under the control of the pituitary gland the adrenal glands produce hormones that regulate salt and water metabolism and the powerful corticosteroids. Another part of each gland produces the hormones adrenaline (in the US epinephrine) and nor-adrenaline (in the US nor-epinephrine).

ADRENALINE (US – Epinephrine)

Adrenaline, produced by the adrenal glands, is commonly known as the 'fright, flight or fight' hormone. It increases the rate of the heartbeat, speeds up the rate and depth of breathing, reduces the blood supply to the intestines so that more blood can flow to the muscles, constricts the anal sphincter and increases the force of muscular contraction generally. In other words the whole body is ready for immediate physical or mental exertion.

AFTER-BIRTH – see PLACENTA

AGORAPHOBIA   130

A condition in which the sufferer has a pathological fear of open spaces.

A.I.D. – see ARTIFICIAL INSEMINATION

A.I.H. – see ARTIFICIAL INSEMINATION

ALCOHOLISM   132

Excessive, persisent consumption of alcoholic drinks of any kind – from the mildest beer to whisky – can lead to alcoholism. It is a physical as well as psychological addiction which causes physical, mental and social damage and may well include loss of employment, friends and money, or family disruption. The quantity of alcohol which seems harmless to one person may have devastating effects on another; women in particular are less able to cope physically with large quantities of drink. The cure is complete abstinence from alcohol, and this can only be achieved if one first admits that one is alcoholic and then seeks help. A number of social agencies have been set up to cope with this problem.

ALIMENTARY TRACT   32

The whole stretch of the digestive tract between the mouth and anus is known as the alimentary tract or canal. It consists of the mouth, the oesophagus, the stomach, the duodenum, the small intestine, the large intestine and the anus. It is also called the Gastro-intestinal Tract (G.I. Tract).

ALKALOSIS

A disturbance of the acid-base balance of the body in which the alkalinity of the body's tissues and fluids is increased. Alkalosis is characterized by apathy, irritability, delirium, dehydration and sometimes tetany. The condition can be caused by loss of acid by vomiting, or the overuse of antacids.

ALLERGEN

An allergen is an antigen that causes an allergy in a person sensitive to it. There are many different types of allergen, among them pollens, dust, house mites, fur, feathers, dyes, cosmetics, drugs, chemicals and food. When the specific allergen has been identified by tests it is possible in some cases to desensitize the person affected and so to reduce the scale of any allergic reaction.

ALLERGY   21,30

A condition in which the body becomes so sensitive to an antigen, or allergen, that an allergic reaction is caused. The allergen reacts with the body's own antibodies to produce histamine and serotonin, causing inflammation and symptoms specific to each allergy. These symptoms can range from hay fever and asthma to very serious shock.

ALOPECIA

The medical term for loss of hair, or baldness. In alopecia areata, hair falls out in small patches – the cause of this condition is unknown; alopecia totalis is a condition in which all body hair, including eyebrows and eyelashes, is lost. Alopecia can be due to serious illness, certain poisons, hormonal disorders, skin disease or age. The term alopecia is also used to cover natural hereditary male baldness.

ALVEOLUS

A tiny sac, in the lungs at the end of the respiratory tract, the alveolus is the site of the exchange of oxygen and carbon dioxide between the blood capillaries and the air.

AMENORRHOEA   100,136,138

The absence of menstrual periods. Amenorrhoea is normal before puberty, during pregnancy and suckling, and after the *menopause*. Sometimes periods fail to start after puberty as a result of a *congenital* defect, but if they stop after that the cause can range from *hormone* deficiency or brain damage to *depression* or *anorexia nervosa*.

AMNESIA
A loss of memory that can be partial or total and may even involve the sufferer not knowing who he is. Amnesia may follow physical injury, disease, drug usage or psychological *trauma*.

AMNIOCENTESIS
A test, that can be used to detect a number of *foetal* disorders, including *spina bifida*. A small sample is taken from the fluid that surrounds the foetus inside its membraneous amniotic sac. It is taken with a syringe, under local *anaesthesia*, before the 16th week of *pregnancy*.

AMOEBIC DYSENTERY – see DYSENTERY

ANAEMIA (US – Anemia) 100,162
A condition in which the *oxygen*-carrying potential of the blood is reduced through a lack of the pigment *haemoglobin*, characterized by tiredness, pallor, poor resistance to infection and breathlessness on exertion. Anaemia may be caused by an underproduction of *haemoglobin* in the body, as in pernicious anaemia where *Vitamin B*^{12} is lacking, or in iron-deficiency anaemia, where iron is lacking. Both are vital for the manufacture of haemoglobin. In *leukaemia* the production of red *blood cells* in the *bone marrow* is inhibited, causing anaemia. Other causes of anaemia are an abnormality in the haemoglobin, called sickle-cell anaemia, an abnormality in the red blood cells, called spherocytosis, and an abnormally large loss of blood, as in *haemorrhoids*, an *ulcer* or excessive *menstrual* bleeding.

ANAESTHESIA (US – Anesthesia)
Strictly anaesthesia is a loss of sensation in the body. More generally the term is applied to the deliberate deadening of sensation in the body to allow medical or surgical procedures to be carried out without the patient feeling any pain. Anaesthesia is said to be general when it involves the whole body and the patient is unconscious, and local

when only one area of the body is affected.

ANAESTHETIC (US – Anesthetic)
An agent that produces *anaesthesia* in a part or the whole of the body. A general anaesthetic is normally a barbiturate drug that produces unconsciousness. The state is then maintained by anaesthetic gases. Local anaesthesia is obtained by an injection of lignocaine or other cocaine derivatives. The use of anaesthetics has become much more sophisticated in the last decade.

ANAL
The adjective meaning 'of the anus', as in 'anal *sphincter*', but also used to denote a pattern of behavior. A person with an anal character is one who is excessively tidy, mean and obstinate and who behaves in an obsessive or compulsive way.

ANALGESIA
A reduced sensitivity to pain – in fact the correct, though little used term for local *anaesthesia*. The condition is induced by pain-killing drugs called analgesics, which can vary in strength from aspirin to morphine.

ANDROGEN
The *hormones* that stimulate the development of male sexual characteristics such as muscle mass, beard growth and the deepening of the voice. Androgens are produced by the *testes* and in small quantities by the *adrenal glands* and the *ovaries*. Too much androgen in women causes masculinization or *virilism*, while too little in men causes a lessening of male sexual characteristics. Synthetic androgens are given to alleviate this – see *testosterone*.

ANEMIA – see ANAEMIA

ANESTHESIA – see ANAESTHESIA

ANESTHETIC – see ANAESTHETIC

ANEURYSM 80,84,94
A localized swelling of the wall of an artery, which may be due to a disease process, as in *syphilis*, a *degenerative disease* like *atherosclerosis* or to a *congenital* defect in the arterial wall. Most congenital aneurysms are found in the brain,

where there is a danger that they will burst and cause a cerebral *haemorrhage*, but the most common aneurysms are *aortic* or *ventricular*. An aortic aneurysm affects the aorta, or main artery of the body. A degenerative disease weakens the muscular lining of the aorta, allowing the blood to force the wall out in a balloon-like swelling. The aneurysm may burst, or alternatively kill nearby tissues by squashing the blood vessels that supply them. A ventricular aneurysm may form in the left ventricle of the heart around the weakened heart muscle left by a *heart attack*, and may lead to heart failure. Surgical treatment is needed for both types of aneurysm.

ANGINA PECTORIS 82
A severe and constricting pain in the centre of the chest which may spread to the shoulders and jaws and down the left arm. The pain, which is often described as the feeling that someone is sitting on the chest, normally starts on exercise and is relieved by rest. It occurs when the heart needs more blood because of an increase in the demands on it, but cannot obtain the blood due to obstruction or disease of the *coronary arteries*. It is one of the warning signs that a *heart attack* may be imminent.

ANGIOGRAPHY 80
The *X-ray* examination of blood vessels. A special dye that shows up on X-rays is injected into the vessels of the system to be investigated and a series of X-ray pictures taken. The progress of the dye through the system can be seen and the size and shape of the vessels judged. The technique can show up obstructions of the blood vessels and so monitor the progress of *degenerative diseases* of the circulation like *atherosclerosis*. Angiocardiography, where the technique is used on the chambers of the heart and the *coronary arteries* can give important information to the heart surgeon before he operates. The *X-ray* films produced are called angiograms.

ANKYLOSIS 112
A *joint* is said to be ankylosed when the bones of the joint are attached to each other, either by bone or fibrous tissue, and become immobile. The condition can be *congenital* or may be the result of an inflammatory disease which has affected the joint

over a long period. Ankylosing spondylitis immobilizes the joints of the backbone; in the United States the term is taken to mean *rheumatoid arthritis* of the spine, whereas in Britain it refers to a spinal disease whose cause is not known.

ANOREXIA   136
A loss of appetite. When the condition cannot be explained by local disease it is called anorexia nervosa. This is a psychological illness that is most often found in female adolescents. It often starts with a simple desire to lose weight. Soon eating becomes abhorrent and loss of weight can lead to starvation and even death. The underlying causes of anorexia nervosa are complex, but often include family problems and a rejection of adult sexuality. Associated symptoms are irritability, melancholia, lethargy, *hysteria* and a completely unrealistic image of the size of the sufferer's body. Treatment is normally by psychiatric therapy.

ANTACIDS   45
Drugs that neutralize the acidic digestive juices of the stomach. Antacids are commonly used to relieve the discomfort and pain of indigestion and *peptic* ulcers.

ANTIBIOTICS
A group of drugs, either natural or synthetic, which are derived from microorganisms and destroy other microorganisms. Specific antibiotics are used to treat infections caused by *bacteria* or *fungi*. Less specific, or broad-spectrum, antibiotics destroy a wide range of microorganisms; they may, in fact, destroy the essential organisms in the intestines and other organs. Though antibiotics are of enormous importance in the treatment of all bacterial and fungal infections, the body becomes resistant to them after a while, so they are rarely given for minor infections which will clear up of their own accord.

ANTIBODY
A *protein* substance developed by the body as a defence against any *antigen* that is present in the circulation. Antibodies attack the antigens in the blood stream and destroy them. They can be passed from mother to baby and also be induced by *vaccination*, or *immunization*,

thus giving *immunity* against some diseases. Antibodies also react to specific antigens called *allergens* to give an *allergic* reaction.

ANTICOAGULANT
An agent which delays or prevents the clotting of blood. Anticoagulants are used to break up blood clots in the body or in blood vessels when *thrombosis* or an *embolism* are diagnosed. Heparin is a natural anticoagulant found in the blood, but synthetic drugs are also used.

ANTICONVULSANT
A drug that prevents or reduces the severity of convulsions, especially in *epilepsy*.

ANTIDEPRESSANT
A drug used to moderate the symptoms of depression.

ANTI-EMETIC
A drug that prevents vomiting.

ANTIGEN
Any substance that causes the production of *antibodies* when recognized by the body as foreign or dangerous.

ANTIHISTAMINE
A drug used to counteract the effects of histamine, usually in *allergy*. Antihistamines are sometimes used as sleeping pills, because one of their side effects is drowsiness.

ANTISEPTIC
A chemical that prevents the growth or arrests the development of *bacteria* and other microorganisms, but does not harm the skin and *mucous membranes* – see *sepsis*.

ANURIA
Literally a lack of urine, anuria implies either *kidney failure* or an obstruction in the *ureter*. The former is extremely serious and the patient may need *dialysis*; the latter is relatively easily remedied.

ANXIETY   130,153
A sense of dread, fear and distress over a threat to the things that one holds dear. Low levels of anxiety, over a real but minor threat, are actually beneficial and normal; they stimulate the body to action. Sometimes anxiety becomes acute, extremely unpleasant and all-pervading. This condition is called an anxiety state, or anxiety *neurosis*,

and produces physical as well as mental symptoms – a rapid, pounding heart-beat, trembling, dry mouth, a frequent desire to pass water or faeces, nausea and tension. Occasionally a condition that appears to be anxiety state is actually a sympton of an organic disease such as *thyrotoxicosis* and is treated as such. More usually the problem is psychological.

AORTA
The main artery of the body, which starts in the left *ventricle* of the heart and runs down the body in front of the spine to end in the iliac arteries that supply most of the blood to the *pelvis* and lower limbs. Throughout its length, small and large arteries branch off from the aorta to supply the rest of the body.

APHASIA
The inability to express oneself through speech and sometimes to understand the meaning of words. It is usually caused by disease in the speech areas of the brain or by a *cerebrovascular accident* (C.V.A.).

APPENDICITIS   52
An acute inflammation of the *appendix*. The first signs of appendicitis are usually a severe pain in the center of the abdomen, fever and vomiting. Later the pain moves to the lower right-hand side of the abdomen, and the area is extremely tender to the touch. The inflamed appendix is removed in a simple operation called an appendicectomy, because if it is allowed to burst *peritonitis* can result.

APPENDIX   52
A small worm-like appendage to the large intestine which has no known function, but may become inflamed – see *appendicitis*.

APPETITE   45,136,138,153
The desire to eat food. Appetite may be increased or decreased by a number of conditions and factors. There is no such thing as a 'normal' appetite; this depends on the type of person, his build, his *metabolism* and his work. A building labourer, for example, will generally need many more *calories*, and therefore much more food, than a clerk.

At certain stages during life a large appetite is normal. During pregnancy women eat more than usual, and so does a child during peak periods of growth. The child's appetite may fall off dramatically after a spurt of growth, or sometimes as an expression of independence that soon passes. Appetite can also increase as a result of a disease such as *thyrotoxicosis*, where metabolism is raised, or to relieve the pain and discomfort of *ulcers* and *dyspepsia*. Psychological reasons often play their part in creating a large appetite; sometimes young girls eat out of *hysteria*, while excessive amounts of food are frequently eaten as a comfort or consolation. Worms are thought by many to be the cause of a large appetite, but are rarely found in the western world.

The taste buds are normally affected in fevers or a cold, and the result is commonly a loss of appetite. The desire to eat may also be lost as a result of more serious disorders of the *stomach*, *heart* and *liver*, and also for psychological reasons, including fright, *shock*, *depression*, *hysteria*, psychosis and *anorexia* nervosa.

ARRHYTHMIA
An irregularity of the rhythm of the heart.

Normally the beat of the heart is controlled by a natural *pacemaker*, called the sino-atrial node, initiating electrical impulses. If these impulses are disturbed, either in their initiation or during their passage through the heart tissue, the pattern of heart muscle contraction will alter. A slow heartbeat is called a *bradycardia*; a fast heartbeat a *tachycardia*. Probably the most common arrhythmia is atrial *fibrillation*. Most arrhythmias can be treated with drugs but sometimes an artificial pacemaker is needed.

ARTERIOSCLEROSIS   80
A thickening of the arteries that is one of the natural consequences of the ageing process. The causes are still obscure, but are thought to include high *blood pressure*, *diabetes* and a family disposition to the condition. The term is often used loosely as an alternative to *atherosclerosis*.

ARTERITIS
A disease in which the walls of the arteries become inflamed and swollen. It may be the result of an *infection* or of a disease of the *connective tissue*.

ARTERY
A blood vessel carrying oxygenated blood under pressure from the heart to the organs and tissues of the body. The exception to this rule is the pulmonary artery, which carries deoxygenated blood from the heart to the lungs.

ARTHRITIS   112
The inflammation of a joint, causing swelling, redness of the skin over it, pain, immobilization and a sensation of heat inside the joint. Arthritis can be caused by a large number of diseases and infections, including diseases of the *nervous system*, *degenerative* and *metabolic* diseases. Rheumatoid arthritis, whose cause is not known, is probably the most serious form of arthritis and can lead to crippling deformity, while osteo-arthritis, where bone can overgrow the joint, is perhaps the most common form. There is no cure for arthritis as such, though the condition may clear up for a time on its own. Simple *analgesics* like aspirin may be used to counter the inflammation and relieve pain.

ARTHROPLASTY
An operation in which a diseased joint is surgically repaired, sometimes with the help of an artificial replacement for a badly damaged part.

ARTIFICIAL INSEMINATION
The introduction by another agent of male *semen* into the female *womb* in order for conception to take place. When the husband's semen is used, the procedure is called artificial insemination husband, or A.I.H.; when the husband is sterile the semen of an anonymous donor may be used. This method is known as artificial insemination donor, or A.I.D., and is only undertaken after lengthy *counselling*.

ASCITES
A collection of fluid in the abdomen which leads to *abdominal swelling* and may cause shortness of breath. Ascites can be caused by *liver* or *kidney* disease, *heart failure*, chronic *peritonitis*, or by various *cancers*.

ASPHYXIA
An increase in the amount of *carbon dioxide* in the body and a decrease in the level of *oxygen* as a result of an obstruction of the *respiratory* system, as in drowning, suffocation or poisoning by gases. If breathing does not resume very quickly, the victim will become *cyanosed* and the heart will stop beating. Brain damage will occur if the cells of the brain are not given oxygen within about four minutes, so prompt treatment, which may involve artificial respiration, is essential.

ASTHMA   21
A condition characterized by intermittent bouts of wheezing, with the sufferer snatching for air, in which the *bronchi*, or passages of the lungs, become so narrowed that it is almost impossible to get air into them. An attack may be caused by an *allergy*, exercise or worry. In between attacks a sufferer often breathes normally.

ASTIGMATISM
A disorder of vision whereby the image of an object becomes distorted.

Astigmatism can easily be corrected by the use of glasses whose lenses, which are usually thick and cylindrical, produce a distortion that cancels out the existing defect.

ATHEROMA   64
The thickening of the walls of the arteries by deposits of fatty substances, such as *cholesterol*. Eventually the arteries may be blocked by the deposits and a *heart attack* or *stroke* may result. The condition is linked to *obesity*, cigarette smoking, a diet rich in animal fats and a lack of exercise.

ATHEROSCLEROSIS   80
A disease in which *atheroma* occurs, which may be caused by a defect of fat *metabolism*.

ATHLETE'S FOOT – *see* TINEA PEDIS

ATRIUM
The two upper chambers of the heart are called the right and left atria. The right atrium receives deoxygenated blood from the body, and communicates with the right *ventricle*; the left atrium receives oxygenated blood from the lungs and passes it to the left ventricle. When the atria contract irregularly and spasmodically the condition is called atrial *fibrillation*.

ATROPHY
The wasting away of a part of the body. Atrophy is usually caused by an inadequate nutritional supply to it, or by diseases that affect the muscles and nerves.

AURA
A set of symptoms or feelings which precede physical or mental disorders. Different aura can be specific to different conditions, yet vary from patient to patient.

AUSCULTATION
An investigation in which the doctor listens to the sounds made by the organs of the body – mainly the heart, lungs and intestines – to try to detect any abnormalities in their function. The movement of fluid or gas within the body can also be heard.

AUTOIMMUNE DISEASE 112,162
A disease in which the body is unable to distinguish between foreign substances and substances produced by itself. As a result *antibodies* are produced which destroy normal parts of the body. A number of conditions are now thought to be autoimmune diseases – among them several types of *anaemia*, rheumatoid *arthritis*, *myasthenia gravis* and *glomerulonephritis*.

AUTONOMIC NERVOUS SYSTEM – *see* NERVOUS SYSTEM

AVERSION THERAPY
A treatment in which an unpleasant stimulus is paired, and therefore associated in the mind, with an act of behavior that is considered undesirable for social or medical reasons.

B

BACILLUS
A type of *bacterium*

BACKACHE 45,100,114,138
A common complaint with a variety of causes, ranging from *depression* to *cancer*. The most common form of backache is a dull pain felt in the small of the back by people of any age. It is often worse in the morning and improves during the day. This ache is normally due to poor posture and is best treated by sleeping on your back on a hard surface. The

problem is that the spine is not really designed for upright posture; the weights and stresses which, in most other animals, are supported by four limbs are supported by two through the backbone. The spine is a major cause of back trouble and pain for this reason. Some of the more specific structural reasons for pain are a *slipped disc, kyphosis, scoliosis, laudosis, muscle spasms* and *muscle strains*.

Occasionally back pain is an indication of more serious disease. *Osteo-arthritis* is sometimes a cause of pain in the elderly as the spine shows signs of wear and tear, while *ankylosing* spondylitis also affects the back. Various cancers cause back pain at a late stage in the disease when *secondaries* reach the spine. A number of abdominal disorders may also lead to pain in the back such as *duodenal* ulcer or *dysmenorrhoea*.

BACTERIA
Microorganisms that reproduce by cell division, which are found in almost every kind of environment. Bacteria cause disease through the poisons that they excrete, though some are actually beneficial to man and are found in the intestines, the mouth and the *vagina*. They are destroyed by *antibodies, antibiotics* and the white *blood cells*.

BAD BREATH – *see* HALITOSIS

BALANITIS
An inflammation of the glans *penis*, often associated with *phimosis*, or tightness of the *foreskin*. Balanitis usually clears up after treatment with *antibiotics* but, if it recurs, then circumcision may be necessary. It is normally a condition of childhood.

BALDNESS – *see* ALOPECIA

BARIUM ENEMA 34,41
A similar investigation to a barium meal where barium is passed into the *rectum* under pressure. The technique is useful in the diagnosis of *diverticular disease* and *carcinoma* of the colon.

BARIUM MEAL 45,50
A technique by which x-rays can be taken of the *oesophagus, stomach*, small intestine and upper parts of the large bowel. The patient fasts overnight, and may have his

alimentary tract cleared with an aperient. He then swallows a beaker-full of a barium sulphate preparation. This substance is radio-opaque – in other words it shows up on x-rays – and the x-ray films that are taken can demonstrate the presence of *oesophageal strictures*, a *hiatus hernia, gastric* or *duodenal ulcers* and *tumors*.

BATTERED BABY SYNDROME
A syndrome that has gained increasing recognition over the last few years, in which injuries are inflicted on babies and infants by their parents. The parents normally act under considerable emotional, mental and environmental *stress*; they themselves often come from broken homes and an unstable family background. The injuries, which often go unsuspected by friends and neighbours, are sometimes extremely serious.

BEDSORE
An *ulcerated* and sometimes gangrenous area of skin which is due to continual pressure. Bedsores are seen in the bedridden and after the removal of a badly fitted plaster-cast or splint. They can be avoided if the patient's position is frequently changed and the skin kept clean and dry.

BEHAVIOR
The actions and reactions of a person to the circumstances of his environment and relationships. Behaviorists believe that psychological problems are best approached by treating the behavior patterns of a patient by means of a behavior therapy such as *aversion therapy*.

BELL'S PALSY – *see* PARALYSIS

BENIGN
A tumor or growth that is not progressive or *malignant* and rarely grows again if it is removed, is said to be benign.

BICUSPID VALVE – *see* MITRAL VALVE

BILE
A bitter, alkaline fluid that is produced in the *liver* and stored in the *gall bladder*. When fatty food is eaten, the gall bladder releases related quantities of bile which pass down the common bile duct to enter

the intestines just below the *stomach* at the *duodenum*. Bile acts like a detergent, breaking up globules of *fat* so that they can be more easily digested.

BILIARY COLIC – *see* GALL STONES

BILIOUS ATTACK
The term is normally used incorrectly to denote the unpleasant taste of *stomach* fluids in the mouth, as in *acid regurgitation* and *dyspepsia*, associated with *nausea* and *vomiting*. When vomiting is very severe small quantities of yellowy-green *bile* may be brought up, but this is rare.

BILIRUBIN
One of the components of *haemoglobin* which is excreted in the *bile* after the breakdown of red *blood cells* in the *liver*. Bilirubin is a yellow-orange pigment; when its blood level is increased by a malfunction of the liver or by *gall stones* the body may become yellow, or *jaundiced*.

BIRTHMARK
A mark on the skin that is present at birth. The skin is *pigmented*; sometimes the style of the pigmentation and the shape of the area affected is *hereditary* – see *naevus*.

BISEXUALITY
A condition in which a person has *chromosomes* and sometimes genitals which are neither fully male nor fully female (see *hermaphrodite*), or in which a person is sexually attracted to both males and females.

BLACKHEAD – *see* ACNE

BLADDER   96
A muscular expanding sac that acts as a reservoir for *urine*. The bladder receives urine from the *kidneys* through the *ureters*; when it becomes distended, urine is expelled through the *urethra*.
Frequent urination can be caused by many factors. In pregnancy the bulk of the *foetus* in the *womb* may press down on the bladder causing frequent urination; in elderly men an enlarged *prostate* gland may pinch the urethra just below the bladder and cause dribbling and difficulty in urination. Sometimes the bladder cannot release urine at all, normally when there is a fault in

the nerve supply to the *sphincter*. This is called *retention*, when *catheterization* may be necessary.

BLEPHARITIS
An inflammation of the eyelids. Blepharitis may be *ulcerative*, in which case the cause is a *bacterial* infection, or non-ulcerative. In the latter, the cause is often not known, but may be *allergy*, dust or irritant chemicals. Sometimes cosmetics can trigger an allergic reaction that leads to blepharitis. The condition may be relieved when the eyelids are bathed in salty water, but *antibiotic* ointment will probably be needed to clear it up completely.

BLISTER
A swelling just below the skin containing *serum* and caused by pressure, friction or a burn. When small blood vessels are ruptured, the swelling may fill with blood and is called a blood blister.

BLOOD
The fluid that flows through all the organs and tissues of the body. Blood is made up of a liquid called plasma, in which red *blood cells*, white blood cells, platelets and *fat* globules are suspended, as well as a huge variety of chemical substances. It has numerous functions: the nourishment and *oxygen* supply of cells; the transport of wastes such as *carbon dioxide*; the defence of the body against infection; and the control of the body's chemistry and heat. In order to do this the blood carries, apart from red and white cells and platelets, *hormones*, *electrolytes*, *antibodies* and *vitamins*.

BLOOD CELLS – *see* ERYTHROCYTES, LEUCOCYTES

BLOOD CLOTTING
The process, also called coagulation, by which *blood* becomes a solid mass and seals a wound. When blood is exposed to the air the platelets release an *enzyme* that helps to convert the *protein* fibrinogen, found in blood *plasma*, to insoluble fibrin. This forms a mesh over the wound in which blood cells are trapped. The production of fibrin is a very complex procedure, involving a number of other chemicals called clotting factors; the lack of one of these factors may cause a rare disease in which the blood will not clot – see *haemophilia*.

BLOOD CORPUSCLE – *see* ERYTHROCYTES, LEUCOCYTES

BLOOD COUNT
A blood test in which the number of red and white *blood cells* in a fixed volume of blood are counted. A blood count can show up any excess or deficiency in both types of cell and is often used in the investigation of diseases.

BLOOD GASES   10
The main blood gases are oxygen and carbon dioxide, though nitrogen is also found in the blood and excreted from the body in urine. Oxygen enters the blood from the air in the *alveoli* of the lungs in exchange for carbon dioxide; together with *haemoglobin* in the red *blood cells* it forms the substance oxyhaemoglobin, and is carried in this form to individual cells of the body where cellular *respiration* takes place. Carbon dioxide is produced as a waste product of chemical reactions at the cellular level and transported in the blood as a weak acid solution in the blood *serum*.
Normally, in arterial blood, oxygen has a 'partial pressure' of 75 to 100 mm of mercury, while carbon dioxide has a 'partial pressure' that is between 35 and 45 mm mercury. In disorders that affect the lungs, such as severe *asthma*, *bronchitis* and *emphysema*, these values may vary, and the amount by which they deviate from the norm is a good indicator of lung function and capability. The values are determined by a 'blood gases' investigation. A sample of blood is taken from an artery – normally the femoral artery in the groin or the radial artery in the wrist – and analysed immediately, so that the pressures of the blood gases cannot equilibrate with those of the atmosphere.

BLOOD GROUPS
A system of classification of blood types which is based on whether or not particular *antigens* are present on the red *blood cells*. There are over 30 blood group systems, but the ABO system is the most important. Here there are four possible blood groups – A, B, AB, and O. Blood group A has the A antigen, group B the B antigen, group AB both A and B antigens and group O neither A nor B antigens. Each group has an *antibody* in the plasma that corresponds to the antigen that

is missing from the red blood cells – so group A has antibody B, and group B has antibody A. If two types of blood are mixed and their antigens and antibodies clash a blood transfusion will be unsuccessful. Blood group AB is called the universal receiver as it has no A or B antibodies and can receive at a blood transfusion blood of any group; blood group O is called the universal donor because it has neither A nor B antigens and can be given to any blood group. Apart from their use in matching blood for transfusions, blood groups can be used to test paternity suits and for *genetic* studies because the presence or absence of the two antigens is *hereditary* – see *Rhesus factors*.

BLOOD PRESSURE 74

The pressure of the blood on the walls of the blood vessels. The highest and lowest pressures are called the systolic and diastolic pressures respectively. Systolic pressure is seen during *systole*, when the *ventricles* of the heart are contracting; diastolic pressure during *diastole*, when the ventricles are relaxing. By the use of the blood pressure cuff, or *sphygmomanometer*, these two pressures can be measured and expressed in millimeters of mercury. The values are written as a fraction, with the systolic pressure on top; the normal range for a young adult would be 120/80, though there can be a considerable variation in individuals. A consistent diastolic pressure over 100 mm or a systolic pressure over 140 mm of mercury would, however be considered abnormal, though pressures as high as 180/190 are sometimes seen, normally in old people. An increase in blood pressure may be due to physical effort, or to *stress* and emotional factors, and is called *hypertension*. An abnormally low blood pressure, called *hypotension*, may be caused by *shock* or circulation diseases.

BLOOD SERUM

The fluid left behind when clotted blood is allowed to stand. Serum is essentially the same as blood plasma, but does not contain fibrinogen or *blood clotting* agents.

BLOODSHOT EYE 124

The white of the eyes, or sclera, is supplied with blood by many tiny *capillaries*. Normally these cannot be seen, but when they become damaged or dilated, as after a severe fit of coughing, the eye may appear bloodshot. Sometimes the eye seems to be more pink than bloodshot. The cause of this is often *conjunctivitis*.

BLOOD TESTS 94,146,151,153

Blood tests are an important diagnostic tool. Blood may be taken from the body and analysed in order to provide diagnostic information or to confirm a diagnosis on many occasions. Among the most common blood tests are a blood *count*, a '*blood gases*' investigation, an E.S.R. and a *blood group* test. Otherwise the level of sugar in the blood may be tested – see *glucose*, *diabetes*; the blood *urea*, to assess *kidney* function; the blood analysed in liver function tests; *thyroid* function may be tested, to diagnose *thyrotoxicosis* and *myxoedema* and to monitor the treatment of these diseases; the *Wasserman Reaction* can detect *syphilis*; the presence of *Rubella antibodies* in the blood show whether a woman has had German measles; tests can be carried out for sickle cell *anaemia*, or for specific *enzymes* that are found in the blood after a *myocardial infarct*; blood levels of substances such as *calcium*, *cholesterol* and fats can be monitored; *blood clotting* disorders can be investigated, as can *hepatitis* and many other conditions.

Blood is taken from the body by venepuncture or venesection. In the former a vein is punctured by a syringe and blood drawn off; in venesection the vein may be opened surgically. Samples of blood may be obtained from special parts of the body, for example the chambers of the heart, by *catheterization*.

BODY ODOUR

During adolescence the hormonal changes in the body may affect the sweat glands so that a distinctive body odour develops. Though the problem normally passes away within a few years it can be very distressing for the sufferer. The only treatment is scrupulous cleanliness, the use of an *antiseptic* lotion in the bath and proprietory deodorants.

BOIL

Sometimes called a feruncle by doctors, a boil is an *abscess* in the skin. Pus collects when *bacteria* invade the skin through a cut or a hair follicle, and the resulting boil usually responds to treatment with *antibiotics* – though it is often necessary to release the pus by opening the boil with a scalpel.

BONE 108

A form of dense, hard connective tissue that makes up the *skeleton* of the body. It consists of a matrix of fibers impregnated with calcium salts in which bone cells called osteocytes are embedded.

BONE MARROW

The soft tissue in the hollow of bones. Marrow plays an important part in the formation of *blood cells*, though in later life the specialized tissue that produces the cells is replaced by *fat*. If some blood diseases are suspected a sample of bone marrow may be taken, either from the breastbone or hip, with a long needle, and analysis of the tissue can give important diagnostic clues.

BOTULISM

A severe form of food poisoning caused by the toxins produced by the *bacterium* Clostridium botulinum. The poison is destroyed by heat, so is normally only found in raw or badly preserved foods. Botulism attacks the *nervous system* and can be fatal.

BOW LEGS 112

An outward curve of the thighs, a gap at the knees and an inward curve of the calves. Bow legs are quite normal in small children, but when they persist can be caused by *arthritis* or abnormal bone growth. Surgical treatment may be necessary in extreme cases.

BRADYCARDIA

A slow heartbeat. Bradycardia is common, and quite normal, in trained athletes, where the heartbeat may be well below 60 beats per minute; it may also be caused by specific drug therapies. A slow and irregular heartbeat may be due to heart block – a condition in which the impulses from the sino-atrial node, the natural *pacemaker* of the heart, are not properly conducted to the heart muscle; it may also be seen when the pressure inside the skull is raised, by, for example, an expanding brain tumor. Bradycardia is an *arrhythmia*, and the opposite of *tachycardia*.

BRAIN 58
A large mass of nervous tissue that lies within the skull. It is composed of grey and white matter. The grey matter consists of nerve cells, the white matter of extended nerve cells that connect the different parts of the brain. The brain controls and regulates all the activities of the body and is the seat of consciousness, subconsciousness, memory, emotion and reason. It floats in *cerebrospinal* fluid and is contained within three membranes called the *meninges*; there are a number of cavities within the structure of the brain known as *ventricles*.

BREAST CANCER 104
A tumor of the breast which is the commonest form of *cancer* in women. The first sign is a small lump in the breast or the armpit which may easily remain unnoticed unless the breasts are examined regularly and systematically. Such a lump is by no means always a *malignant tumor*, but should always be investigated immediately. A breast tumor will normally be treated surgically, and sometimes a *mastectomy* may be necessary. If untreated the disease will spread through the *lymph* system to the *bones, lungs* and *liver* – see *cancer*.

BREATHLESSNESS – *see* DYSPNOEA

BREECH BIRTH
The presentation during *labour* of the baby buttocks first – as is seen in more than 3% of all births. Sometimes the baby is turned head-first before labour, otherwise it is manipulated during labour.

BRONCHIOLITIS
A *viral* or *bacterial* infection of the bronchioles, the very smallest *bronchi*, which become clogged by *mucus* and *pus* so that *oxygen* cannot be taken up in the *alveoli*. It may be necessary to give oxygen to relieve the problem, which then normally responds to *antibiotics*.

BRONCHITIS 19
An inflammation of the *mucous membranes* of the *bronchi* of the lungs that is more common in Britain than in any other country in the world. The first attack of bronchitis may be caused by a *viral* or *bacterial* infection which enlarges the lubricating glands of the bronchi,

inflames the bronchial membranes and fills the airways with mucus. The sufferer becomes breathless, wheezes and continually coughs up *phlegm*. After several attacks the tiny hairs that sweep debris away become permanently damaged and the inflammation becomes constant. The condition has now passed from *acute* to *chronic* bronchitis and large amounts of phlegm are coughed up each day. The bronchi contract spasmodically and can rarely be relaxed by *bronchodilators*. Bronchitis may lead to *emphysema* and can eventually be fatal. It is exacerbated by air pollution and cigarette smoking.

BRONCHODILATOR 19,21
A drug that relaxes the muscles of the walls of the *bronchi* and thereby opens up the airways of the lungs. Bronchodilators are commonly used in aerosol form to relieve *asthmatic* and *bronchitic* attacks.

BRONCHOSCOPE
An instrument used for the internal examination of the *bronchi*, and sometimes for tissue sampling. The use of *fiber-optics* in modern instruments has made the technique considerably more effective.

BRONCHOSPASM 19,21
A spasmodic contraction that narrows the walls of the *bronchi* in conditions such as *asthma* and *bronchitis*.

BRONCHUS 10
The airways of the lungs are all called bronchi after the *trachea*, or windpipe, branches into the main right bronchus and left bronchus – until the bronchi themselves branch into the smaller bronchioles. Bronchioles in their turn open into the *alveoli*.

BRUISE – *see* ECCHYMOSIS

BULIMIA NERVOSA (also GORGE-PURGE SYNDROME) 138
A recently described syndrome in which bouts of excessive overeating, or gorges, are followed by self-induced vomiting, or purging. The syndrome is seen in young women who have a tendency to weight problems and those suffering from *depression*. Some may over-eat to satisfy their depression and then induce vomiting to assuage guilt; others have found alternate gorging

and purging a method that allows them to lose weight yet continue eating normally. Unfortunately this behavior soon becomes *compulsive* and is ultimately ineffective; it may also cause social problems, while repeated vomiting leads to physical problems.

BUNION
An inflammation and swelling of the joint of the big toe. The *bursa* of the joint is often affected and the big toe may be pushed towards the other toes. Bunions are normally caused by badly fitting shoes. Though painful the condition does not usually merit medical treatment, but when the deformity and the pain are severe surgery may be necessary.

BURSA
A cavity in the fibrous tissue surrounding a joint. The bursa is lined with a synovial membrane and filled with *synovial fluid* which reduces friction and wear between the moving parts of the joint.

BURSITIS
An inflammation of a bursa, which may result from injury or an infection. The joint becomes tender and painful, and movement of the affected joint may be difficult. Treatment is normally by rest and immobilization, while painkillers and heat alleviate discomfort. Tennis elbow and 'housemaid's knees' are both common forms of bursitis.

C

CAESAREAN SECTION (US – Cesarean Section)
Reputedly the method by which Julius Caesar was born, caesarean section is a way of delivering a baby when a normal birth would be too dangerous. The baby is taken from the *uterus* in a surgical operation in which the abdominal wall is cut. The technique is used when either the *pelvic* girdle is too small or the baby too large, when *labour* does not start and cannot be induced, when labour is ineffective, or when the baby cannot be turned in a *breech birth*, or in *placenta praevia*.

CALCIFICATION
The deposit of *calcium* and calcium

salts in the tissues. Calcification occurs naturally during the process of bone development and growth, and also as a gradual process in old age, when *cartilage* and *connective tissue* may become bony. Calcium can be deposited in the walls of arteries and in joints in a number of diseases. Abnormal calcification is called calcinosis.

CALCIUM
A mineral present in the blood that is essential for the support of the body. As well as forming a major part of bones and teeth, calcium is important in many of the body's chemical reactions – so much so that when the level of calcium in the blood drops it is taken from bone to maintain the level. The mineral is found in many foods, but the main sources are dairy products, and *Vitamin D* is necessary for its absorption into the body. Calcium deficiency is marked by dental *caries*, brittle bones, heart problems, irritability and persistent bleeding and is particularly dangerous during pregnancy when more calcium than usual is needed to build up the *foetal* bones.

CALCULUS
A stone made up of mineral salts that is sometimes found in the kidneys or gall bladder – see *gall stones, kidney stones.*

CALLOSITY
A thickening and hardening of the skin that is usually caused by pressure and friction – see *corn.*

CALORIE
Strictly speaking, a calorie is a unit of heat. In medicine it is used to measure the energy value of foods – 1 calorie being the amount of energy needed to raise the temperature of a given volume of water from 14.5 to 15.5°C. The daily calorific requirement varies between 1200 and 4000, depending on age, sex, body weight, activity and pregnancy.

CANCER   26,41,56,104,106
A malignant tumor in which cells grow rapidly and uncontrollably. The tumor may start in any tissue or organ in the body and is generally called a carcinoma, though some tumors may have specific names. Cancer usually spreads, or metastasizes, to new areas of the body through the *lymph* system and the

blood. The first tumor is called a primary cancer; the following cancers are known as secondaries. Each tumor tends to form secondaries according to a specific pattern. The exact cause of cancer is not known and medical knowledge about the way a tumor develops and spreads is still incomplete. As yet there is no certain cure for the disease, but if a tumor is recognized early enough it can be treated successfully with *X-ray* therapy, drugs and surgery. See – *breast cancer, stomach cancer, cervical cancer, lung cancer.*

CANDIDIASIS
An infection that is usually caused by the fungus Candida Albicans. Candidiasis affects the skin and *mucous membranes* of the mouth, throat, lungs and *vagina.* When the vagina and mouth are affected the condition is commonly called *thrush,* and can be one of the side-effects of broad-spectrum antibiotics and the oral contraceptive pill. The condition normally responds to specific anti-fungal agents.

CAPILLARY
The smallest blood vessels of the body that form a network in tissue to link arterioles and venules and allow the exchange of oxygen, *carbon dioxide* and other chemicals between cells and the blood.

CARBOHYDRATE
A group of substances that contain only carbon, oxygen and hydrogen. Carbohydrates are one of the three main constituents of food (the others are *fat* and *protein*) and are broken down by the body to *glucose,* which can either be stored or used immediately to provide energy.

The main sources of carbohydrates in western society are bread and potatoes – see *metabolism.*

CARBON DIOXIDE – *see* BLOOD GASES

CARBUNCLE
A collection of *boils* under a single area of inflamed skin. A carbuncle may need to be lanced, but normally responds to *antibiotics.*

CARCINOGEN
A substance that may cause cancer. Cigarette smoke, for example, contains carcinogens.

CARCINOMA
A *malignant tumor;* the word is often used as a synonym for *cancer.*

CARDIAC ARREST – *see* MYOCARDIAL INFARCT

CARDIOVASCULAR SYSTEM   74
The circulation, consisting of the heart and the network of blood vessels.

The cardiovascular system is divided into the systemic and pulmonary circulations; the former is the web of veins and arteries that carries blood between the tissues and the heart – the latter the system that carries blood to and from the lungs.

CARIES
A condition in which bones and teeth decay and crumble away. Dental caries is commonly seen in western society, and is associated with poor dental hygiene and high levels of sugar in the diet. The condition can also be a symptom of a deficiency in *Vitamins D* and *C.*

CAROTID ARTERY
As the principal suppliers of blood to the head and neck the two carotid arteries rise up to the head on either side of the neck. The carotid *pulse* can be felt just below the point of the jaw on the right and left of the neck.

CARTILAGE
Dense *connective tissue* that forms part of the skeleton. Cartilage is found in the nose, the *larynx,* the ribs, between the vertebrae, and covers the moving surfaces of joints.

C.A.T (Computer Axial Tomography)
A recently developed diagnostic technique in which an image of the organs and tissues of the body can be obtained from any plane of the body that is desired. A horizontal plane can be chosen, for example, through the chest and the lungs and heart so that the various regions and organs can be seen in section.

CATARACT   122
A loss of transparency of the lens of the eye.

Initially vision becomes blurred, but eventually all sight in the eye that is affected will be lost. Vision can be restored by a relatively simple operation.

CATARRH
A general term used to indicate the over-production of mucus by the nose and *sinuses*, usually as a result of an inflammation of the *mucous membranes*.

CATATONIA   140
A type of abnormal behavior in which the sufferer either becomes violent without motive, repeats complicated actions over and over again and is overactive, or becomes totally unresponsive and inhibited, refuses to move or talk and remains in a stupor. Catatonia is normally associated with *schizophrenia* but can also be the result of other conditions, such as *hysteria*. Drugs can help in the short term, but *psychiatric therapy* and possibly *electroconvulsive therapy (E.C.T.)* may be necessary.

CATHETER
A tube that is passed into the body for the purpose of removing fluid, injecting fluids or examining the inside of an organ. Cardiac catheterization is used to give doctors information about the condition of the heart and the *coronary arteries* – a tube is placed in a blood vessel of the arm and fed through the vessels until it reaches the heart. Sometimes catheterization is necessary in problems of the urinary system, such as *retention*. A tube is passed through the *urethra* and into the *bladder*

CELIAC DISEASE – *see* COELIAC DISEASE

CELLULITIS
An inflammation of cellular and *connective tissue* that is caused by *bacteria*. The area affected can become coarse and puffy, but the condition is normally responsive to *antibiotics*.

CEREBRAL HAEMORRHAGE   64
A rupture of a blood vessel in the brain. A cerebral haemorrhage is normally caused by *degenerative disease* of the circulation and is associated with high *blood pressure*; it can result in a *stroke*, *coma*, death or just a passing dizziness, depending on the part of the brain that is affected.

CEREBRAL PALSY
A developmental defect of the brain that usually causes *spastic* paral-

ysis. Cerebral palsy can be congenital; sometimes it is caused by *virus* infections, *meningitis*, a lack of *oxygen* during pregnancy or by birth injuries. Treatment, which aims to improve the disability rather than cure it is by *physiotherapy*, speech therapy and special care.

CEREBRAL THROMBOSIS
An obstruction of one of the blood vessels of the brain by a blood clot, or *thrombus*, which may lead to a *stroke*.

CEREBRAL TUMOR
A term used to denote any mass in the brain. Sometimes the mass may be a *cyst*, an *abscess* or a *syphilitic gumma*; otherwise it is a *tumor*, or a growth of abnormal tissue that may be *benign*, or a *malignant carcinoma*. All cerebral tumors take up space normally occupied by brain cells, so either the pressure inside the skull is increased or brain cells are actually destroyed. Mental changes are often the result, with *epileptic convulsions*, giddiness and increasing impairment of the nervous system. Surgical treatment is usually necessary.

CEREBROSPINAL FLUID (C.S.F.)
A clear fluid that surrounds and flows through the brain and spinal cord. Its main function is to cushion the brain from shock, and to keep a constant pressure inside the skull. Sometimes viral or bacterial infections in the cerebrospinal fluid cause meningitis, an inflammation of the meninges. A number of conditions that affect the brain and spine leave traces in the fluid, which can be detected when a sample is taken by means of a cerebrospinal puncture – see *lumbar puncture*.

CEREBROVASCULAR ACCIDENT (C.V.A.) – *see* CEREBRAL HAEMORRHAGE, CEREBRAL THROMBOSIS

CERVICAL CANCER   106
Cancer in the *cervix*, or neck, of the womb. Cervical *cancer* is the most common type of cancer of the womb, but there is a good chance of successful treatment if the condition is detected early enough. Routine smear tests, where cells are scraped from the cervix and examined under a microscope to see if abnormal cells are present, make

this possible.

CERVIX   106
The word means 'à neck', and is normally used to denote the neck of the *womb*, though it can also be applied to many other organs. 'Cervical' may refer to the womb, as in '*cervical cancer*', or to the neck itself, as in 'cervical vertebrae'.

CESARIAN SECTION – *see* CAESARIAN SECTION

CHANCRE   94
The first sign of *syphilis*, which appears two or three weeks after the disease has been contracted. A chancre may appear almost anywhere, but is most commonly seen on the *penis*, mouth, *urethra* or eyelid. It is a scooped out, slightly *ulcerated* red area which may ooze a little but is not painful. The chancre, or chancres, heal without leaving a scar.

CHANGE OF LIFE – *see* MENOPAUSE

CHEILOSIS
A reddening, thickening and cracking of the lips that is seen in *Vitamin B* deficiency.

CHEMOTHERAPY
The treatment or control of disease by the use of drugs, as opposed to surgery, *radiotherapy* etc.

CHEST PAIN   14,19,26,68,138
Most diseases of the chest, from *bronchitis* to *cancer*, cause chest pain at some stage in their progress. With most of these conditions, however, pain is not a major symptom and is often variable. There are usually many more obvious problems, such as *weight loss*, *fever*, *night sweats* and so on, which point more clearly towards a diagnosis.

Some conditions do have chest pain as their main symptom. The most common of these is *ischaemic heart disease* and its symptom *angina*, which is the warning sign that a *heart attack* may be imminent. Severe bouts of coughing may leave a very sore feeling in the chest, and any injuries to the ribs, especially fractures, can cause considerable pain which improves with rest and time.

Pericarditis, or inflammation of one of the membraneous sacs that surround the heart, may cause a severe sharp pain in the chest which is worse in some body positions than in others. *Pleurisy* causes a stabbing pain in the peripheral areas which is made worse by deep breathing and coughing, while *herpes zoster*, or *shingles*, may cause chest pain even before the characteristic spots of the condition have appeared, and it may continue for a while after they have gone. *Pneumonia* is sometimes a cause of chest pain, but the pain is not the primary diagnostic feature of the disease.

Occasionally the small joints between the ribs and the breastbone ache and become tender in a condition known as *Tietze's Syndrome*. Often there is no physical cause for pains in the chest; they may be associated with *depression*, a *heart attack* in the family or with *hypochondria*.

CHICKEN POX – *see* VARICELLA

CHILBLAIN
Swelling and inflammation of the toes or fingers caused by cold and damp. When the area affected becomes warm, the chilblain starts to itch and burn.

CHOLECYSTITIS 43
An inflammation of the *gall bladder*, which may be either *acute* or *chronic*. Acute cholecystitis is normally the result of a *bacterial* infection, while chronic cholecystitis is usually caused by *gall stones*. If the bacterial infection does not respond to *antibiotics*, or if gall stones are present, a surgical removal of the gall bladder, or *cholecystectomy* may be necessary. The gall bladder can be examined by means of *cholecystography*.

CHOLECYSTOGRAPHY
(Cholecystogram) 43
An examination of the *gall bladder* in which a substance that shows up on *X-rays* is taken by mouth. When the substance has passed into the gall bladder from the *liver* an X-ray photograph is taken and the presence of any *gall stones* detected.

CHOLELITHIASIS 43
The formation of *gall stones* in the *gall bladder*, which may lead to *cholecystitis*.

CHOLERA
A disease contracted through water

or food that has been contaminated by the *faeces* of a sufferer in which there is an *acute bacterial* infection of the small intestine. Severe and persistent vomiting follows, with violent *diarrhoea* and characteristically watery stools. The result is extreme *dehydration* and a great thirst which may lead to death within one or two days. Treatment is by replacement of the body fluids and *antibiotics*. Cholera is rare these days in the western world because standards of hygiene and sanitation are much higher than in the past, but cholera *epidemics* still often follow natural disasters where proper sanitation is impossible. An epidemic can be avoided by mass *vaccination*, which needs to be repeated in six months.

CHOLESTEROL 80
A substance similar to *fat* that is found in many dairy products and is also synthesized in the *liver*. Cholesterol is important for the body's chemistry and found naturally in the *bile*, *blood* and tissues. In *atherosclerosis* cholesterol is a major constituent of the *atheroma* that thickens the wall of the blood vessels, but there is still much discussion among the experts about whether an increase in the dietary intake of cholesterol necessarily makes atherosclerosis more likely. Tests designed to prove or refute the theory have so far given variable results.

CHOREA
An involuntary twitching of the muscles of the limbs and face that is caused by disease of the areas of the brain that control subconscious voluntary movements. In elderly people senile chorea is sometimes seen, while Sydenham's Chorea may make sedation necessary; it is associated with rheumatic fever during childhood. The most serious form of the condition is *Huntingdon's Chorea* – a hereditary disease which appears, between the ages of 30 and 50, to attack the neurones of the brain and cause *dementia* as well as chorea. Huntingdon's Chorea is progressive and fatal; there is no effective treatment for it.

CHROMOSOME
A structure in the nucleus of a cell that carries *hereditary* factors called *genes*. Each cell contains 46 chromosomes, of which 23 derive

from the father and 23 from the mother; the exceptions are the *ova* of the female and the *sperm* of the male which contain 23 chromosomes. In the sperm and ova 22 chromosomes are called somatic – that is they are concerned with hereditary factors other than sex – and the one other chromosome is the sex chromosome. After fertilization a female *foetus* will have two sex chromosomes in each cell – XX, while a male foetus will have an X sex chromosome and the male Y sex chromosome. When cells divide during growth each chromosome duplicates itself exactly so that each new cell carries the same hereditary factors. Sometimes abnormal sex chromosome configurations, such as XXY, are found – see *Klinefelter's Syndrome*.

CHRONIC
A term that describes a prolonged disease process that progresses slowly. 'Chronic' is opposed to 'acute', and does not necessarily mean that the disease is severe.

CIRCULATION – *see* CARDIOVASCULAR SYSTEM

CIRRHOSIS 132
A chronic disease of the *liver*. In the first stage of the disease *fat* infiltrates the structure of the organ, then fibrous tissue forms a network through it. Liver cells lose their ability to function properly and the organ becomes enlarged and lumpy as groups of cells regenerate. There is increasing resistance to the flow of blood through the organ and a build-up of fluid in the abdomen called *ascites*. Eventually liver failure leads to death, as there is no effective treatment for cirrhosis other than the removal of its cause – which may range from *chronic alcoholism* with impaired nutrition to *hepatitis*, poisoning by substances such as carbon tetrachloride, *heart failure* or *bile* duct obstruction.

CLAUDICATION 80
A severe pain in the calf and leg muscles that is felt after walking but which disappears after rest. Claudication is the result of an insufficient supply of blood to the muscles, caused normally by *atherosclerosis*.

CLEFT PALATE
A congenital defect in which there is a fissure of varying size and shape

in the palate, or roof of the mouth. Most cleft palates can be repaired surgically. The condition is often associated with a *hare lip*.

CLUBBING   10
A thickening and rounding of the ends of the fingers and sometimes toes so that they resemble clubs. The condition may be a harmless congenital abnormality, but it is also seen in long-standing diseases of the *respiratory system, endocarditis* and *lung cancer*; in young children it may indicate the presence of *congenital* heart disease.

CLUB FOOT – *see* **TALIPES**

COELIAC DISEASE (US – Celiac)
A condition in which the cells of the small *intestine* degenerate so that food can no longer be digested and absorbed properly. Coeliac disease is caused by a sensitivity of the cells to gluten, which is found in wheat germ and rye, and results in malnutrition and stunted growth; the *stools* have an offensive odour and characteristic appearance. The condition can be remedied by a gluten-free diet.

COITUS INTERRUPTUS – *see* **CONTRACEPTION**

COLIC
A severe pain in the abdomen that comes and goes, and is sometimes called colicky pain – see *abdominal pain*.

COLITIS   37
An inflammation of the colon, which may be caused by *bacterial* infection of the lining and is called infective colitis, or can be ulcerative colitis, for which the cause is not known. Colitis causes *abdominal pain*, with *diarrhoea* and blood and mucus in the *stools*.

COLLES FRACTURE
A fracture of the forearm just above the wrist in which the hand and wrist are twisted backwards in the shape of a table fork. It is usually caused by a fall on the outstretched arm, and is one of the commonest fractures, especially amongst the elderly.

COLOR BLINDNESS
A general term for a number of conditions in which one or more

colors are confused with other colors. See *protanopia, deuteranopia, tritanopia*.

COLOSTOMY   37
A surgical procedure in which a part of the colon is connected to an artificial opening called a stoma in the abdominal wall. Colostomy becomes necessary when the gut can no longer perform its functions in conditions such as *cancer* of the bowel and ulcerative *colitis*. *Faeces* are collected in a colostomy bag that is attached to the *stoma*. The colostomy may be permanent, but if the original problem is solved the procedure can be reversed.

COMA   146
A deep, unconscious stupor from which the sufferer cannot be aroused. A coma can result from injury to the head, alcohol, carbon dioxide poisoning, ·vascular accident in the brain and a number of diseases such as *diabetes, meningitis* and *fevers*.

COMMON COLD – *see* **CORYZA**

COMMUNICABLE DISEASE
A term for a disease that can be caught by one person from another. Communicable diseases are also sometimes called infectious diseases.

COMPLICATION   155
A disease or injury superimposed upon another condition which changes and complicates the outcome and treatment of that condition. *Meningitis*, for example, is occasionally a complication of *mumps*.

COMPULSION
A repetitive stereotyped act – such as hand washing – which is performed as a result of obsession.

CONGENITAL
An abnormality that is present at birth that may be caused by inherited factors or developmental problems.

CONJUNCTIVITIS   124
Commonly called pink eye, conjunctivitis is an inflammation of the conjunctiva, or *mucous membrane*, that lines the eyelids and the front of the eyeball. It can be caused by *bacterial* infection, *allergy* or oc-

casionally by irritating chemical fumes; the eyeball becomes red and sore and there may be a discharge. The condition usually clears up on its own after a few weeks, though *antibiotics* may hasten a cure if bacteria are the cause of the problem.

CONNECTIVE TISSUE
The tissue that holds the various structures of the body together. It consists of a matrix of fibers of several different types interspersed with cells. There are a number of kinds of connective tissue, including *ligaments, tendons, cartilage* and *bone*.

CONSTIPATION
The passing of hard stools infrequently – the opposite of *diarrhoea*. Constipation is normally overemphasized as a problem, because the frequency of bowel movements varies considerably from person to person. Some people have even been known to open their bowels only once a week. As long as the stool is fairly soft and is passed without too much effort and discomfort, the frequency of bowel movements is irrelevant.

Constipation may be indicative of intestinal disease if the stool is very hard and painful to produce, or if it appears as small pellets like rabbit droppings. Intermittent constipation and diarrhoea is more unusual and demands immediate investigation – especially if blood and mucus are present in the stools.

CONTACT DERMATITIS – *see* **DERMATITIS**

CONTRACEPTION   98
The prevention of conception as a result of sexual intercourse. Probably the oldest method of contraception is coitus interruptus, or withdrawal of the *penis* before ejaculation. As some *semen* seeps from the penis prior to ejaculation, coitus interruptus is a very unreliable method; it also leads to *psychosexual* problems.

Another well known method of contraception is the use of a sheath, or condom, over the penis. This forms a mechanical barrier round the penis so that semen cannot reach the vagina. This method is reliable, but care must be taken when the condom is removed. It may also cause a loss of sensation for the male.

The female equivalent of the sheath is the diaphragm, or dutch cap, which forms a barrier over the *cervix*. It is inserted, covered with spermicidal jelly prior to intercourse, and removed a couple of hours later.

A rather more modern contraceptive method is the use of an oral contraceptive, popularly known as 'the pill'. The usual preparation is a combination of *oestrogen* and *progesterone* which prevents *ovulation* when it is taken regularly for 21 days. Without ovulation there is no possibility of *fertilization* and pregnancy. The pill is effective, but some women find that is has unsettling side-effects, and prefer an alternative method.

Recently a 'mini-pill' has been developed. This is a progesterone preparation that is taken continuously. It does not prevent ovulation, but makes the mucus of the cervix hostile to sperm. As the mini-pill does not inhibit *lactation* it is the most suitable pill for nursing mothers.

Intra-uterine devices (I.U.D.s) are small objects placed in the *uterus* which do not prevent fertilization, but stop the fertilized *ovum* from becoming implanted in the womb. A method based on the same principle has been known for many years – in the desert stones are placed in the womb of a camel to prevent pregnancy.

There is only one method which avoids pregnancy and satisfies the majority of religious and ethical objections to contraception. This involves planning sexual intercourse for those times in the *menstrual cycle* when fertilization is impossible – see *rhythm method*.

CORN

A callosity, or hard thickened area of the skin on or between the toes. Corns are normally caused by pressure or friction on the affected parts by badly fitted shoes; proprietary remedies are often used, but the only effective treatment is the purchase of shoes that fit properly.

CORONARY ARTERIES   74

The blood vessels that supply the muscles of the heart with blood. The right and left coronary arteries, the two main vessels, branch off the aorta and form a network of ar-

terioles around the heart. If the flow of blood is interrupted a *myocardial infarct* may result.

CORONARY ARTERY DISEASE – see ISCHAEMIC HEART DISEASE

CORONARY THROMBOSIS – see MYOCARDIAL INFARCT

CORTICOSTEROIDS (US – Corticoids)

A group of *hormones* that are produced by the *adrenal glands*. Some corticosteroids control salt and water balance, but most, such as hydrocortisone (also called cortisol), play an important part in the *metabolism* and in the chemistry of stress. They are also used as drugs in the treatment of inflammatory conditions, by mouth or as an ointment.

CORTISONE

A corticosteroid that is used to treat a lack of production of corticosteroid hormones by the *adrenal glands* in conditions such as *Addison's Disease*. Cortisone must be used with great care because it can have a number of serious side-effects.

CORYZA

A common virus infection of the upper *respiratory tract* in which the *mucous membranes* become inflamed, the nose is either blocked with *catarrh* or runny, and there is normally a sore throat, headache and cough. The common cold is extremely contagious; the symptoms appear about 48 hours after infection. The condition lasts for seven or eight days, but the only treatment possible is for the relief of symptoms rather than the infection itself.

COUNSELLING

A technique in which the counsellor listens to the patient's problems and encourages him or her to identify them and work out their solution on his or her own.

CRAMP

A spasmodic contraction of a muscle that can be painful and alarming. Sometimes it becomes impossible to perform one particular task without cramps, but the same muscles can carry out all other actions. This is known as occupa-

tional cramp, the most common example being writer's cramp. The cause of cramp can vary from an abnormal salt balance in the body to tiredness and· stress; treatment is normally by flexion and extension of the muscle, with heat and massage.

CREPITATIONS   14

A crackling sound in the lungs that can be heard through a stethoscope in certain diseases. It is normally caused by fluid in the *alveoli* and may be heard in infections such as *pneumonia*. Crepitations are also an early sign of *heart failure*.

CRETINISM   153

A congenital deficiency in *thyroid hormones* that causes retarded growth, or *dwarfism*, mental retardation and coarse features. The condition can be improved by the early administration of thyroid hormones.

CROHN'S DISEASE (US – more usually Regional Ileitis / Enteritis)   39

A *disease* of unknown cause in which parts of the intestines become swollen and inflamed, eventually blocking the passage of the contents of the bowel. Crohn's Disease may affect most parts of the intestine, but usually attacks the ileum.

CROSS EYES – see STRABISMUS

CROUP

A disease of young children in which breathing is difficult and painful, and the resulting respiratory inadequacy leads to a fast heart beat and sometimes *cyanosis*. The condition is the result of a *viral* infection which makes the *larynx* inflamed and swollen and obstructs the airways. Croup can be relieved by the application of heat to the throat and by steam inhalations, but in severe cases a *tracheotomy* may be necessary.

CUSHING'S SYNDROME

A condition in which over-production of *corticosteroid hormones* by the *adrenal glands*, either as a result of an adrenal *tumor* or the malfunction of the *pituitary gland*, causes fatness, fatigue, excess hair growth, reddening of the face and neck, *diabetes*, high *blood pressure* and often mental changes.

CYANOSIS

A bluish or slate-like tinge to the skin that is caused by a lack of *oxygen* in the blood. Properly oxygenated arterial blood is red in color, while deoxygenated venous blood is bluish. Cyanosis is caused by respiratory failure, *heart failure* and *congenital* heart disease, as in 'blue babies'.

CYST

A closed pouch that contains either fluid or solid material. Many different kinds of cysts are found in different areas of the body. They may be blocked *glands*, such as *sebaceous* cysts, *tumors* or the result of a *parasitic* infection. Occasionally a cyst is the result of abnormal development of the *foetus* and is *congenital*.

CYSTITIS   92

An inflammation of the *bladder* that causes a burning pain on urination, frequency of urination and abdominal pain.

It is normally caused by a *bacterial* infection that is treated with *antibiotics*.

CYSTOCELE   48

A *hernia* of the *bladder* that is sometimes seen in women after childbirth when connective tissue is in a weakened state. The condition may need to be repaired surgically.

CYSTOSCOPY

A technique in which the *bladder* can be examined by means of a small fiber-optic instrument that is passed up through the *urethra*. Cystoscopy is usually performed under *anaesthetic* and is useful in the investigation of *haematuria* and the management of conditions such as *carcinoma* of the bladder.

D

DANDRUFF

A scaling and flaking of the superficial layers of the scalp. A small amount of dandruff is quite normal, but when the problem becomes more severe and causes distress it may be necessary to wash the hair in a special shampoo – see *seborrhea*.

D. & C. - *see* DILATATION & CURETTAGE

DEAFNESS   116

The inability to hear, which may be partial or total, and has numerous causes. Most commonly, deafness is the result of an accumulation of hard wax, or cerumen, in the ear – the wax can easily be softened with eardrops and removed with a syringe. A degree of deafness is quite often experienced during the course of infections of the mouth, nose and throat such as head colds, *adenoids* and *tonsillitis* in children, because the middle ear and throat are connected by the *Eustachian tubes*. A more specific infection of the middle ear which is an important cause of deafness in children is called *otitis* media, and is treated with *antibiotics*.

Sometimes deafness is caused by a malfunction of the nerves that supply the ear. This may be a side-effect of some drugs when used in large quantities, or due to neurological disease. An injury that jars the delicate bones of the inner ear, such as a fracture of the base of the skull, may cause deafness; as may constant exposure to loud noise. The condition may have a *hereditary* cause, as in otosclerosis, where the bones of the middle ear become hardened, or may be *congenital* as a result of an attack of *rubella* in the mother. When associated with a buzzing in the ears, called tinnitus, and *vertigo*, deafness can be the result of *Menière's Disease*. Hearing deteriorates with age, but the cause is unknown; the use of a hearing aid helps to alleviate the problem.

DEFAECATION (US–Defecation)

The passing of solid wastes, called *faeces*, from the body through the *anus* in the form of *stools*.

DEFIBRILLATOR

A machine that gives a measured electric shock to a patient through electrodes placed on the chest. It is used to restore the heart to its normal rhythm – sometimes during *atrial fibrillation*, but more usually during the *ventricular* fibrillation that is associated with a heart attack.

DEGENERATIVE DISEASE 80,110

A general term used to describe those diseases in which tissue tends to lose its essential nature and functions, such as *osteoarthritis* and *atherosclerosis*. Tissue degeneration is always a feature of the ageing process, but in the degenerative diseases the process is speeded up.

DEHYDRATION

A state in which the body becomes dangerously short of fluids, which can be the result of vomiting and *diarrhoea*, as in *cholera* and *gastroenteritis*, or the inability to take fluids by the mouth. Fluid replacement solves the problem, but if this is not possible orally a weak salt solution is given directly into a vein in an *intravenous drip*.

DELIRIUM   132

A state in which normal conscious thought and speech is lost that often results in great physical and mental restlessness. Delirium is seen in severe illnesses, high *fevers* and withdrawal from drug addiction. When withdrawal is from alcohol the delirium is known as delirium tremens (D.T.s).

DELUSION   140

A firmly held belief that is either totally false or exaggerated and does not change in response to logical argument. Delusions are seen in *paranoia*, *schizophrenia* and a number of *psychoses*.

DEMENTIA   128

A form of mental illness in which *cerebral atrophy* causes the progressive loss of normal thought and reasoning processes. Forgetfulness is common, as is a deterioration in appearance and life-style. A certain amount of cerebral atrophy is a natural part of ageing and when dementia is seen after the age of 65 it is called senile dementia; presenile dementia, seen before this age, is usually caused by diseases that affect the brain.

DEPRESSION   138

A mental state in which normal feelings of mild depression turn into an overwhelming sensation of blackness and despair which may even lead to suicide. It is characterized by early morning waking, poor *appetite*, *insomnia* and loss of *libido*; there may also be *psychosomatic* symptoms.

DERMATITIS

An inflammation of the skin. Sometimes the word is used loosely to cover a number of skin conditions, including *eczema*. Contact dermatitis is an *allergic* reaction of the skin to certain substances that may be held against it.

DETACHED RETINA
A condition in which the *retina* becomes separated from the back of the eye by fluid, usually because the fluid has leaked through a tear in it. Unless the retina is being pushed forward by a *tumor* or a blood clot it can usually be replaced surgically and vision restored.

DETOXICATION
The removal of poisonous substances from the body. In the body detoxication is the function of the *liver* and *kidneys*; the term is also used to denote a specialized hospital in which alcoholics and drug addicts can 'dry out' – a detoxication center.

DEUTERANOPIA
A form of color blindness in which the color green cannot be distinguished.

DEXTROSE – *see* GLUCOSE

DIABETES INSIPIDUS
A condition, sometimes inherited, in which the *pituitary gland* does not produce enough antidiuretic *hormone*. Normally this hormone limits the production of *urine*, so consequently large volumes of dilute urine are passed; the sufferer feels thirsty and drinks quantities of water. The condition, which is sometimes called nephrogenic diabetes, can be treated by *hormone replacement therapy*.

DIABETES MELLITUS   146
A disease, often known as sugar disease, which results from a relative lack of the *hormone insulin*. As insulin reduces the level of sugar in the blood, diabetes causes a very high blood sugar level. If untreated this may cause thirst, frequent passing of water, skin infections and weight loss. In extreme cases the diabetic may go into a *coma*. The condition can be controlled by insulin administered by injection or by special tablets taken by mouth, depending on the type of diabetes.

DIAGNOSIS
The eventual determination by a doctor of a patient's disease, in the light of a discussion of the patient's symptoms, the case history, a physi-

cal examination, and sometimes further tests.
See You and Your Doctor, p.6

DIALYSIS
A procedure used in *kidney* failure to take over the function of the kidney in cleansing the blood. In haemodialysis the patient's circulation is connected to a machine that pumps the blood over a membrane which imitates the filtering action of the kidney, and then pumps it back into the body. Patients with renal failure may need to dialyse for about 30 hours each week, but once learnt the procedure can be carried out overnight at home.

In peritoneal dialysis a tube is introduced into the *peritoneum* through the abdominal wall and the cavity filled with fluid. By the process of osmosis waste products are transferred across the membranes of the peritoneum into the fluid, which is then pumped out of the cavity. This technique is used when a dialysis machine is not available.

DIAPER RASH – *see* NAPPY RASH

DIAPHRAGM
A strong muscular sheet that separates the chest, or thorax, from the abdomen. The diaphragm contracts downwards each time a breath is taken, to increase the volume of the thorax; on expiration it relaxes back into its normal domed shape. 'Diaphragm' is also the term for a female contraceptive device – see *contraception*.

DIARRHOEA (US–Diarrhea)
The frequent passage of semi-formed *stools* in *defaecation*. Diarrhoea may lead to *dehydration* if it is severe and prolonged; it is normally caused by infective *colitis*, but can be a symptom of a number of other diseases.

DIASTOLE
The part of the heart's pumping cycle in which the heart muscle is relaxed and the chambers are filling with blood.

DILATATION & CURETTAGE (D. & C.)
A gynaecological operation where the *cervix* of the *womb* is dilated with a special instrument and the inside of the womb scraped. A D. & C. may be performed to remove a growth, to remove tissue after a

miscarriage or to take a sample of tissue for microscopic examination.

DILATION (DILATATION)
The enlargement of a hollow structure such as a blood vessel – see *vasodilation*.

DIPHTHERIA
An infectious disease of the upper respiratory tract and throat that is caused by bacteria. Diphtheria is a serious disease that can cause death within a few days unless treated; luckily since the widespread adoption of *vaccination* against the disease it has become extremely rare in western society.

DIPLOPIA
Double vision. Diplopia is seen in disorders of the nerve supply of the eyes and in diseases that affect the brain, such as *meningitis*.

DISC   114
A pad of fibrous tissue between the vertebrae, properly known as an intervertebral disc. Occasionally an intervertebral disc may rupture when under stress; more commonly it projects backwards in the condition known as a slipped disc. Both conditions are painful and may require long periods of bed-rest.

DISCHARGE   94
An abnormal seepage of fluid from the orifices of the body. There may be a discharge from the ears when the outer ear is infected, while a *urethral* discharge in men may be an indication of *venereal disease*. Some discharge from the *vagina* is normal in women after *puberty*, but when the amount of the discharge increases or causes irritation an infection such as *thrush* or *trichomonias* may be the cause.

DISLOCATION
A process, normally caused by injury, by which a joint becomes disrupted. The two articulating surfaces of the joint are forced out of position so that they are no longer adjacent to each other. A dislocation is normally treated, or reduced, by manipulation.

DISSEMINATING SCLEROSIS – *see* MULTIPLE SCLEROSIS

DIURETIC
A substance that acts on the kidneys to increase the production of urine.

A diuretic drug is usually prescribed in cases of *heart failure* and shortness of breath in order to prevent a build up of fluids in the tissues, called *oedema*, and in the treatment of *hypertension*. There are a number of naturally occurring substances that have a diuretic effect, such as coffee.

DIVERTICULAR DISEASE   34

A condition in which diverticula cause *diarrhoea* or *constipation* and *abdominal pain* without any infection or inflammation – see *diverticulitis*.

DIVERTICULITIS   34

An inflammation of the diverticula, usually in the large bowel, which is common in the west in people over 50 and causes *diarrhoea* or *constipation* and *abdominal pain*.

DIVERTICULUM   34

An outpocketing or pouch in the wall of the *intestine*, most commonly in the *colon* or large bowel. Diverticula may be associated with disease, but more usually are a symptomless consequence of age. Sometimes these pouches become infected and cause *diverticulitis*.

DIZZINESS   118

A sensation of spinning or whirling. When accompanied by *deafness* and a ringing in the ears dizziness may be caused by *Menière's Disease* – see *vertigo*. Dizziness is common in the elderly, but can be avoided by steady, deliberate movements and rest. Sometimes it is a symptom of diseases of the *cardiovascular system* and *hypertension*; dizziness can also be caused by an infection of the middle ear called labyrinthitis.

DOUBLE VISION – *see* **DIPLOPIA**

DOWN'S SYNDROME – *see* **TRISOMY 21**

DRIBBLING   72,96

When from the mouth, dribbling is a spill-over of *saliva* which is often a sign of teething in a baby, but in adults can be a symptom of *Parkinson's Disease* or indicate poor coordination between the nerves and muscles of the mouth and *pharynx*. Dribbling of urine can be a sign of urinary tract problems in women when it is called stress *incontinence*; in men it is often a sign of a problem in the *prostate gland*. Dribbling of urine

can usually be corrected surgically – see *incontinence*.

DRIP – *see* **INTRAVENOUS DRIP**

DROOPING EYELIDS – *see* **PTOSIS**

DUCTUS ARTERIOSUS

A part of the *foetal* circulation that connects the *pulmonary artery* to the *aorta*, because foetal blood does not circulate through the lung. The vessel normally closes off at birth, or slightly afterwards; when it does not it is called a patent ductus arteriosus and may need to be closed surgically – otherwise the baby's circulation will not be able to function properly and the baby may become *cyanotic*.

DUODENAL ULCER   45

An *ulcer* of the *duodenum* that typically causes *abdominal pain* a few hours after eating and often wakes the sufferer in the early hours of the morning. It is usually relieved by milk and antacids and is normally treated by drugs instead of surgery.

DWARFISM   151

Abnormally small stature. There are a number of causes for dwarfism, including poor nutrition in infancy due to *malabsorption*, an underactivity of the *thyroid gland* in childhood leading to *cretinism*, a *Vitamin D* deficiency that leads to *rickets* and an underactivity of the part of the *pituitary gland* that produces growth *hormone*. Perhaps the most common type is called achondroplastic dwarfism, in which the long bones of the arms and legs fail to grow properly. Achondroplastic dwarfism is a *hereditary* disorder.

DYSENTERY

A severe *diarrhoea*, in which there may be blood and mucus, which can either be caused by a *bacterial* infection of the *intestines*, called bacillary dysentery, or by *parasitic* infection as in amoebic dysentery. Serious fluid loss may occur.

DYSLEXIA

Difficulty in reading and writing. The condition often goes unnoticed until progress at school is found to be unusually slow. Typically people with dyslexia confuse certain letters – especially d, b and p.

DYSMENORRHOEA   100

Period pains, usually in the form of

lower abdominal cramps and pains which come on a few days before the period is due but disappear when *menstruation* starts. In some women dysmenorrhoea can be so severe that *hormonal* treatment is required.

DYSPAREUNIA

Pain during sexual intercourse. Dyspareunia may have a physical cause, such as an inflammation of the *cervix* or the scars of an *episiotomy* performed during childbirth; more commonly the causes are psychological and point to a *psychosexual* problem.

DYSPEPSIA   45

A term for a collection of symptoms, including *abdominal pain*, *heartburn*, a feeling of fullness, belching and sometimes nausea and vomiting, which are also called indigestion. Dyspepsia may be caused by *stress*, but is also characteristic of *gastric* or *duodenal ulcers*.

DYSPHAGIA

Difficulty in swallowing, which can be due to painful infections of the mouth, teeth and throat, an obstruction or to badly fitted dentures. Occasionally, dysphagia is the result of a lack of coordination between the nerves and muscles of the *pharynx* or a *stricture* of the *oesophagus*.

DYSPNOEA (US – Dyspnea)   19,21

Breathlessness or breathing difficulty. Dyspnoea is normal when caused by physical exercise, but when present at rest or when excessive and prolonged after exercise it is an indication that a disease process is affecting the *respiratory system*. In dyspnoea the sufferer gasps for *oxygen*: sometimes because air cannot flow freely in the lungs, as in *chronic bronchitis* and *asthmatic* attacks; sometimes because the amount of lung tissue available for *oxygen-carbon dioxide* exchange has been reduced by *emphysema*, *tuberculosis* or *cancer*. Dyspnoea can also be caused by problems that do not directly involve the lungs, such as a deficiency of *haemoglobin* in the blood, or heart disease.

DYSURIA   92,94

Pain or difficulty in passing urine, which may be caused by *cystitis*, *urethritis*, a *venereal infection* or *prostatism* in older men.

E

EARACHE 118
A very common complaint, especially in childhood, earache is normally caused by an infection of the ear – see *otitis*. An infection of the throat and *pharynx* may also cause earache because of the link between the ears and throat called the *Eustachian Tubes*. For the same reason tooth decay or a dental *abscess* may cause earache. Occasionally earache is caused by *mastoiditis*, or more seriously by acute *meningitis*.

ECCHYMOSIS
A bruise. An ecchymosis is caused when pressure forces blood into the skin or *mucous membranes*, discoloring the tissues in a characteristic blue-black way. As the blood is broken down into its constituents the color changes to a greenish-brown, or yellow. A tendency to bruise unusually easily, or the appearance of spontaneous bruises, may be an indication of some blood diseases; it may also be a natural consequence of old age.

E.C.G. – *see* ELECTROCARDIOGRAM

ECLAMPSIA
A rare but serious complication of pregnancy whose cause is still unknown. Eclampsia sometimes causes the death of the *foetus* in the *womb*, and is characterized by high *blood pressure*, *proteinurea*, *kidney* and *liver* damage and *oedema*; these may progress to *convulsions* and *coma*. Eclampsia affects about 1 in 1000 pregnant women and can be prevented by routine examinations.

E.C.T. – *see* ELECTROCONVULSIVE THERAPY

ECTOPIA
Literally 'out of place', ectopia, or its adjective ectopic, is used to describe two particular circumstances. An ectopic heartbeat, also called extrasystole, is an extra heartbeat that may be present quite normally or may be induced by smoking or drugs such as caffeine. In an ectopic pregnancy, the fertilized egg implants and grows in the *Fallopian tubes* instead of the *uterus*.

ECZEMA 30
An itchy skin complaint in which the outermost layer of the skin, or epidermis, becomes inflamed. Eczema is sometimes due to an *allergy* to some external agent – see contact *dermatitis*. It may, on the other hand, be constitutional – that is, an eczema that often occurs in families and is sometimes associated with *hay fever* and other allergies. Treatment is by the local application of *steroid* creams and, if possible, the identification and removal of the cause of allergy. The condition may be made worse by constant washing in soap and water. Varicose eczema is seen around the ankles and is caused by poor circulation in the legs.

EDEMA – *see* OEDEMA

E.E.G. – *see* ELECTROENCEPHALOGRAM

EGO
A term used in *psychoanalysis* to denote the self, the conscious part of the mind that mediates between the subconscious, or *id*, and the moral conscience, the *super-ego*.

ELECTRA COMPLEX
A *Freudian* concept in which the repressed sexual love of a daughter for her father is said to be responsible for some aspects of personality and behavior. The term derives from classical Greek legend.

ELECTROCARDIOGRAM (E.C.G.)
A trace of the electrical activity of the *heart*. Usually known as an E.C.G., the trace is obtained by the use of an electrocardiograph, in which electrodes are placed on the limbs and chest wall. The E.C.G. gives information about the rate and rhythm of the contractions of the heart and shows the damage sustained during a *heart attack*, or whether one is imminent. The procedure is quite painless and takes about five minutes; sometimes it may be repeated after a short period of exercise, so that the doctor can see how the heart reacts to increased demands upon it.

ELECTROCONVULSIVE THERAPY (E.C.T.) 138,140
A treatment that acts in an unknown way, in which electrodes are attached to the temples and an electric current passed between them. The technique may be beneficial in severe *depression*, and in *schizophrenia*, but the side-effects can include a transient headache and loss of memory.

ELECTROENCEPHALOGRAM (E.E.G.)
A recording of the electrical activity of the brain that is obtained by placing electrodes on the scalp, which are linked to an electroencephalograph. An E.E.G. can show up any bursts of abnormal electrical activity in the brain – as is seen, for example, in *epilepsy* or a brain *tumor*.

ELECTROMYOGRAM (E.M.G.)
A recording of the electrical activity of muscle, normally after stimulation of the muscle fibers. An electromyogram, or E.M.G., is used to investigate disorders of the muscles and to assess their recovery after a *paralytic* illness.

ELEPHANTIASIS
A disease, rare in the northern hemisphere, in which the channels of the *lymph* system become blocked so that the limb or area affected floods with tissue fluids and becomes massively enlarged. Elephantiasis is normally caused by a *parasitic* invasion of the lymph ducts and usually affects the lower limbs and *scrotum*.

EMBOLISM
An arterial blockage that is caused by an embolus, or piece of material – usually a blood clot – that is carried around in the blood. Other types of emboli are those made of fatty material, balls of fungus, foreign bodies or air. The blockage prevents blood from reaching the part of the body beyond the embolus and may cause a *stroke* or *gangrene* in the affected limb. Occasionally the embolus can be dissolved by *anticoagulant* drugs, but more often it has to be removed surgically.

EMBRYO
The fertilized *ovum*, or egg, from the moment of conception to the eighth week of pregnancy.

E.M.G. – *see* ELECTROMYOGRAM

EMPHYSEMA 19
A chronic lung condition in which the *alveoli*, or small air sacs of the lungs, become distended and

cannot deflate. Breathing becomes difficult and the oxygen-carbon dioxide exchange in the lungs inefficient. The condition is associated with longstanding *bronchitis* and smoking, and may cause a *barrel chest*. There is no specific treatment for emphysema, though the sufferer sometimes needs to be given oxygen.

When air escapes from the lungs into the surrounding tissues – either after an operation or a penetrating injury of the chest – the condition is called surgical emphysema. The surrounding skin puffs up and has a characteristic crackling feel to the touch.

EMPYEMA

An accumulation of *pus* between the two layers of *pleura*, the inner lining of the chest wall and the outer covering of the lungs. Empyema is similar to a pleural effusion, except that the fluid that accumulates is full of *bacteria* and cells and normally follows an infection in the lungs. It is usually necessary to drain the pus away surgically.

ENDEMIC

A term that describes a disease or infection that occurs so frequently in an area that most people have at some time suffered from it – unless they have some special resistance or immunity to it. *Malaria*, for example, is endemic in some parts of West Africa.

ENDOCARDIUM

A membraneous lining of the inside of the *heart* and the heart valves. Endocarditis is an infection of this membrane and may be *viral* or *bacterial* in origin. The condition may also be due to rheumatic fever and can seriously damage the heart valves so that surgical repair is necessary – see *valve replacement*.

ENDOCRINE GLANDS   144

Ductless glands that make *hormones* and secrete them into the bloodstream, including the *thyroid*, *parathyroid*, *pituitary* and *adrenal* glands and the *testes* and *ovaries*.

ENDOMETRIUM   100

The membrane that lines the *womb*. The endometrium goes through a cycle of changes each month in response to the female *hormones*, that prepares the womb for the im-plantation of a fertilized *ovum*, or egg. If no egg implants, the endometrium is shed in *menstruation*. Sometimes the endometrium becomes inflamed in a condition called endometritis that is one of the causes of *dysmenorrhoea*.

ENEMA

A preparation given through the *rectum* which clears the rectum and *colon* of *faeces*, either before an operation or childbirth, or as a treatment for constipation. In a barium enema, barium is introduced into the lower bowel so that *x-ray* films can be taken of the area. This technique is commonly used in the investigation of *rectal bleeding*.

ENLARGED GLANDS   155,158

Any visible or palpable swelling or tenderness of one or more of the *glands* of the body, which may be due to a number of causes. *Mumps*, for example, results in a swelling of the parotid glands under the jaw, and is caused by a *virus* infection. Other common diseases that affect the glands directly are *tonsillitis* and *glandular fever* (in America called infectious mononucleosis). Sometimes lymph glands, or nodes, become swollen as a response to infections in other parts of the body; when a finger becomes infected the glands in the armpit may become enlarged. Occasionally glands become enlarged because of the action of a malignant disease such as *leukaemia* or *Hodgkin's Disease*. If any gland in the body is persistently swollen, a doctor should be consulted.

ENTERIC FEVER

Those *fevers* that affect the gut and cause *enteritis*, including *typhoid* and *paratyphoid* fever.

ENTERITIS   37,39,54

An inflammation of the small intestine. Enteritis may be caused by *viral* or *bacterial* infection or by disease processes, as in *Crohn's Disease* – see *gastroenteritis*, *enteric fever*, *colitis*.

ENURESIS

The involuntary and unconscious passing of *urine* – usually at night, when it is known as nocturnal enuresis. Nocturnal enuresis, or bedwetting, is normal during the first few years of life, but usually stops after 'potty training'. If it continues into later childhood or adolescence enuresis may be a considerable problem. Occasionally it is due to an infection of the *urinary tract*, or to minor anatomical abnormalities; more usually it is the result of *psychological* difficulties.

ENZYME

A substance that acts as a catalyst in the body – in other words it speeds up and facilitates one of the reactions in the chemistry of the body without being used up in the reaction. The most important group of enzymes in the body are secreted by *glands* into the gut, where they help to break down complicated chemical structures in food into simpler forms that can be absorbed. Sometimes, often in *hereditary* disorders, one enzyme may be missing. This can have serious consequences on the metabolism – see *phenylketonurea*.

EPIDEMIC

The sudden eruption of a disease or infection in a community that spreads with great speed and involves a large proportion of the population.

EPIDIDYMITIS

An inflammation of the epididymis, the long tube that connects each *testis* to the *vas deferens*, in which sperm is stored and matures. The inflammation is usually caused by *bacteria* and may result in pain and a redness and swelling of the scrotum, but normally responds to *antibiotics*.

EPIDURAL

A form of *anaesthesia* that is now widely used to relieve pain during labour. A small catheter is passed into the epidural space surrounding the spinal cord in the small of the back, under local anaesthesia, and an anaesthetic substance injected through it. Pain is relieved by this method, but the baby's *respiration* is not affected and the mother remains wide awake.

EPILEPSY

A condition caused by abnormal electrical discharges in the brain that generally manifests itself in one of two ways. Grand Mal is the most serious kind of epileptic seizure, in which the sufferer falls to the ground, his limbs twitch, and he may foam at the mouth and pass water involuntarily. This 'fit' may be preceded by an *aura* and followed by a deep sleep or trance-like condition. In Petit Mal the sufferer experiences a short period of altered consciousness in which he seems to be in a world of his own. The eyes stare and thought and actions are interrupted, but there is no 'fit' as in Grand Mal. Both these forms of epilepsy have no known cause and are therefore called *idiopathic*. They can be treated with special *anticonvulsant* drugs that must be taken regularly.

Sometimes fits follow brain damage – either as the result of an accident, as in post-traumatic epilepsy, or as part of a disease that attacks the structure of the brain. The fits may affect the whole body, or just one limb, depending on the area of the brain damaged. Any fit that occurs for the first time late in life should be investigated, because it may indicate brain damage – as in a brain *tumor*.

EPINEPHRINE – *see* ADRENALINE

EPISIOTOMY
A cut made in the *perineum* during the last stage of labour to facilitate the easy birth of a baby. The incision is made under a local *anaesthetic*, starting at the *vulva* and running up at an angle at either 5 or 7 o'clock from the midwife's viewpoint. After the birth the cut is sewn up and the mother encouraged to take frequent hot salt baths to prevent infection.

EPISTAXIS
Nose bleeding. The most common cause of nose bleeds is injury to the blood vessels resulting from over-enthusiastic picking of the nose. Sometimes, especially in adolescents, nose bleeds may be spontaneous and without much significance; when seen in middle age, or later, they are usually a sign of a more serious problem such as high *blood pressure*, or *blood clotting* disorders. In old age epistaxes may be the result of a general weakening of the blood vessels of the nose. Throughout life nose bleeds can be the result of conditions as varied as the common cold and nasal *polyps*.

ERYSIPELAS
An infection of the skin by streptococcal *bacteria* that results in areas of red, hot and swollen skin,

with associated *feverishness*. The condition usually responds to *antibiotics*.

ERYTHEMA
A redness of the skin caused by *dilation* of the small blood vessels, sometimes as a result of a nervous mechanism of the body; at other times a sign of infection or inflammation.

ERYTHROCYTE 162
A red blood cell. An erythrocyte is formed in the bone marrow and spends about 120 days in the blood stream before being broken down in the *liver*. It contains the iron-based protein *haemoglobin* that combines with *oxygen* to form oxy-haemoglobin, thus allowing the transport of oxygen around the body. There are a number of abnormalities of red blood cells that cause disease – see *anaemia, thalassaemia*.

ERYTHROCYTE SEDIMENTATION RATE (E.S.R.)
A common blood test which measures the rate at which the red blood cells settle to the bottom of a tall tube in a sample of blood. The process takes longer in acute infections, *connective tissue diseases* and sometimes in *neoplasia*.

ESOPHAGUS – *see* OESOPHAGUS

E.S.R. – *see* ERYTHROCYTE SEDIMENTATION RATE

ESTROGEN – *see* OESTROGEN

EUSTACHIAN TUBES 116
Two tubes that link the middle ears to the *pharynx* and act as a pressure regulating device. Infections can spread along the tubes (sometimes called audio-meatory tubes), which is the reason why some people with head colds and upper *respiratory tract* infections may suffer from *deafness* or *earache*.

EXHIBITIONIST
Commonly the term is taken to refer to anyone who enjoys showing off; specifically it refers to someone, usually male, who derives sexual gratification from the exposure of his genitals.

EXOPHTHALMOS 151
Protruding eyes. The condition is most commonly a sign of *Grave's Disease* or *thyrotoxicosis*, when the

eyes protrude more than usual and the upper eyelid is abnormally retracted. Occasionally exophthalmos is the result of a *tumor* of the eye socket – when it only affects one eye – or a *thrombosis* of the sinuses of the brain.

EXPECTORANT 19
A substance, usually a linctus, that is given in conditions such as *bronchitis* to encourage the coughing up of *phlegm*.

EXTRASYSTOLE – *see* ECTOPIA

EXTRAVERT (or EXTROVERT)
A cheerful, outgoing person who tends to be uninhibited and more interested in outside activities than in introspection. The opposite of *introvert*.

EXUDATE
A fluid rich in *white blood cells* that slowly oozes through the walls of blood vessels at the site of infection.

EYELID NODULES 146,153
Small lumps on the eyelids. They may be chalazion or meibomiam *cysts* – that is swellings of the *sebaceous glands* of the eyelid – which may be painful if infected. Sometimes an eyelid nodule is a *stye*, or hordeolum, an inflammation of a gland or hair follicle at the base of the eyelash, which becomes red, swollen and painful. When the nodules are fatty, yellow and just below the skin they are known as *xanthelasma*. They are not serious in themselves, but may be an indication of high blood *cholesterol* levels, and are sometimes seen in a number of *chronic* diseases, such as *diabetes mellitus* and *myxoedema*.

F

FACIAL PAIN 28,68
Pain in the face can have a number of causes. Sometimes a dull throb in the jaw can be caused by toothache or a dental *abscess*. In *sinusitis* there is an ache and local tenderness over the *sinuses* which is often associated with a headache. A severe continuous facial pain can be caused by *herpes zoster*, or shingles, and may be felt before the characteristic spots of the disease appear. Sometimes, especially in old

people, it continues after the spots have gone, and is called post-herpetic *neuralgia*.

Probably the most severe facial pain of all is called trigeminal neuralgia. Its cause is not known, though it normally affects older people, and at one time used to be called 'Tic Douloureux'. The pain is very sharp and only lasts a few seconds, though it may be followed by a continuous dull ache. It can be started by a touch on a 'trigger zone' when the face is being washed or the hair brushed. Trigeminal neuralgia can be treated by drugs, but sometimes it is necessary to destroy a part of the affected nerve surgically or with an alcohol injection.

FACIES   153
A facial appearance that is characteristic of specific diseases. Sufferers from *myxoedema*, or an under-activity of the *thyroid* gland, usually have coarse dry skin, puffiness around the eyes, scanty eyebrows and dullness and apathy in their expression. This combination of facial characteristics is known as the facies of myxoedema.

FAINTING – *see* SYNCOPE

FALLOPIAN TUBES (US – Oviducts)   98
The tubes that connect the two female *ovaries* with the *uterus* or *womb* through which the eggs, or *ova*, travel to the womb. The tubes are fairly delicate structures and may become swollen and clogged up if there is any infection in the pelvis – a condition called *salpingitis*. Sometimes an ovum that has been fertilized implants in one of the tubes instead of the wall of the womb. This is known as an ectopic pregnancy, and may cause considerable pain and bleeding as the *foetus* tries to grow in a space that is too small for it.

FALLOT'S TETRALOGY
The most common form of *congenital* heart disease, in which there are four linked deficiencies in the heart. Children born with Fallot's Tetralogy are normally small and sickly, tend to squat on their heels, are short of breath and become *cyanotic*, or blue. The defects can be corrected by surgery.

FALLS
A common problem in the elderly, falls are usually caused by a combination of failing eyesight and poor balance. They are especially common at night, when elderly people often have to get up to pass water. An irregular pulse, or cardiac *arrhythmia* may cause a transient loss of consciousness and so a fall. Sometimes a fall is a by-product of *syncope*, or a faint, or the severe convulsions of Grand Mal *epilepsy*. In older people some drugs may not be *metabolized* and excreted from the body as quickly as in youth; as a result a sleeping pill taken at bedtime may still have effects the morning afterwards and so cause a fall.

FASTING
An abstention from food. Fasting is usually necessary before an operation, in case the *anaesthetic* causes vomiting. It may also be necessary before certain

FATIGUE   17,100,138,153,162
A feeling of excessive tiredness. Fatigue is quite common, and usually fairly innocent – when it is experienced, for example, after strenuous exercise. When fatigue is felt after minimal exercise, or rest, it may be a sign of underlying disorder.

Most commonly fatigue is felt with *influenza* and other *viral* illnesses – sometimes before other symptoms become apparent. It may be a sign of *anaemia*, particularly of iron-deficiency anaemia in association with heavy periods, or *menorrhagia*, in women. Pregnancy also causes tiredness and the expectant mother will need extra rest.

Fatigue is usually seen in *myxoedema*, when the *thyroid* gland is underactive; it is also a common symptom of *depression*.

FATS
A group of organic compounds that are the principal form for the storage of energy in the body. In the digestive process, ingested fats are emulsified by *bile* and broken down by the *enzymes* of the intestine. They enter the blood stream and are either stored in cells or oxidized to carbon dioxide and water, with the formation of *ketones* as a by-product, in the release of energy.

FEARS   130
The majority of fears are quite normal; fear is a natural human emotion and is an important part of the body's defence mechanisms. When a fear becomes excessive or *obsessional*, however, it is abnormal and is then known as a *phobia*.

FEMINIZATION
A condition in which men develop female sexual characteristics such as breasts and lose facial and body hair, as a result of *liver disease*, *hormone therapy* – as in sex change therapy – or *endocrine* and *chromosomal* abnormalities – see *Klinefelter's Syndrome*.

FERTILITY   98
An ability to reproduce easily. Fertility is not usually a problem these days as there are artificial methods of curbing it – see *contraception*. An inability to conceive is not uncommon – see *infertility*. The most fertile time of the reproductive or *menstrual cycle* is *ovulation*, which occurs about 14 days before the start of a period. The best time for conception is therefore between the 10th and 20th day of the cycle, where day one is the first day of the period.

FERTILIZATION   99
The joining together of the *sperm* and *ovum* after intercourse. After fertilization the egg implants in the wall of the *womb* and the *foetus* starts to grow.

FETUS – *see* FOETUS

FEVER – *see* PYREXIA

FIBER-OPTICS
A scientific development which is now widely applied and has made the internal examination of the body and its organs relatively simple. A light shone down a rod made of a special type of glass fiber is reflected internally along the rod, with minimal leakage, and illuminates the area at the end of the rod. The light continues to be reflected internally as the rod twists and turns on its passage through the vessels and tubes of the body. By this means many of the organs and passages of the body can be investigated – see *cystoscopy*, *bronchoscopy*, *gastroscopy*.

FIBRILLATION
The uncontrolled and spasmodic contraction of muscle fibers. The term is usually applied to an abnormal contraction of the heart

muscles, in which the heart loses its regular pumping rhythm and contracts, in the classic description, 'like a bag of worms'. Fibrillation most commonly affects the muscles of the *atria* of the heart. Atrial fibrillation is not usually serious, because the heart can still pump blood efficiently. The condition sometimes clears up spontaneously, but more often requires drug therapy. Ventricular fibrillation is much more serious, because if the *ventricles* fail to contract properly very little blood is pumped into the arteries. A lack of oxygenated blood causes *cyanosis* and unconsciousness that may quickly lead to brain damage. This is one of the mechanisms of a *heart attack* and needs immediate . treatment – either by electric shocks or drugs.

FIBROID   102
Benign tumors of *connective* or muscular tissue that are sometimes found in the *uterus*. Fibroids may cause pain, heavy periods and infertility; occasionally they are symptomless. The tumors may need to be removed surgically.

FIBROSITIS – *see* RHEUMATISM

FISSURE
A narrow crack or breech in the normally intact skin or *mucous membrane*. Fissures are most commonly seen in the corners of the mouth in a condition known as angular *stomatitis*, which may be caused by *vitamin* deficiencies, and in the *anus*, where they are called anal fissures. Fissures can be very painful and provide a site for *bacterial* invasion of the tissues.

FISTULA   39
A tunnel-like connection, either between two internal organs or between one organ and the surface of the body. Fistulae may be *congenital* – most commonly between the *rectum* and the *vagina* in a recto-vaginal fistula. They may also be caused by a bursting abscess or be a side-effect of abdominal surgery. Fistulae are sometimes a *complication* of *Crohn's Disease* and usually need to be repaired surgically.

FITS – *see* EPILEPSY

FLAT FEET
Normally the weight of the body is supported on the front and back part of the feet. The arch of the instep does not directly support weight, but adds bounce and spring to the step. In flat feet the arch flattens out, usually because of a loss of muscle tone and a softness of the *ligaments* that support the arch. The condition is normally a result of standing for long periods without actually exercising the muscles and is linked with *obesity*; occasionally flat feet are a sign of poor nutrition. Flat feet, or fallen arches, cause the feet to tire and ache more easily and make walking painful. The condition can be relieved to a certain extent by exercises and the use of artificial arch supports inside the shoe.

FLATULENCE
The presence of gases in the stomach or bowels. Stomach gases are expelled by belching, or eructation; bowel gases are expelled through the *anus* as flatus. Stomach gases sometimes build up from the small amounts of air that are swallowed with food, but some people, especially those who are nervous or who suffer from *dyspepsia*, swallow large amounts of air. This tendency is known as aerophagy. Gases are produced in the bowel as a result of the *bacterial* fermentation of partly digested foods. Some foodstuffs, such as beans, onions and eggs, are more prone to this than others.

FLOATING STOOLS
Stools which have a tendency to float on the surface of the water in the lavatory and smell foul. They have a high content of undigested *fat* and indicate *malabsorption* of food into the body, which may be a sign of *coeliac disease*.

FLOODING   100
A term that is sometimes used to describe very heavy periods, or *menorrhagia*, but also describes a type of behavior therapy in which the patient is 'flooded' with stimuli. Instead of a gentle re-conditioning process over a period of time, the patient is exposed to the most anxiety-provoking situation possible at once. A sufferer from agoraphobia, for example, would be taken to a large supermarket and left on her own.

FLUSHING – *see* BLUSHING

FOETUS (US – Fetus)   98
An unborn baby that is developing inside the *womb*. The foetus is considered to have a legal status as an individual from the 28th week of pregnancy.

FOLIE A DEUX
A condition in which the interaction between two apparently normal people produces a mutual *psychosis*. The term is sometimes used by criminologists to explain otherwise inexplicable homicides. The activities of 'Bonnie and Clyde' are a classic example, but often the patients are sisters.

FONTANELLE
Soft areas between the bones of the skull that allow for growth and the moulding of the baby's head as it is born. There are two main fontanelles – the anterior, which is the larger and can be felt as a soft patch on the top of the baby's head, and the smaller posterior fontanelle at the back of the head. The fontanelles disappear as the baby grows; the soft areas become bony and knit together with the other bones of the skull.

FOOD POISONING
An acute illness characterized by abdominal pains, stomach cramps, vomiting and diarrhoea which follows the consumption of contaminated food. The food may be contaminated by *bacteria* or by toxic chemicals; depending on the cause of contamination symptoms appear anything from one to 24 hours after eating. Sometimes food poisoning is caused by the *toxins* that the bacteria produce and by cooked meats that have been incorrectly canned – see *salmonella*.

FORAMEN OVALE
A hole between the left and right *atria* of the *foetal* heart which allows blood to flow from one atrium to the other. The foramen ovale usually closes at or soon after birth, as part of the change from the foetal circulation that is linked to the mother to the baby's independent circulation. Sometimes it does not close off completely, and the baby is said to have a 'hole in the heart'. The hole causes a characteristic cardiac *murmur* and may require surgical treatment.

FRACTURE
A break in a bone. In a simple fracture the break is clean and the

skin remains intact; in a compound fracture there is a wound that leads to the skin, or parts of bone actually project through the skin. In a complicated fracture the broken bone interferes with an internal organ, while in a comminuted fracture the bone is broken into a number of pieces. A fracture is usually the result of direct pressure on the bone, but sometimes a result of indirect pressure. In children, whose bones are soft, the bone may bend rather than snap – this is called a greenstick fracture. Fractures are a common hazard of old age, when bones become increasingly brittle.

FREE ASSOCIATION
A technique used in psychoanalysis in which the patient speaks his thoughts out loud as soon as they come into his head,

FREQUENCY – *see* MICTURITION

FREUDIAN
A branch of psychiatry based on the teachings of the Austrian psychoanalyst Sigmund Freud (1856–1939). Freud stressed the existence of the subconscious mind, the importance of dreams, the effect of subconscious drives, motivations and taboos on behavior and the importance of childhood experiences associated with sex on later life. Freud believed that the liberation of subconscious motivations through *psychoanalysis* could cure *neurosis*.

FRIGIDITY
A lack of sexual desire and inability to reach *orgasm* in women. Frigidity may be caused by a number of factors. Everyday stresses and strains may result in a lack of libido, or relative frigidity, while physical pain on intercourse, called *dyspareunia*, may lead to frigidity if untreated. Other causes include a fear of becoming pregnant in unmarried women who have no form of *contraception* and a generalized illness and lethargy, in which the sufferer does not feel like doing anything – let alone having intercourse. Usually frigidity has a *psychogenic* cause – this is a cause that is in the mind rather than the body – which often responds to *psychosexual counselling*.

FUGUE
A mental state in which the sufferer is separated both mentally and physically from his normal environment. It is associated with *hysteria* and some mental diseases.

FUNCTIONAL
Diseases are called 'functional' when they are *psychosomatic* or due to emotional factors rather than physical illness.

FURUNCLE
A *boil*. Furunculosis is a condition in which a number of boils occur together and is normally the result of a *bacterial* infection. It is treated with *antibiotics*, as well as local creams and dressings.

GALL BLADDER 43
A three to four inch long pear-shaped sac in which *bile* is stored. The gall bladder lies underneath the *liver* on the right side of the body; it receives bile from the liver through the hepatic duct and delivers it to the duodenum through the common bile duct. The most common problems affecting the gall bladder are *cholecystitis* and *gallstones*.

GALLSTONES 43
Hard masses, generally composed of *cholesterol*, *bile* and *protein*, that may form in the gall bladder. Gallstones sometimes cause no pain at all, but when they block the bile duct – often in association with *cholecystitis* – the severe pain of gallstone colic may be felt. This can be one of the most crippling forms of *abdominal pain*; it may radiate to the back and the right shoulder. The condition can be treated surgically by a cholecystectomy.

GANGRENE
The death of tissue in part of the body when its blood supply is interrupted – for example by an *embolism* or a wound. The affected part mav stay dry and mummify, i.e. turn black and fall off, or become wet and putrify.

GAS GANGRENE
A serious infection of a wound by gas-forming *bacteria* called clostridia, which are found in the soil. The bacteria thrive where there is little oxygen and so tend to infect deep wounds that have a poor blood supply. Gas is formed as part of the decomposition process that spreads along the tissue planes of the body. The condition is treated by strict cleansing of the wound to admit air to the site of infection and by *antibiotics*, but sometimes amputation of the affected part is necessary. Oxygen under high pressure can also be used, as well as gas gangrene antitoxins.

GASTRECTOMY 45,56
An operation in which either part or all of the stomach is removed. A gastrectomy is sometimes performed when all other treatment has failed to cure a *gastric ulcer*, or in *cancer* of the stomach. After the operation the patient has to eat small meals very frequently, because the remainder of the intestines cannot cope with large masses of food.

GASTRIC ULCER 45
An *ulcer* in the stomach that causes a gnawing pain, especially after a meal. The ulcer, which is a break in the *mucous membrane* that lines the organ, may also cause vomiting and bleeding – which makes the *stools* appear black and tarry – see *melena*. The condition may be relieved by antacids, but surgery is sometimes necessary.

GASTRITIS 45
An inflammation of the stomach that may result from an excess of alcohol or irritant foods and can cause *vomiting*. In some forms of gastritis the lining of the stomach *atrophies*, sometimes as a result of drugs or *stress*, and *gastric ulcers* form.

GASTROENTERITIS 54
Vomiting and *diarrhoea* as a result of a *bacterial* or *viral* infection of the stomach and intestines, or of food poisoning. The problem usually clears up after a few days, but it may be necessary to replace any fluid loss, especially if small children are affected.

GENES
The basic units of *hereditary* information that are carried on the *chromosomes*. A gene is made up of a substance called D.N.A. (Deoxyribonucleic acid) which is arranged in a double helix. The arrangement of the genes is called the

genetic code; this reproduces itself exactly in the process of cell division, so that every cell in the body contains the same genetic code.

When the *sperm* fertilizes the *ovum* in the reproductive process two genetic codes are brought together. The eventual genetic information carried by the baby depends to a certain extent on the character of the genes – dominant genes are always carried from parent to child; recessive genes only pass on their characteristics if they are present with another recessive gene. Very occasionally a part of the code is deleted or changed in a genetic mutation. This is thought to be the mechanism by which new species evolve.

The theory of genetics is often used in medicine in the investigation of diseases that are hereditary.

GERMAN MEASLES – *see* RUBELLA

GINGIVITIS
An inflammation of the gums. Gingivitis is most commonly a sign of poor dental hygiene, but may be a result of *vitamin* deficiencies.

GLAND   144
An organ or group of cells that produces a *hormone* or other secretion. There are a huge number of glands in the body, but generally hormones are produced by the endocrine, or ductless glands while exocrine glands secrete *mucous* and *serous* substances through ducts.

GLANDULAR FEVER (US – Infectious Mononucleosis)   158
An acute infectious disease, thought to be caused by a *virus*, that affects the *lymph* nodes and *spleen*, making them swollen and sore. Other symptoms are a *fever*, headache and *anorexia* and an overproduction of special 'mononuclear' *leucocytes* that can be detected in a blood test. Often liver function is also impaired and *hepatitis* may be seen. There is no specific treatment for glandular fever. The symptoms may persist for several weeks.

GLAUCOMA   126
A serious eye condition in which the pressure of the fluid within the eye is raised so that the eye becomes red, painful and may eventually lose its sight. Glaucoma is treated by the reduction of the fluid pressure, either by drugs or by surgery.

GLOMERULONEPHRITIS
An infection of the glomeruli of the *kidney*. The glomeruli are clusters of blood *capillaries* surrounded by renal tubules at which filtration of wastes from the blood takes place. The cause of glomerulonephritis is unknown, but the infection often follows conditions of the upper *respiratory tract* and may cause *haematuria*, *proteinuria*, *hypertension* and sometimes *convulsions* and *coma*.

GLUCOSE (US – Dextrose)   146
A sugar that is manufactured by the body from ingested *carbohydrates* during digestion. Glucose is an important source of energy for the body; it can be converted to carbon dioxide and water, to *fat* or stored in the *liver* and muscles as glycogen. The level of glucose in the blood is controlled by the *hormone insulin*; when too much or too little insulin is produced the blood glucose level changes in either *hypoglycaemia* or *hyperglycaemia* respectively, the latter being a symptom of *diabetes*.

Deficiencies in glucose *metabolism* can be dangerous, because the nervous system and the brain are especially dependent on glucose as a source of energy. Glucose metabolism can be investigated in the glucose tolerance test, in which the blood glucose level over a period of time is measured after a known quantity of glucose has been administered.

GOITRE   149
A swelling of the *thyroid* gland in the neck. Goitre is normally caused by a deficiency of iodine in the diet. Iodine is important in the production of the thyroid *hormone*; when less of the hormone than normal is being produced the *pituitary gland* tries to stimulate the thyroid gland, thus increasing its size. The thyroid gland may also become swollen as a result of infection, over-activity – as in *thyrotoxicosis* – or a *tumor*. Goitre is seen in association with *exophthalmos* in a condition called Graves' Disease.

GONAD
The reproductive glands that produce the cells, or gammetes, that are necessary for sexual reproduction. In the male the gonads are the *testes*, which produce *sperm*; in the female they are the *ovaries*, which produce the *ova*, or eggs.

GONORRHOEA (US – Gonorrhea)   94
A *venereal disease* that is transmitted by sexual contact, gonorrhoea is an infection of the *mucous membranes* of the genital tract that may cause a yellow discharge and frequent, painful urination. In women the disease may only cause minor symptoms, or in some cases no symptoms at all. If untreated gonorrhoea may cause complications such as *arthritis* and *endocarditis*, and may lead to *infertility*. The condition is treated by penicillin and *antibiotics*.

GORGE-PURGE SYNDROME – *see* BULIMIA NERVOSA

GRAFT
A piece of tissue that is used to replace another piece of tissue that is diseased or misfunctioning. The most common type of graft is a skin graft, where a piece of skin is taken, normally from the upper thigh, and used as a replacement for an area of skin that has been burnt or scarred. Bone grafts are less common, but sometimes small chips of bone are grafted onto existing bone to strengthen it. The corneas of recently dead donors can be transplated to a damaged cornea to restore vision in a corneal graft. For organ grafts see *transplantation*.

GRAND MAL – *see* EPILEPSY

GRAVES' DISEASE – *see* THYROTOXICOSIS

GRIEF
A normal response to bereavement and personal misfortune. In some societies grief is formalized into elaborate ceremonial; in western society it is usually sustained more quietly, but nevertheless plays an important role in the psychological adjustment to bereavement.

GRIPE
An intermittent but severe type of colicky *abdominal pain* that is often caused by wind in babies.

GROIN ITCH – *see* TINEA CRURIS

GROIN PAIN   34,48,52
A pain in the groin may have a number of causes. A femoral or inguinal *hernia* causes groin pain, especially on straining. Sometimes an *abscess* develops in the psoas

muscle that helps to flex the hip joint and is associated with *tendinitis*, an inflammation of the muscle tendon. This is particularly a problem for athletes; in professional athletes the pubic symphisis, at which the two pubic bones join, may also become strained and weakened and so cause groin pain. *Appendicitis* pain is sometimes felt in the right groin, while *diverticulitis* occasionally causes pain in the left groin.

GROUP THERAPY

A form of *psychotherapy* in which there are a number of participants who all discuss and analyse their problems. The various members of the group interact, and stimulate discussion and sometimes conflict with each other. This form of psychotherapy is particularly useful in the treatment of problems such as *alcoholism*. The same group usually meets regularly over a long period of time.

GUTHRIE TEST

A simple blood test performed on all new babies to test for the metabolic disease *phenylketonuria*.

GYNAECOMASTIA (US – Gynecomastia)   146

The growth of breasts in a man, which may be caused by abnormalities of the *endocrine* glands, including *diabetes* mellitus and *acromegaly*; *Klinefelter's Syndrome*; *cirrhosis* of the *liver*; *carcinoma*; or drugs such as digitalis or artificial sex *hormones*.

H

HAEMATOMA (US – Hematoma)

An accumulation of blood resulting from an injury or operation – almost an internal bruise. A haematoma may develop after a head injury when blood accumulates underneath the dura, one of the *meninges* of the brain. This is called a subdural haematoma, and may be dangerous unless treated surgically.

HAEMATURIA   96

The presence of blood in the *urine*, which may have a number of causes – including trauma to the *kidneys*; a kidney stone; *carcinoma* or *papilloma* of the *bladder*; an enlarged or cancerous prostate gland; infectious

glomerulonephritis; renal T.B.; *cancer* involving the kidneys; or *polyarteritis nodosa*. Small amounts of blood in the urine can only be detected with a microscope, but large quantities make the urine smoky and red.

HAEMOGLOBIN (US– Hemoglobin)

A substance composed of a pigment and a *protein* that is carried by the red blood cells, or *erythrocytes*, and is the medium by which oxygen is transported in the blood.

HAEMOLYTIC DISEASE OF THE NEWBORN (US – Hemolytic Disease of the Newborn)   162

A condition in which a Rhesus blood group mismatch between mother and child leads to the destruction of the baby's red blood cells, called haemolysis. The haemolysis causes *anaemia*, *jaundice* and *kernicterus*. The problem is usually detected before birth – see *Rhesus Factors*. Sometimes an exchange transfusion is necessary, in which the blood of the baby is completely changed. The condition is also known as Icterus Gravis Neonaturum or Erythroblastosis Foetalis.

HAEMOPHILIA (US – Hemophilia)

A disorder of the blood clotting process which is caused by a deficiency in one of the necessary factors – see *blood clotting*. The disease, which is *hereditary*, is carried by women, who are not themselves affected. Though actual wounds can usually be avoided, blood is continually lost into the skin and tissues as a result of minor bumps and knocks. Haemophilia can be treated by the administration of the missing factor, which is purified from donated blood, and sufferers can live a long and fairly normal life – though contact sports are inadvisable.

HAEMORRHAGE (US – Hemorrhage)   45,84

Loss of blood from a blood vessel. A haemorrhage may be caused by external trauma or wound, gastric or intestinal *ulceration*, a ruptured *aneurysm*, *blood clotting* diseases or drugs. When a large amount of blood is lost the *blood pressure* drops, consciousness is lost and eventually the victim may die unless the blood is replaced. It is often difficult to diagnose the prob-

lem when bleeding is internal – for example when a *Fallopian Tube* ruptures in an *ectopic* pregnancy – but the sufferer is cold and sweaty, and in some pain, with a rapid pulse, and a low blood pressure.

HAEMORRHOIDS (US – Hemorrhoids)   77

Otherwise called piles, haemorrhoids are large *varicose veins* found in the *rectum* which tend to occur in middle age and are often associated with constipation. Sometimes they are seen for the first time during pregnancy.

Generally, uncomplicated piles are treated with special soothing creams and suppositories, though the sufferer must make sure that he avoids constipation. When these remedies fail the piles may be injected with a substance that thromboses them; if this is unsuccessful they may be removed in a surgical operation.

HAIR LOSS

A loss of between 60 and 100 hairs from the head each day is quite normal, but when hair loss becomes excessive the condition is known as *alopecia*.

HALITOSIS

Bad breath. The most common cause of halitosis is poor dental hygiene, leading to decaying teeth and gum disease, but constipation may also cause bad breath. More serious causes of the problem are *chronic suppurative* diseases of the lungs and *liver* disease.

HALLUCINATION   140

A false sensation that may be visualized, tasted, smelt or heard. Hallucinations can be caused by the hallucinogenic drugs (such as L.S.D.) or may occur in illnesses such as *schizophrenia*, where they are often of the auditory type. Hallucinations also sometimes accompany *epilepsy* when it involves the temporal lobe of the brain.

HARE LIP

A *congenital* abnormality, sometimes associated with a *cleft palate*, in which there is a defect in the upper lip. A hare lip may be relatively minor and cause no problems other than through its unsightliness; when more severe it may interfere with eating. The defect is normally repaired surgically during childhood, usually with good cosmetic effects.

HAY FEVER   30

Sometimes called pollen *asthma*, hay fever is an *allergic* response to pollen.

Sufferers are normally allergic to the pollen of grasses and trees and to the spores of fungi. Pollen acts as an *allergen*, and the allergic reactions include runny eyes, a snuffly nose and sometimes wheezing and shortness of breath. The most effective treatment is to avoid pollen, but *antihistamine* and other drugs may help to relieve the problem. Sometimes courses of injections are given to try and desensitize the sufferer to the pollen to which he is allergic.

HEADACHE   28,70,138

An ache or pain felt within the skull that may have a number of causes. The commonest type of headache is associated with tenseness of the muscles of the head and neck and is called a tension headache. A headache may be caused by 'eye strain' and indicate a need for glasses – or just that the sufferer has been reading for too long in a poor light. Sometimes *sinusitis* causes a headache; typically the sufferer wakes up feeling congested as well as having a headache.

In *migraine* a headache is associated with visual disturbances and sometimes vomiting, while *meningitis* causes a severe headache together with a stiff neck, *photophobia* and *earache*. Rarely, a headache is a sign of a brain *tumor* or *abscess* – but this is one of the least common causes of the condition.

Various drugs may give rise to a headache, in particular G.T.N. (Glycerol Trinitrate), which is given to relieve *angina*. A headache may also be a result of high blood pressure, but it is normally relieved when the condition is treated. A fairly serious cause of a headache in one side of the head in the elderly is temporal *arteritis*, an inflammation of the temporal artery. It is associated with a very high E.S.R. and if not treated, usually by *steroid* drugs, may lead to blindness.

A headache may be an expression of a *psychogenic* disorder, ranging from *depression* to *hysteria*; it is also common after a head injury, with or without a skull fracture or *concussion*.

HEAF TEST

A skin test used to determine whether a child has any resistance to *tuberculosis*. Small pricks are made in the skin and a small quantity of purified tuberculin is introduced. A week later a small ring of red dots shows that the body does have resistance to T.B.; if there is no reaction the child will be vaccinated against the disease.

HEART   74

A muscular organ lying beneath the chest wall. The top of the heart is immediately underneath the breastbone at the level of the second rib and the bulk of the organ extends about 3 ins. (7.5 cms.) to the left of the breastbone, down to the level of the fifth rib.

The heart muscle, or *myocardium*, beats on average about 72 times a minute throughout life to pump blood through the *circulatory system*. The organ is divided into two sides – the right and the left – by a wall, or septum, and each side is subdivided into an *atrium* and *ventricle*. The left atrium is divided from the left ventricle by the bicuspid, or *mitral*, valve; the corresponding valve on the right side of the heart is known as the tricuspid valve – see *heart failure, myocardial infarct, ischaemic heart disease, valvular heart disease, arrhythmia, fibrillation, murmur.*

HEARTBURN – *see* PYROSIS

HEART FAILURE

Heart failure does not, as the term implies, mean that the heart has ceased to beat. The condition is normally secondary to *hypertension* or *ischaemic* heart disease and can best be described in two parts. In right-sided heart failure the right side of the heart does not pump efficiently and the resultant back pressure means that *venous* return is held up. Fluid tends to stagnate in various parts of the body, leading to *oedema*, especially in the ankles and lower back.

Left-sided heart failure is caused by the inadequate pumping of the left *ventricle*. As the pressure builds up blood tends to accumulate in the lungs and *serous* fluid seeps out of the blood vessels to cause pulmonary oedema, leading to severe shortness of breath and sometimes *cyanosis*.

Heart failure is primarily treated

by diuretic drugs which increase the flow of urine and so help to remove the excess fluid. Digitalis is sometimes used to increase the strength of contraction of the heart muscles.

HEMATOMA – *see* HAEMATOMA

HEMIPLEGIA

A *paralysis* of half the body that usually results from a *stroke* or *cardiovascular accident*. The arm and the leg on the affected side are very weak and ineffective – though this may improve with time and *physiotherapy*. Speech may be lost altogether or become slurred, and the sufferer often has difficulty in finding the right word to express himself. After an initial period of bed-rest the patient is mobilized and *physiotherapy*, speech and *occupational therapies* are used to improve his condition and help him.

HEMOGLOBIN – *see* HAEMOGLOBIN

HEMOLYTIC – *see* HAEMOLYTIC

HEMORRHAGE – *see* HAEMORRHAGE

HEMORRHOIDS – *see* HAEMORRHOIDS

HEPATITIS

A *viral* infection of the *liver* that causes inflammation of the organ and results in *jaundice*. Infectious hepatitis has an incubation period of 15 to 40 days and is spread by *faecal* contamination of food or drink. Serum hepatitis is spread through contact with the blood or blood products of a carrier – who may not himself be affected by the disease. It is common among drug addicts and has a much longer incubation period, which can be from 30 days to about four months.

Sufferers from hepatitis are usually yellow, from jaundice, feel very ill and have a fever associated with headaches, vomiting and sometimes pains in the joints. Serum hepatitis can be fatal, and a small proportion of those with the disease die. Because of the liver damage caused by the disease it is important to abstain completely from alcohol for at least three months.

HEREDITY

The mechanism by which some

physical, mental and behavioral characteristics are handed down from parents to their children. The basic unit of heredity is the *gene*.

HERNIA   48,50
The protrusion of an organ or tissue through the tissue that normally bounds it. The commonest form of hernia is an inguinal hernia in the groin, where a weakness of the muscle layers allows the underlying bowel or fat to protrude through them. An inguinal hernia may be treated by the use of a truss or by surgery.

An umbilical hernia is sometimes seen in young babies – especially African or West Indian children – where the abdominal contents bulge out around the navel. The condition usually rights itself within a few years, but if it persists, or is distressing for the mother and child, it may be repaired surgically – see *hiatus hernia.*

HERPES   68
A common *virus* of the chicken pox family, which can occur in three distinct forms. Herpes simplex, or cold sores, are the common lesions that appear around the mouth and in the nose in association with colds and viral illnesses. Although uncomfortable and unsightly they are not normally dangerous and there is no really effective treatment for them.

Herpes zoster, or shingles, is a painful condition in which red spots erupt over the body – usually in a band that starts under the armpit and swings across the chest, though sometimes the face is affected. The spots follow the course of a nerve, because the virus attacks the nerve's point of origin at the spinal cord, and normally last for a few weeks before subsiding. When the face is the major site for the spots the problem may be more serious and eyesight may be affected. After the spots have disappeared there may still be some pain, which is called post-herpetic *neuralgia.* Herpes Zoster usually affects older people who have had chicken pox during childhood; children who come into contact with shingles occasionally develop chickenpox - see *varicella.*

Herpes genitalia shows itself as a collection of small blisters on the genitalia which may affect the *cervix* and cause pain on inter-

course. The condition may appear and disappear spontaneously and is difficult to treat.

HETEROSEXUAL
A person who has sexual feelings that are directed exclusively towards members of the opposite sex.

HIATUS HERNIA   50
A type of *hernia* in which a portion of the stomach protrudes through a gap in the *diaphragm*. A hiatus hernia can cause *oesophageal regurgitation* and *heartburn*; the symptoms become more severe when the sufferer is bending down or lying flat. The condition is seen more often in women than in men, is associated with age and is treated by drugs, rest and support, though an operation may be necessary.

HICCOUGH   52,132
A condition in which the *diaphragm* gets out of step with the epiglottis, the cartilage that closes off the windpipe during swallowing. The result is a spasmodic and repeated cough as breath is being taken in. Hiccoughs are normally harmless, and the result of indigestion, over-eating, wind or faulty swallowing. Occasionally they are indicative of more serious disorders such as *pleurisy, appendicitis, liver, kidney* or brain disease, or *alcoholism.* Hiccoughs in babies, especially after food, are quite normal and no attempt should be made to stop them.

HIP REPLACEMENT   112
An operation in which the head of the femur, the long bone of the thigh, is replaced by an artificial part made of metal or strong polythene. The technique may be used when *arthritis* or another disease, or a serious fracture following a fall, has made use of the joint impossible.

HIRSUTISM
The excessive growth of hair, especially in unusual places, which sometimes affects women and may run in families. Generally, the cause is not known, but sometimes the condition is due to a *hormonal* imbalance, or glandular disease or certain drugs.

HOARSENESS   24,153
A soreness of the throat associated with a partial or complete loss of

voice. Hoarseness is normally the result of over-use of the voice, for example as in shouting at a football game. Sometimes hoarseness is caused by *laryngitis,* and very occasionally by growths on the vocal cords or an increasing coarseness of the cords in *myxoedema.* The growths may be caused by *cancer* or by harmless growths, but should always be investigated, especially if the hoarseness is persistent.

HODGKIN'S DISEASE
Also called lymphadenoma. Hodgkin's Disease is a malignant disease of unknown cause in which the *lymph* nodes become progressively enlarged; the *spleen* and *liver* are also involved. The condition causes a characteristic sporadic fever, weight loss, night sweats and itching. In the early stages *radiotherapy* may be a successful form of treatment; later on the condition is treated by drugs, radiotherapy and sometimes surgical removal of the spleen or splenectomy.

HOLE IN THE HEART – *see* FORAMEN OVALE

HOMEOPATHY
A system of medicine in which extremely small quantities of those drugs that produce the same symptoms as a disease are used to treat that disease.

HOMOSEXUAL
A person who has sexual feelings that are exclusively directed towards members of his or her own sex. Female homosexuals are known as lesbians.

HORMONE   144
A substance produced by an *endocrine gland* that is secreted into the bloodstream and then circulates throughout the body to have its main effect at some distance from the original gland. Hormones are chemical messengers which stimulate activity in the tissues, organs and sometimes other glands of the body – see *testosterone, androgen, oestrogen, insulin, progesterone, adrenaline.*

HUNTINGDON'S CHOREA
A type of *chorea* associated with *dementia* that is hereditary and usually attacks between the ages of 30 and 50. The disease is progressive and incurable.

HYDRAMNIOS

An excess of amniotic fluid during pregnancy. Amniotic fluid surrounds the developing *foetus* inside the amniotic sac in the womb, and in hydramnios the pregnant woman seems to be larger than expected and becomes breathless and may develop *varicose veins*. The condition is commonly associated with twins.

HYDRONEPHROSIS

A condition in which the *kidney* becomes distended with fluid because of an obstruction to the flow of urine away from it, often a stone in the *ureter* or an enlarged *prostate* gland. It is usually necessary to remove the cause of the blockage surgically, before permanent damage has been done to the kidney.

HYMEN

A fold of membrane that covers the entrance to the *vagina*. The hymen usually perforates before puberty, but if the perforation is small it may tear the first time sexual intercourse is attempted. Occasionally the hymen is too strong and needs to be removed by a doctor.

HYPERGLYCAEMIA (US – Hyperglycemia) 146

An increase of the level of sugar in the blood. Hyperglycaemia is a product of *diabetes* mellitus, in which a deficiency in the supply of the hormone *insulin* from the *pancreas* removes the limiting controls on sugar in the blood. The condition causes dehydration and may eventually result in *coma*; it can be relieved by the administration of fluids and insulin.

HYPERHIDROSIS 153

Excessive sweating. An overactivity of the sweat glands may be caused by fevers, drugs or diseases such as *thyrotoxicosis*. Occasionally the condition is so severe that an operation is necessary, in which sweat glands are removed or their activity reduced.

HYPERTENSION

High *blood pressure*. Hypertension may be caused temporarily by emotions such as anger, but when it is permanent there may be a number of reasons for it. Sometimes hypertension is a product of *endocrine gland* disorders, particularly of the adrenal glands as in *Cushing's Disease* or a type of adrenal gland *tumor* called a *phaeochromocytoma*. The condition may also be caused by a coarctation, or narrowing, of the *aorta*, or a *stenosis* of the renal artery.

The most common form of hypertension is called essential hypertension. It is *idiopathic* – that is, its cause is unknown. The condition is to an extent *hereditary*, is more common in males and rarely seen under the age of 40. Essential hypertension is associated with *arteriosclerosis* and often leads to strokes and heart attacks, but can be treated with hypotensive drugs that lower the blood pressure.

HYPERTHYROIDISM – *see* THYROTOXICOSIS

HYPNOSIS

A trance-like state that is induced by a trained therapist or hypnotist. The technique is sometimes used in medicine in psychotherapy and for the treatment of drug addiction.

HYPOCHONDRIA 138

A condition in which an individual is abnormally preoccupied with his health and is constantly becoming convinced that he is the victim of disease. Hypochondria may be associated with underlying *depression* and is extremely difficult to treat.

HYPOGLYCAEMIA (US – Hypoglycemia) 146

A lack of sugar in the blood, that is usually seen in *diabetics* who have had too little to eat or have given themselves too much *insulin*. Hypoglycaemia causes an abrupt onset of sweating, weakness, dizziness and nervousness, with eventual loss of consciousness and *coma*. Diabetics in this condition must be given sugar – either by mouth, if they are still conscious, or intravenously if they are in a coma. A lesser degree of hypoglycaemia is sometimes seen after fasting or in severe hunger; it can be checked by drinking a glass of milk or by eating food.

HYPOMANIA – *see* MANIA

HYPOTENSION

Low blood pressure. Hypotension is seen after a *haemorrhage*, a heart attack or a pulmonary *embolism* and may be seen in untreated Addison's Disease. The blood pressure is also lower than normal during pregnancy.

HYPOTHALAMUS

The part of the forebrain that is responsible for control of primitive functions of the body such as water balance, *carbohydrate* and *fat metabolism*, sleep, body temperature, hunger, thirst and sexual activity. It also acts as a center for integrating nervous and hormonal functions.

HYPOTHERMIA

A condition in which body temperature is well below normal. In babies and old people especially, a lack of adequate heating and clothing may lead to severe hypothermia that can cause *coma* and eventually death.

The term is also used to describe a surgical technique in which body temperature is deliberately lowered in order to reduce the body's oxygen requirements so the blood vessels can be clamped off for a longer period than would otherwise be safe.

HYPOTHYROIDISM – *see* MYXOEDEMA, GOITRE

HYSTERECTOMY 102,106

The surgical removal of the womb, or *uterus*, that is normally performed because of *fibroids* or *cancer* of the *cervix* or uterus itself. The operation may be total – when the whole womb is removed – or subtotal – when the neck of the womb, or cervix, is left. In either case, after recovery from the operation the woman should be able to enjoy a normal sex life; she will not, however, have any more periods, or be able to have any more children.

HYSTERIA

Contrary to its popular usage, hysteria when used in a medical sense, refers to a neurotic condition in which the nervous system overreacts to stress by converting normal emotions into bodily symptoms that mimic those of organic disease. The symptoms may range from loss of sensation to derangement of joints, *paralysis*, and blindness – though more commonly they include aches and pains, dizziness, fainting and palpitations. Although hysteria is more common in women (the term is derived from the Greek word for the womb), it affects both sexes, especially during adolescence.

I

IATROGENIC DISEASE

Any disease or condition that is induced by medical treatment. The side-effects of drugs, for example, may occasionally be worse than the original problem that they were given to combat.

ID

A term used in psychoanalysis to denote the subconscious mind, containing the primitive and instinctive drives that relate to birth, life and death. Through the mediation of the *ego*, or conscious mind, the potentially violent forces of the id are balanced by the *super-ego*, or moral conscience.

ILEOSTOMY   37,39,41

An operation in which the ileum is joined to a hole, or *stoma*, in the abdominal wall so that the contents of the ileum may be excreted and collected in a bag that is attached to the stoma. An ileostomy may be performed to allow the colon to rest, following severe *colitis* or in *Crohn's Disease*; it may also be necessary if the colon has been damaged by a wound or parts of it have been removed following *cancer* of the *colon*.

IMMUNITY

The body's resistance to disease. When an *antigen* is recognized by the body *antibodies* are produced to combat it, in an immune reaction. Sometimes the antibodies are already present in the body – this is called natural immunity, where certain animals and races have an inbuilt resistance to some diseases or poisons.

Immunity may be acquired naturally when the body retains its ability to produce antibodies after a disease has passed; this condition can be artificially induced in *immunization*. A temporary immunity can be achieved by an injection of *blood serum* taken from a person who is already immune, because the antibodies that are needed will be present. In the same way new-born babies are immune to a number of conditions because they have received antibodies from the maternal blood, but this immunity does not last longer than a few weeks.

IMMUNIZATION

A process in which protection against disease, or *immunity*, is given by means of *vaccination*, or inoculation. The vaccine, which is usually given by injection, consists of small quantities of live or specially treated *viruses* or toxins; it sets up a reaction within the body in which antibodies specific to the micro-organism are produced, providing resistance against the diseases that this causes. Immunization is commonly performed against diseases such as *diphtheria*, *tetanus*, *polio*, *pertussis* (or whooping cough), *tuberculosis*, *measles* and *rubella* (or German measles) – the last mainly in the case of young girls so that they do not contract the disease during a pregnancy. Immunization has almost eradicated *smallpox*, and it is nowadays only considered necessary to vaccinate against the disease in special circumstances.

IMPETIGO

A *bacterial* infection of the skin, usually on the face, in which yellow, crusted lesions are formed. The condition is extremely contagious and spreads over the face and to the limbs. Impetigo is usually treated by *antibiotic* creams.

IMPLANTATION

A method of giving drugs, in which pellets of the drug, which is usually a *hormone*, are implanted in the tissue beneath the skin. The pellets release small amounts of the drug into the bloodstream over a period of time. The technique is sometimes used to replace female hormones that may be lost after a *hysterectomy* that removes the *ovaries* as well as the *womb*.

IMPOTENCE   132,146

A male inability to achieve complete sexual intercourse. Sometimes the impotent man may be able to have and sustain an erection but be unable to ejaculate; commonly he ejaculates prematurely; sometimes he is unable to maintain an erection. Impotence can be caused by physical diseases, such as *alcoholism*, *neuropathy*, *liver disease*, *diabetes* and spinal injuries; more commonly it has psychological causes and is treated by *psychosexual therapy*.

INCONTINENCE   60

Dribbling of *urine* or leakage of *faeces*. Some degree of urine incontinence is fairly common in the elderly, who may lose tone in the *perineal muscles* that control urination; the condition is also sometimes seen after some gynaecological operations and as a consequence of *prolapse* of the womb. Incontinence may be seen in women after childbirth whose pelvic muscles have been weakened and also as a result of spinal injuries or advanced multiple sclerosis where the nerves of the *bladder* are damaged. Incontinence during the night is called *enuresis*.

INCUBATION PERIOD   17

The time between the contraction of an illness and the appearance of the first symptoms. Some diseases have very long incubation periods – serum *hepatitis* may become evident up to six months after it has been contracted, and *leprosy* five years afterwards. Different infections have different and characteristic incubation periods, for example *influenza* takes two to four days, and *measles* 12 to 14 days.

INDIGESTION – *see* DYSPEPSIA

INFANTILISM

The retention during adulthood of childlike physical and mental attributes. The term is commonly used to denote a problem in which the sexual organs remain small and childlike even after puberty. Infantilism may be caused by *gland* disorders or sometimes associated with *chronic* disease – see *dwarfism*.

INFARCTION

A term used to describe the changes in tissue when the blood supply to it is cut off – usually by a blood clot, or *thrombus*. The word is commonly used to describe the consequences of a coronary thrombosis – a *myocardial infarction*.

INFECTION

A general term that describes the acquisition of certain types of illness which can be spread from person to person. Infections are normally caused by an invasion of the body by *bacteria* or *viruses*, but may be due to other micro-organisms such as *parasites* or fungi. (An infection by lice or worms is sometimes called an 'infestation'.)

An infection can be contracted in several different ways – by direct contact, as in a kiss from a person with a cold or *influenza*; by the oral-faecal route, in which an infective agent is excreted in the *faeces* of a carrier and due to contamination of cutlery or food is ingested by another person, as occurs in diseases such as infective *hepatitis* and *typhoid*; by airborne droplets of saliva that are spread by sneezing or coughing; through a vector, or carrier, such as mosquitoes which carry *malaria* and *yellow fever*; by drinking contaminated fluids, such as water, which may be contaminated by *cholera*, or milk, which may carry bovine *tuberculosis*; by direct contact with animals or animal skins, as in *psittacosis*.

Infection may be prevented in several ways – by *immunizing* a population against diseases, as has been done with great success against *smallpox*; by keeping infected people in isolation, or quarantine; by disinfecting clothes, crockery etc.; by the control of vectors such as mosquitoes.

INFERTILITY
An inability to conceive and reproduce. In man infertility may be caused either by a lack of sufficient quantities of *sperms* or a defect in them. In women the condition may be due to an abnormality or disease of the *uterus*, a defect in the mechanism of *ovulation* or an infection that has resulted in a blockage of the *Fallopian tubes*. There are a number of techniques which can increase the likelihood of conception if the problem is not caused by disease; if a couple cannot conceive because of male infertility *artificial insemination* may be considered.

INFLAMMATION
A tissue reaction to infection or injury in which the affected area becomes red and swollen, the inflammatory response involves *dilation* of the local blood vessels and the passage to them of white blood cells, or *leucocytes*, to fight the infection.

INFLUENZA   17
Commonly called 'flu', influenza is an illness caused by a group of *viruses* which is characterized by symptoms of the upper *respiratory tract*, *fever*, headache and muscular aches and pains. Influenza typically occurs in an *epidemic* during the winter and has a short *incubation*

period of two to four days. The disease normally lasts for about a week and then passes, though there may be periods of malaise and depression for a few more weeks. Complications of influenza may include broncho-*pneumonia*, usually as a result of a secondary infection by other viruses or *bacteria*. There is a common misconception that influenza can be treated by *antibiotics*. This is not so; antibiotics are only effective against bacterial infections, and influenza is a viral infection. In fact there is no effective treatment for influenza, and doctors concentrate on relieving the symptoms of the disease rather than curing it.

Occasionally a very severe outbreak of influenza may be responsible for a number of deaths, especially of elderly and infirm people. Nowadays these groups are often offered an injection that confers a degree of *immunity* against the most likely strains of the influenza virus. Unfortunately this has only a limited success, because the strains of virus seem to change nearly every year.

INGUINAL HERNIA – *see* HERNIA

INSOMNIA   130
Sleeplessness – an inability to go to sleep and remain asleep for a normal period of time. Insomnia may be caused by stimulants that have been taken too close to bedtime, such as coffee or tea, and by physical disease, but the most common causes of insomnia are anxiety, stress and *psychological problems*.

INSULIN   146
A hormone secreted by the *pancreas* that controls the level of sugar in the blood. Insulin is either deficient or entirely absent in *diabetes*; those affected with the disease have to take tablets to top up their level of naturally occurring insulin, or administer purified pork or beef insulin by injection. Insulin cannot be taken by mouth as it is a *protein*, and would be digested in the *alimentary tract*. An overdose of insulin causes *hypoglycaemia*, while too little insulin causes *hyperglycaemia*.

INTESTINE   32,37,39,54
Commonly called the gut, the intestines are the coils of bowel inside

the abdomen in which the major part of the digestion of foods takes place. The small intestine consists of the duodenum, jejunum and ileum; the large intestine of the caecum, *appendix*, colon and *rectum*. The muscular walls of the intestine contract rhythmically to move the bowel contents towards the rectum in a motion known as *peristalsis*. The intestines may become infected and subject to disease in a number of conditions – see *coeliac disease*, *Crohn's disease*, *colitis*, *enteritis*, *gastroenteritis*.

INTRAUTERINE DEVICE (I.U.D.)
A contraceptive device that is fitted inside the *uterus* to prevent pregnancy by causing a small degree of inflammation which kills *sperm* and prevents implantation of any fertilized egg in the uterine wall. I.U.D.s are placed in position by specially trained doctors and may be left there for a period of two years or more, depending on their type.

I.U.D.s, commonly called coils, may on rare occasions cause complications in their users. Very occasionally, the I.U.D. fails and the user becomes pregnant: usually the pregnancy continues normally and the coil is found embedded in the *placenta* after the delivery of the baby. There is a fractionally higher incidence of uterine infection, which may cause *infertility*, in coil users, who may also tend to have heavier periods and *dysmenorrhoea*.

INTRAVENOUS DRIP (I.V. DRIP)
A technique for giving measured quantities of fluid over a period of time direct into the blood stream through a needle that is fixed inside a vein. A drip can be used for *parenteral* feeding, for the controlled administration of drugs, to give saline solutions or *plasma* in cases of severe *haemorrhage* or *shock*, or to give a blood transfusion.

INTROVERT
An individual who is shy and retiring, and more interested in himself than in the outside world – the opposite of *extravert*.

INTUBATION
A procedure in which a tube is passed into the windpipe during general *anaesthesia* or deep unconsciousness – as in a drug overdose -

so that the person can breathe artificially by use of a *ventilator*.

IRIS 120

The colored part of the eye that surrounds the pupil. The iris is always dark blue in new-born babies but may change color later. The iris expands and contracts in response to light stimuli to control the amount of light that enters the eye through the pupil; it may become inflamed in iritis, which is associated with *uveitis*.

ISCHAEMIA (US – Ischemia)

A deficiency in the blood supply to an area of the body. Ischaemia may be caused by *trauma*, by the constriction of a blood vessel or by *thrombosis*; when it affects a limb ischaemia may cause *gangrene*. In the brain or lungs it may cause an area of *infarction* and when there is ischaemia in the muscles of the heart – ischaemic heart disease – the result may be *angina* and possibly a *myocardial infarct*.

ISOMETRICS

Exercises in which a muscle, or group of muscles, is not made to contract but in which the muscle tension is alternately increased and relaxed – for example when the two fists are pushed together in front of the chest.

ITCHING – *see* PRURITUS

J

JAUNDICE

A yellowish coloration of the skin and tissues directly caused by the presence of excessive amounts of *bilirubin*, or bile pigment – one of the breakdown products of *haemoglobin* – in the blood. Jaundice is indirectly caused by *hepatitis*, *gallstones* (where the jaundice is called 'surgical' or 'obstructive') and the excessive breakdown, or haemolysis, of red blood cells. Haemolysis may be caused by poisons, certain micro-organisms and some forms of *anaemia*; haemolytic jaundice is seen when the *liver* becomes unable to cope with the large amounts of bilirubin that the breakdown of the red cells produces. Haemolytic jaundice is treated by removing the cause of the haemolysis – see

haemolytic disease of the newborn.

In babies, especially those born prematurely, the liver is sometimes not sufficiently developed to cope with the normal breakdown of red blood cells. The result is a form of jaundice known as neonatal jaundice, which normally clears up within a few days.

JOINT 110,112

An articulation between two bones. Joints can be classified according to the type of articulation and possible movement. A wide range of movements is possible in the 'moveable' joints, such as the ball and socket joints of the hip and shoulder, the hinge joints of the knee and elbow and the gliding joints of the wrist and ankle. 'Fixed' joints allow no movement – examples are the sutures of the skull and the joints between the three bones of the pelvis.

In a joint the two bones are separated by a layer of *cartilage* and *synovial* membrane while the joint cavity is filled with synovial fluid. These structures reduce the amount of friction between the bones and cut down on 'wear and tear'. Muscles attached to various points on the bones around the joints contract and relax to produce movement through the joint; sometimes the movement is limited to flexion and extension, while in more sophisticated joints rotation is also possible.

Joints may be subject to a number of diseases and problems. A joint may be *dislocated*, or dislodged from its correct articulation, by injury and need to be reduced by manipulation. A *degenerative disease* such as *osteoarthrosis* may cause a loss of joint space, especially in the hip, knees or shoulders. *Rheumatoid arthritis* tends to affect the smaller joints, causing marked swellings and deformities. The joint cavities may also become infected, in *bursitis*; in gout, crystals of uric acid are deposited in a joint, often the joint of the big toe, and cause heat, tenderness and pain. A large number of *viral* illnesses can cause aches and pains in the joints.

JUGULAR

The jugular veins are among the largest in the body; in two paired branches – the internal and external jugular veins – they drain blood from the head and neck. The jugular vein acts as a sort of pressure gauge

and by looking at the level of the column of blood in it the doctor can obtain important information about the activity of the right *atrium*. This pressure is called the J.V.P., or jugular venous pressure, and may be raised in a pulmonary *embolism*.

K

KELOID

An ugly, lumpy form of scar tissue that may form at the site of a surgical incision, wound or burn and is more common in dark-skinned people.

KERATOPLASTY

A replacement of the *cornea* in which clear corneas from recently dead donors are grafted onto the eye.

KERNICTERUS

A potentially dangerous condition in which the *bile* circulating in the blood in *haemolytic disease of the newborn* affects the brain and may cause fits and severe brain damage.

KERNIG'S SIGN

An indication of *meningitis* in which the leg cannot be straightened when the thigh is at an angle of 90 degrees to the body without great pain.

KETONES 147

Chemical compounds that are formed as products of *fat metabolism*. Under normal circumstances sugar rather than fat is metabolized to produce energy. In starvation, however, and some *diabetic* states, fat is metabolized. When this is happening a ketone called acetone can be smelt on the breath as a sweet sickly odour and ketone bodies can be detected in the urine in a condition called ketonurea. Starvation, diabetes mellitus and severe *diarrhoea* and vomiting all cause ketonurea.

KIDNEY 90

A paired organ 4 ins. (10cms.) long that lies against the back wall of the abdomen. The kidneys filter fluid wastes from the blood and excrete them through the *ureters* to the *bladder* in the form of *urine*. Each kidney is made up of thousands of tiny filtration units called nephrons.

In a secondary function the kidneys, or renal glands, secrete a *hormone* called renin that plays a part in the control of *blood pressure*.

The kidneys may become infected in a condition called *pyelonephritis* or *pyelitis*, or distended if the passage of urine is held up – in *hydronephrosis*. Sometimes small deposits of calcium salts or uric acid, which are normally in solution in the urine, lodge in the kidneys and cause considerable pain. They may dissolve of their own accord, but occasionally have to be removed surgically. Kidney damage may be caused by a number of drugs, a persistently high blood pressure, toxins and poisons and some infectious illnesses, such as *malaria*. *Polycystic disease* of the kidney is congenital and may cause kidney damage. When damage to the organs is so severe that they can no longer function, the sufferer is said to be in *renal failure*, and *dialysis* or a kidney *transplant* may be necessary.

KIDNEY FAILURE – *see* RENAL FAILURE

KIDNEY STONE – *see* RENAL CALCULUS

KLINEFELTER'S SYNDROME
A disorder of the *chromosomes*, which instead of being either XX (female) or XY (male) are XXY. Sufferers are usually male in appearance and tall and thin with small *testes* that do not produce *sperm*. Breasts may also be present, in a condition called *gynaecomastia*.

KOPLIK SPOTS
Small bluish-white spots found in the *mucous membrane* of the mouth in *measles*, usually before the normal rash of the disease appears.

KYPHOSIS
A hunched back. The condition can be caused by poor posture and weak muscles, but sometimes it is a symptom of a disease that affects the spine – such as · osteoporosis in which the vertebrae collapse, or *ankylosing spondylitis*, where the joints between the vertebrae fuse to form a rigid deformity. Severe kyphosis may interfere with movements of the chest, and therefore breathing, and may predispose the sufferer to chest infections.

L

LABOUR
The final stages of pregnancy, about 40 weeks after conception, that result in the delivery of the baby. Labour usually starts spontaneously – the first sign is the 'breaking of the waters' when the amniotic sac ruptures to release the amniotic fluid – and is divided into three stages. In the first stage the muscles of the *uterus* contract, causing labour pains, while at the same time the *cervix*, or neck of the womb, widens to allow the baby through. Next, the contractions become stronger, the cervix is fully dilated and the baby's head can be seen just poking through it. The baby is then delivered through the vagina, after much pushing, and the umbilical cord cut.

Occasionally an *episiotomy* is necessary to facilitate this second stage, and sometimes forceps may be needed. In the third stage of labour the *placenta*, or afterbirth, is delivered – the contractions then cease and the uterus returns to its normal size about six weeks later.

There are various ways of making labour as pain-free as possible. These include the deep breathing and relaxation techniques that are taught in antenatal clinics; an *anaesthetic* that is local to the area involved, called a spinal, or *epidural*, anaesthetic; a gas that the mother breathes to help relieve pain; pain-relieving drugs such as pethidine.

LACTATION
The production of milk by the mammary glands, or breasts, that begins at the end of pregnancy in response to *hormonal* changes and is released by the action of the baby sucking at the nipple. Milk is produced for as long as breast-feeding continues.

LAPAROSCOPY
A small investigative operation in which a *fiber-optic* instrument is introduced into the abdomen through a small incision just below the umbilicus, or navel. The surgeon, who is usually a gynaecologist, is able to examine the pelvic organs. The examination is particularly useful in the investigation of *infertility*, when the *Fallopian tubes*

can be seen and any blockage detected.

LAPAROTOMY
An exploratory operation in which a surgeon opens up the abdomen and examines the organs and structures that it contains in an attempt to find the cause of an abdominal mass or pain when all other methods have failed. A laparotomy may also be performed to check on the spread of an abdominal *tumor* or *Hodgkin's Disease*.

LARYNGITIS 24
An inflammation of the *larynx* or vocal cords. Laryngitis makes the voice hoarse and husky, and may, if very severe, cause breathing difficulty. The condition is treated by resting the voice completely, avoiding smoky or dusty atmospheres and taking steam inhalations.

LARYNX 13
The voice box. An apparatus at the top end of the *trachea*, or windpipe, that produces variations of sound as a result of the passage of exhaled air over the vibrating vocal cords. The vocal cords are two folds of tissue that stick out from the sides of the larynx, which is itself made up of a number of *cartilages*, including the epiglottis, thyroid and cricoid cartilages as well as muscle and ligaments.

LASER
Light Amplification by Stimulated Emission of Radiation. The laser is a very narrow and concentrated beam of light energy that can be focused with great precision. In medicine it is used when an operation needs to be performed on a very small area of tissue without touching the surrounding tissue – for example in the welding of a detached *retina* back to the eye.

LASSA FEVER
A serious *virus* disease first reported in West Africa in 1969, which seems to be confined to that area. The first symptoms are a headache, *fever*, and muscular pains and vomiting; eventually death may result from *heart* or *kidney* failure.

LAXATIVE
A drug or proprietary remedy that is given to help the bowels to evacuate. Some laxatives, such as senna

and castor oil, act by irritating the gut; others, like liquid paraffin, soften the bowel contents. Bulking agents have a laxative effect because they create a softer and more bulky stool that is easier to pass. Laxatives are often abused and taken far too frequently, with consequent ill-effects on the bowel. It is important to remember that not all people need to pass a bowel motion every day – see *constipation*.

LEGIONNAIRE'S DISEASE
Named after an outbreak at an American Legion convention in 1976, Legionnaire's Disease is a severe and infectious *bacterial* lung disease, whose symptoms include malaise, muscular aches and pains, *fever*, cough, pain and breathlessness. The *kidneys* are slightly affected and *protein* tends to be lost in the *urine*, while characteristic changes can be seen on a chest *X-ray*. Treatment is by specific antibiotics, but as with many diseases of the lungs the condition is significantly more serious in smokers.

LEPROSY
Also called Hansen's Disease, leprosy is a *chronic* disease caused by *bacterial* infection that develops gradually over a long period, mainly in the tropics. It affects the skin and the nervous system to cause gross disfigurement and distortion of the *joints*. The condition can be treated, but not cured, by specific drugs.

LEUCOCYTE (US – Leukocyte)
A white blood cell. There are several different types of leucocyte, each of which has its own particular function, but generally the cells are manufactured in the *bone marrow*, the *lymph* nodes and the cells lining the capillaries of certain organs; they move through the blood stream and into tissue to destroy *bacteria* and foreign bodies. When leucocytes are themselves destroyed by invading bacteria *pus* is formed, which may collect in an *abscess*. Normally in Caucasians there are between 4,000 and 10,000 leucocytes in each cubic centimeter of blood; this quantity increases, in a process known as leucocytosis, as a response to *viral* and *bacterial* infections, or in *leukaemia*. Leucocytes may be counted in an investigation of possible disease, or before an operation, in a white blood cell count (W.B.C.).

LEUCOTOMY
A brain operation, sometimes called a prefrontal lobotomy, in which some of the nerve connections of the frontal lobe are severed. The operation is rarely performed these days, because of its serious side-effects, but used to be a treatment for *psychopathy* and very serious *depression*.

LEUKAEMIA (US – Leukemia)
A cancer that affects the areas in which *leucocytes* are formed and leads to a huge overproduction of them. There are a number of different types of leukaemia, depending on the area that is affected and the type of leucocyte that is over-produced. Leukaemias can be either *acute* or *chronic* according to the cell type involved and the rate of disease's onset and course.

As a result of leukaemia the production of *red blood cells* and other blood constituents is suppressed, causing *anaemia* and bleeding problems; the *spleen*, *liver*, and *lymph* nodes become enlarged and the sufferer becomes tired and listless. Nowadays leukaemia can be controlled, although it cannot be totally cured. Periods of *remission* may be induced by drugs, blood transfusions and sometimes *radiotherapy*.

LEUKOCYTE – *see* LEUCOCYTE

LIBIDO   72,132,138
The natural sex urge. Libido may be increased by certain drugs – notably L-dopa, which is used to treat *Parkinson's Disease* – and decreased by age, *alcoholism*, drug addiction, *chronic* illness, *depression* and *psychosexual problems*.

LIGAMENT
Bands of strong connective tissue between the bones of a *joint* that strengthen the joint and limit its movements to those for which it was designed. Ligaments may occasionally become torn as a result of the extra demands imposed on them by sports.

LIPID
A descriptive name for fats or fat-like substances that are insoluble in water – see *fat*.

LIPOMA
A *benign*, fatty *tumor* which never becomes malignant and appears as a

soft lump, or collection of lumps, just beneath the skin.

LITHOTOMY
Strictly, the surgical removal of a stone from the *bladder*. The term is more commonly used, however, to describe a position that is commonly assumed by a patient to facilitate a gynaecological examination. The patient lies on her back with her legs parted and her knees drawn up to the stomach; the legs are normally supported by stirrups.

LIVER   33,158
The largest gland of the body that is situated in the upper right portion of the abdomen, just beneath the lowest ribs, and has a large number of functions.

The liver manufactures *bile*, which is collected in the bile ducts and stored in the *gall bladder*; it helps in the *metabolism* of *carbohydrates*, *proteins* and *fats*; it helps to regulate the level of sugar in the blood by converting *glucose* to glycogen, and shares the storage of the glycogen with the muscles; it manufactures the *blood clotting proteins* fibrinogen and prothrombin; it breaks down, or detoxifies, certain poisons, such as alcohol; it breaks down worn out *red blood cells*; it manufactures the fat-soluble A *vitamins* and stores vitamins B_{12}, D and K.

The liver can be affected by a number of conditions, including: *hepatitis*; *cirrhosis*; *virus* infections such as *glandular fever* and *yellow fever*; an *abscess* caused by *bacteria* or protozoa; by *cancer* (a *tumor* in the liver is called a hepatoma) or by a number of poisons and drugs.

LOBOTOMY – *see* LEUCOTOMY

LOCAL ANAESTHETIC – *see* ANAESTHETIC

LOCHIA
The odourless reddish-brown discharge that leaks from the *vagina* after childbirth. After a week or so the quantity decreases and eventually the discharge stops.

LOUSE
A parasite that affects man, usually by clinging to hair and sucking blood from the skin. There are several different types of lice – Pediculus Humanus Corporis usual-

ly infests clothing, and is called a body louse, while head lice, or nits, which are properly called Pediculus Humanus Capitus, live in the hair of the head. Pubic lice, or Phthirus pubis, usually infest the pubic hair, but may be found in other body hair. Lice are passed on by direct contact, which may be sexual, and are treated by various solutions.

LUMBAR PUNCTURE 60,94

An investigation in which a sample of *cerebrospinal fluid* is taken from the body and analysed. The patient curls up in a ball while lying on his side and after a local *anaesthetic* has been applied and skin cleansed a needle is inserted into the back, usually between the fourth and fifth lumbar vertebrae. A small quantity of the fluid is drawn off, to be measured, cultured for *pathogenic* organisms and examined microscopically. The patient is usually asked to lie on his back and keep still for about 12 hours, and he may experience a slight headache. The technique is useful in the investigation of *meningitis*, advanced *syphilis*, *multiple sclerosis* and subarachnoid *haemorrhage*.

LUNG CANCER 26

Probably the most common form of *cancer*, lung cancer is closely associated with cigarette smoking and air pollution. In the early stages it is symptomless, but later there may be shortness of breath, loss of weight, coughing up of blood and occasionally pain. If untreated lung cancer spreads, or *metastasises*, to other parts of the body through the *lymph* system. Depending on the type of cancer cell and the site of the growth treatment may either be by drugs, by *X-rays* in *radiotherapy*, or by surgical removal.

LYMPH 145

A clear colorless fluid, similar to *blood plasma*, which bathes the tissues of the body and circulates in the vessels of the lymphatic system. Lymph is moved through the body by the pressure of the muscles; valves prevent it from flowing in the wrong direction. It plays an important part in the transport of *leucocytes* and nutrients around the body and is filtered by the lymph nodes, which are found principally in the groin, armpit and neck; the lymph nodes also produce special types of leucocytes.

Because of its role as one of the transport systems of the body, lymph also plays a part in the spread of infection or disease – especially of *cancer*. The lymph system may itself be affected by disease in lymphoedema, where a limb or part of the the body becomes swollen due to an accumulation of lymph in it. This condition may be caused by an injury to the lymphatic vessels, an abnormality in them, a blockage caused by parasites – as in elephantiasis – or a *tumor*, or constriction of the vessels by other tissues, as in pregnancy.

M

MALABSORPTION

A condition in which *fats* and fat soluble *vitamins* in particular are inadequately absorbed in the gut. Malabsorption may be due to the presence of organisms in the intestines, *atrophy* of the the lining of the jejunum – as in *coeliac disease* – or *enzyme* deficiencies such as *chronic pancreatitis*. An individual suffering from malabsorption is thin, wasted, often *anaemic*, with *floating stools* that have an offensive odour.

MALAISE

A general term that describes a state of poor health in which a person is tired and has no energy.

MALARIA

A tropical disease that is carried by a *parasitic* organism called Plasmodia. The organism is carried by mosquitoes, and enters the human blood stream as a result of a mosquito bite. Malaria causes a *fever*, shivering, headache, sweats, *malaise* and *anaemia*. Typically the attacks of fever recur at intervals that are specific to the exact type of parasite. The condition is treated by a short course of drugs, but can be avoided if anti-malarial tablets are taken in areas where the disease is *endemic*.

MALIGNANT

A term used to describe a *tumor* that is *cancerous*, which is likely to spread rapidly and for which the outlook is poor – the opposite of *benign*. Any tumor may be either malignant or benign, depending on the type of cell involved.

MAMMARY GLANDS 104

The two female breasts that produce milk in *lactation*. Sometimes the breasts may be the site of a *tumor* – see *breast cancer* – and they can be examined by *x-rays* or other processes in an investigation called mammography. If this investigation shows cancerous growths it may be necessary for a surgical operation to be performed; occasionally it may be necessary to remove the whole breast in a procedure called a mastectomy, after which a prosthetic breast is fitted – see *mastitis*.

MANIA

A disorder characterized by increased mental and physical activity, in which there are an excessive number of movements and gestures, the sufferer is very voluble, tends to be out of touch with reality and sometimes has delusions of grandeur. The condition is seen in *psychosis* and *manic depression*; a milder form of it is known as hypomania.

MANIC DEPRESSION

Also called manic depressive *psychosis*, the condition is a *psychiatric* disturbance in which severe *depression* alternates with bouts of *mania*. Manic depression is more severe than chronic depressive *neurosis*, and is treated with drugs and sometimes E.C.T.; the chemical Lithium, in particular, may be used to reduce the severity and frequency of the attacks.

MASOCHISM

Named after the Austrian nineteenth-century novelist Leopold von Sacher-Masoch, masochism is an abnormal state of sexuality in which one receives sexual pleasure and gratification from being the object of physical or mental cruelty or domination.

MASTECTOMY – *see* MAMMARY GLANDS

MASTITIS

An inflammation of the breast tissue. Mastitis is commonly the result of a *bacterial* infection that has gained access to the breast through the cracked nipples that may result from breast feeding. *Antibiotics* are usually given, but if the infection does occur during breast feeding it is important that milk continues to be expressed –

otherwise the breast will become engorged and even more painful. Other causes of the condition are a *hormonal* imbalance, as when the breasts become sore and the nipples sensitive before a period.

MASTOIDITIS
An infection of the mastoid *sinuses* of the head, which are situated just behind the ears. Mastoiditis is often the result of a spread of infection from the middle ear, and is felt as a general pain in the area, associated with a headache. The condition is treated with *antibiotics*, but if these are unsuccessful, or the problem recurs frequently, the mastoid sinuses may be removed in an operation called a mastoidectomy.

MASTURBATION
The stimulation of a man or a woman's sexual organs by him- or herself in order to achieve an orgasm.

At one time it was thought that masturbation was a dangerous activity, a sign of moral degeneracy and likely to cause madness; it is now generally recognized that it is a harmless activity with no physical or mental ill-effects and one that is perfectly normal – though excessive or continual masturbation may be a sign of mental illness.

MEASLES   14
A common, highly infectious illness of childhood. Following contact with a sufferer and transmission of the *virus* there is a 12 to 14 day *incubation period*; then symptoms of the upper *respiratory tract* are seen, including a cough, runny nose, *malaise* and *fever*. At this time white spots may appear on the mucous membranes of the mouth. The typical rash of measles is seen around the fourth day. It usually starts behind the ears and spreads to the body and limbs; it is characteristically pink, raised and blotchy, but it does not itch. After a further four or five days the rash disappears and the temperature subsides.

Complications of measles may include infections of the middle ear, or sometimes *pneumonia*. Both of these usually respond to *antibiotics*, but the only effective treatment for measles itself is bed rest and fluids, combined with aspirin to reduce the temperature. *Vaccination* against measles is now available, and is usually given at about 13 months.

MECONIUM
A substance that is excreted by the baby shortly after birth consisting of *bile* from the liver and intestinal debris. Staining of the amniotic fluid by meconium is an indication of *foetal* distress during labour.

MEGALOMANIA
A psychiatric illness in which the sufferer has extraordinarily exaggerated delusions of grandeur.

MELANIN
A pigment found in the skin, hair, *iris* and choroid coat of the *retina* which gives these tissues a dark color.

Sunlight causes an increase in the production of melanin by the body, and the skin becomes darker, or tans, because the pigment forms a protective layer for the tissues underneath. Races who traditionally have lived in areas exposed to strong sunlight have a permanent protective layer of melanin in their skin and are black.

Sometimes *tumors*, called melanoma, occur in the melanin forming cells – usually in the skin, though they may also be found elsewhere. Melanoma are often *malignant* and may spread rapidly, causing *secondaries* in the *liver*.

MELENA   45
The foul-smelling black tarry stools that are excreted after bleeding high in the *gastro-intestinal* system, indicating, for example, the presence of a *peptic ulcer*.

MENARCHE   98
The first *menstruation*, or monthly period, which may be seen between the ages of 10 and 17.

MENIERE'S DISEASE   116
A progressive disease of the inner ear, of unknown origin, in which there is increasing deafness associated with attacks of severe *vertigo* and *nausea*, and *tinnitus*. There is no specific treatment for the condition.

MENINGES
The three layers of tissue that cover the brain and spinal cord, with the *cerebrospinal fluid* circulating between the inner two of them. The outer and strongest layer is called the dura mater. When blood accumulates beneath it as a result of a head injury the condition is known

as a subdural *haematoma*. The meninges become inflamed in *meningitis*.

MENINGITIS
An inflammation of the *meninges* that may be caused by either *viral* or *bacterial* infection. Meningitis can be a very severe illness, causing headache, vomiting, *photophobia*, the presence of *Kernig's Sign* and pain on moving the neck; if untreated, bacterial meningitis may lead to convulsions, *coma* and even death. The bacterial form of meningitis is usually treated with specific antibiotics. These are not necessary in the case of viral meningitis, which normally clears up after a period of bed-rest and painkillers. In order to find out what type of meningitis is causing the problem a sample of *cerebrospinal fluid* may be taken in a *lumbar puncture*.

MENOPAUSE (also CLIMACTERIC)   98
The time of life in a woman at which a number of changes take place with the result that she can no longer bear children, usually between the ages of 40 and 50. The *ovaries* produce less of the female *hormones* and no longer release eggs into the *uterus*, or womb; the womb itself becomes smaller and the walls of the *vagina* thinner and dryer. The change in the normal balance of hormones also leads to a number of general bodily symptoms, such as hot flushes and palpitations.

The menopause may be a very difficult time of life for many women and often causes *depression*. The physical and mental symptoms may be relieved, however, by replacement of female *hormones*.

MENORRHAGIA   100
Excessive *menstruation*, which may either take the form of very heavy bleeding during a period, or of a very prolonged period. The condition may be the result of *hormonal* problems, *fibroids* in the womb or an infection in the *womb* and often results in *anaemia*.

MENSTRUATION   98
The monthly periods in women that start at the *menarche* and finish at the *menopause*. The menstrual cycle repeats itself about every 28 days; in the first part of the cycle an

ovum, or egg, develops in the *ovary* and half-way through the cycle, at about day 14, the egg is shed from the ovary to travel down the *Fallopian tube* into the womb in a process called *ovulation*. At this stage the *endometrium*, or lining of the womb, becomes thicker as a preparation for the implantation of the fertilized egg. If the egg is not fertilized the endometrium is shed in a flow of blood through the *vagina* at day one of the cycle.

METABOLISM
The chemical changes of the body in which food substances are broken down to their simple constituents to provide the energy that is required for body processes and in which chemicals used in the body are built up from the basic chemical ingredients. *Carbohydrates*, for example, are broken down to sugars such as *glucose*, which can then be utilized to produce energy; compounds called amino acids, which are the product of the breakdown of ingested *proteins*, are themselves used in the synthesis of specific proteins in the body. Metabolic diseases are those in which the basic problem is the failure of one of the chemical reactions of the body.

MICTURITION   90
The voluntary process in which *urine* is passed from the *bladder* through the *urethra* to the outside. Micturition is made possible by the coincidental relaxation of the *sphincter* below the bladder and the contraction of the muscles of the bladder wall. When the process passes from voluntary control the condition is called *incontinence*.

MIGRAINE   70
A severe throbbing *headache* that may be one-sided and is associated with *vomiting*, visual disturbances and occasionally temporary speech defects or paralysis of the limbs. Migraine tends to affect women more than men and may begin at puberty and stop at the *menopause*; it is caused by a spasm of the blood vessels of the brain followed by their dilation. An attack may be brought on by certain foodstuffs, such as coffee or chocolate, anxiety or *menstruation*. Treatment is by rest in a darkened room, pain killers, and antiemetics; specific drugs that cause the affected blood vessels to constrict may also be used.

MITRAL VALVE (US – Bicuspid Valve)   86
The valve that separate the left *atrium* and left *ventricle* in the *heart*. The mitral valve is commonly affected in *rheumatic fever* and endocarditis. Small deposits form on the valve causing it to stiffen up and close slightly; the condition is called mitral *stenosis*. The pumping action of the heart is impeded and the result may be a heart *murmur*, breathlessness and sometimes atrial *fibrillation*. The valve may need to be opened surgically, or replaced by an artificial valve.

MOLE – *see* NAEVUS

MONGOLISM – *see* TRISOMY 21

MONONUCLEOSIS   158
An increase in the number of *leucocytes* which are mononuclear in the blood. Infectious mononucleosis is more commonly known as *glandular fever*.

MUCOUS MEMBRANES   45
Tissue that lines many hollow organs as well as the alimentary and respiratory tracts and secretes viscous mucus, usually from special mucus-secreting glands in the epithelium, or outer layer, of the membrane. In some parts of the body the mucous membrane has a specialized function: in the respiratory passages, for example, it contains small hairs, or cilia, which waft particles of dust and debris out of the system. The membrane may become inflamed in response to infection and over-secrete mucus; in fevers, shock and as a result of the action of some drugs it becomes dry. When the continuity of the membrane is broken an *ulcer* is formed.

MULTIPLE SCLEROSIS (also DISSEMINATING SCLEROSIS) 60
A *chronic* disease of unknown origin that affects the *nervous system*, usually begins in young adulthood and is more common in women than men. The disease runs a slow and gradual course which is interrupted by characteristic *remissions* and exacerbations. In the beginning the symptoms may be double vision, clumsiness or unsteadiness, numbness and a tingling in the hands and feet. Later on there may be spastic weakness of the limbs and a loss of *bladder* control. Often the disease progresses very

slowly and the sufferer lives a normal life-span; there is no cure for multiple sclerosis. but *steroid* drugs and *physiotherapy* may help.

MUMPS   155
A *viral* illness that affects the parotid glands – between the angle of the jaw and the ears – causing them to swell and resulting in *malaise*, *fever* and pain. Mumps usually affects children of school age, usually in the winter and spring, but may also be caught by adults. There is an *incubation period* of 15–20 days, after which time the swelling appears, commonly on one side before the other.

The virus may also affect the *testes*, *ovaries* and *pancreas*, causing *abdominal pain* and vomiting. Occasionally mumps causes *orchitis*, or an inflammation of the testicles, which may lead to sterility when the sufferer is an adult male; rarely mumps causes *meningitis*. There is no specific treatment for the condition apart from rest and isolation until the swelling has disappeared.

MUNCHAUSEN'S SYNDROME
Named after Baron Munchausen, a notorious liar, Munchausen's Syndrome is a psychiatric disorder in which an individual constantly feigns illness, often mutilating himself to do so, and demands hospital admission and treatment.

MURMUR
An abnormal sound that can be heard by a doctor when he listens to the heart through a stethoscope, that commonly indicates either a thickening, or *stenosis*, of the heart valves, or that they are not shutting properly. A heart murmur may also be heard in cases where there is a defect in the septum, or division, between the right and left *ventricles*, or when there is a patent *ductus arteriosus*. Some murmurs are quite harmless and termed 'innocent'; others point to a disorder that may require treatment.

MUSCULAR DYSTROPHY
A group of inherited muscle diseases characterized by weakness and wasting of the muscles involved, due to *atrophy* and degeneration. Different diseases in the group are inherited in different ways, affect different muscles and become apparent at varying ages.

Generally, muscular dystrophy appears at an early age and is more common in men than women. *Electromyography* and muscle biopsy are often used to check the diagnosis. There is no cure for muscular dystrophy, but sometimes orthopaedic surgery and *physiotherapy* are helpful.

MYALGIA

A general term denoting pain or tenderness in the muscles.

MYASTHENIA GRAVIS   112,151

A disease of unknown origin that is thought to be associated with a disorder of the *thymus* gland and may be associated with other diseases such as *thyrotoxicosis*, pernicious *anaemia*, *rheumatism* and *arthritis*. Women are affected by myasthenia gravis more frequently than men and symptoms usually appear between the ages of 15 and 50, consisting of abnormal tiredness of the muscles and an inability to sustain muscular activity. Consequently muscular movements such as speech and blinking, while normal at the beginning of the day rapidly deteriorate during the day. The cause of this problem is a failure of the transmission of the nerve impulse at the junction between the nerves and the muscle fibers; drugs can be given that restore this transmission.

The course of myasthenia gravis is variable. Sometimes the disease is mild, while at other times extremely serious; prolonged *remissions* are also seen. Sometimes removal of the thymus gland in a surgical operation leads to a permanent cure, or an amelioration of the symptoms.

MYELITIS

An inflammation of the spinal cord. Myelitis causes a mild fever, followed by a pain in the back that spreads to the limbs. The pain becomes worse and appears to constrict the body at the level of the inflammation; *paralysis* may follow, which may spread upwards to the respiratory muscles and prove fatal. Fortunately this condition is rare – see *osteomyelitis*, *poliomyelitis*.

MYELOGRAM

An *x-ray* procedure in which the outline of the spinal cord and the space surrounding it can be seen, that is performed to show up the presence of *tumors* or a compres-

sion of the cord. A radio-opaque dye is injected into the *cerebrospinal fluid*, in a *lumbar puncture*.

MYELOMA

A malignant *tumor*, or proliferation, of abnormal cells in the bone marrow, that causes changes in the composition of the blood, *anaemia*, *kidney* damage and a characteristic *x-ray* appearance of the skull, ribs, pelvis and vertebrae. The symptoms of a myeloma – which may be multiple, when it is called myelomatosis – start with back pain and may be followed by the collapse of a vertebra, causing *paraplegia*. The condition can be diagnosed by examination of a sample of bone marrow, but the condition is progressive and usually fatal.

MYOCARDIAL INFARCT (also CORONARY THROMBOSIS; HEART ATTACK)   82

A blockage of one or more of the *coronary arteries* that causes an area of *infarction* in the *myocardium*, or muscle of the heart. The condition normally follows a period of weeks or months of *angina* after exercise and sometimes rest – but may also occur without warning.

A myocardial infarct, or heart attack, is felt as a severe and constricting pain like a clenched fist behind the breastbone, which may spread into the jaw or the left arm. Sometimes it is felt between the shoulder blades, in the right arm or even in the hand. Associated with the pain are a shortness of breath, cold sweats and a feeling of doom. Immediate medical care is essential.

A heart attack causes characteristic changes in the E.C.G. trace and in the blood, where increases in the level of certain *enzymes* can be detected. The condition is usually treated with bed-rest, either at home or in a specialist coronary care unit – depending on the size of the infarct and the age and circumstances of the patient; the presence of any complications such as *congestive heart failure* or irregularities of the rhythm and rate of the heart, called *arrhythmias*, will also be taken into account.

MYOCARDIUM   74

The muscle of the heart. The myocardium is a specialized muscle that contracts on average 80 times a minute for the duration of life. It may become inflamed in a *viral*

infection called myocarditis, or in *rheumatic fever* or *diphtheria*. Myocarditis causes chest pain and an irregularity of the heartbeat; it is treated by bed-rest and painkillers.

MYOPATHY   151

A general term denoting any diseases of the muscles, either inherited like *muscular dystrophy*, or due to *carcinoma* or *endocrine* diseases such as *thyrotoxicosis*.

MYOPIA   120

Short sightedness. Distant objects appear blurred because of a defect in the refractive qualities of the lens of the eye, but near objects can be seen clearly. The fault can be corrected if special concave lenses are used.

MYXOEDEMA (US – Myxedema)

An under-activity of the *thyroid* gland that produces a characteristic appearance or *facies*. Myxoedema may have several causes: an *auto-immune* disorder, or defect in the body's own *immunity* systems; drug treatment for *thyrotoxicosis*; surgical removal of the thyroid gland; a defect in the *pituitary gland* that controls the activities of the thyroid gland; or an iodine deficiency, as in *goitre*.

The condition is more common in women than men and tends to first appear at the age of 45, though it may also affect young people – when it is known as juvenile myxoedema. The symptoms include a hoarse voice, puffiness around the eyes, mental and physical lassitude, weight gain, constipation, sparse coarse hair and eyebrows and *menorrhagia*. Diagnosis is by blood tests and treatment by the administration of the thyroid hormone thyroxine in tablet form. Occasionally a *psychotic* state with *delusions* called myxoedematous madness is seen in association with the disease, but this usually remits on treatment.

N

NAEVUS (US – Nevus)

A raised, red *birthmark* caused by dilated blood vessels in the skin – also known as a strawberry naevus. Surgery is not usually necessary and the mark fades as the child becomes older. Other types of naevus are the 'port-wine stain', which does not usually fade, the naevus pilosus, or 'hairy' naevus and the spider naevus, where a small area of red pigmentation is surrounded by tiny dilated blood vessels.

Common moles are also a form of naevus; they are usually benign and not normally treated unless for cosmetic reasons. Some types of mole may become *malignant* and require surgical treatment.

NAPPY RASH (also NAPKIN RASH; US – Diaper Rash)

Properly called ammonical *dermatitis*, nappy rash is a rash on a baby's bottom caused by the wearing of wet nappies. Sometimes the rash becomes infected with candida albicans, or *thrush*. The condition can be helped by frequent changes of nappies, thorough washing and drying of the affected area and the application of soothing creams such as zinc and castor oil cream.

Nappies should not be washed in strong soap powders – the ordinary household detergents should be quite adequate. After washing they should be rinsed in clear water only.

NARCOLEPSY

A chronic condition in which the sufferer has recurrent and uncontrollable sleep and drowsiness, but can easily be roused. Narcolepsy is sometimes associated with auditory hallucinations and passing *paralysis*; cataplexy, where the sufferer loses muscle tone, falls to the floor and loses consciousness, is also a common *complication*.

NARCOSIS

A state of deep sleep and unconsciousness that is caused by narcotic drugs, or is sometimes the result of an accumulation of poisons or metabolic products as in *uraemia*, following terminal *kidney* failure.

NASO-GASTRIC TUBE

A polythene tube that is passed into the stomach through the oesophagus and the nose, either to feed a patient after an operation, to aspirate the contents of the stomach, as after drug overdoses or poisoning, or to test the composition of the gastric juices.

NAUSEA

A feeling of sickness and that vomiting is imminent. Nausea is a symptom of a large number of illnesses, but it is commonly experienced during the first three months of pregnancy when it is known as morning sickness, or hyperemesis gravidarum. Nausea may also be felt as a result of the motion of cars or boats, when it is popularly called travel sickness. It can be treated by proprietary remedies, or drugs called antiemetics.

NECROSIS

The medical term that describes the death of tissue. *Myocardium*, for example, the muscle of the heart, may become necrosed after a *myocardial infarction*.

NEONATE

A term that describes the newborn baby until the fifth week after birth.

NEPHRECTOMY   90

The surgical operation in which a *kidney* is removed. The term is derived from the name of the tiny filtration units inside the kidney, called nephrons.

NERVE   58

A component of the nervous system that connects the tissues of the body with the brain or spinal cord. Nerve fibers are classified according to their function, and either carry sensation to the brain, in which case they are sensory nerves, or motor impulses to the muscles and glands, when they are called motor nerves. Large nerves contain a mixture of these fibers and serve particular limbs or organs. Nerves are susceptible to damage from trauma and infections – see *neuritis, neuropathy*.

NERVOUS SYSTEM   58

The network of *nerves* and nerve cells that covers the whole body, regulating and coordinating its activities and sensing and responding to changes in environment and internal and external stimuli.

The central nervous system or C.N.S., comprises the nerve fibers and cells of the brain and spinal cord and is linked with the peripheral nerves that control voluntary actions, the sensory and motor nerves; it includes the parts of the brain and spinal cord that supply muscles and organs under voluntary control, and the parts of the brain that are involved with conscious thought and sensation.

The autonomic nervous system controls the involuntary functions of the body – those functions that continue without conscious control, such as the contractions of smooth muscles, in *peristalsis* and the activity of the heart muscle. The system is subdivided into the sympathetic nervous system and the parasympathetic nervous system.

The former governs responses that are usually associated with fright or the utilization of energy, such as constriction of the blood vessels, speeding up of the heart, a rise of *blood pressure*, the erection of hairs on the skin and a slowing down of activity in the *alimentary tract*. The sympathetic nerve fibers mainly originate in the thoracic and lumbar portions of the spinal cord.

The parasympathetic nervous system causes *dilation* of blood vessels, a fall in blood pressure, contraction of the pupils of the eyes, a slowing of the heart, increased activity in the *alimentary tract* and increased glandular secretion. The parasympathetic nerve fibers mainly originate in the cranial and sacral areas of the spinal cord.

NETTLE RASH – *see* URTICARIA

NEURALGIA   68

A pain, usually of unknown cause, that is felt in the whole area supplied by an individual *nerve*. The commonest form of neuralgia is called trigeminal neuralgia – see *facial pain* – while post-herpetic neuralgia is sometimes seen after shingles – see *herpes*. The term is often used loosely to describe pains of unknown origin.

NEURITIS   60,94,146

An inflammation of a *nerve* or nerves, which may have a large number of causes including *vitamin* deficiencies; alcohol in excess; *diabetes*; poisoning; infections, such as *toxoplasmosis, malaria, measles, syphilis* and *multiple sclerosis*; or pressure on a nerve or a wound involving it. Neuritis generally causes *neuralgia*, but may have more serious effects, depending on the nerve that is involved and the degree of inflammation – see *neuropathy*.

NEUROPATHY   132,146

A disease of the peripheral *nerves* that may be caused by *neuritis, leprosy, sarcoidosis, alcoholism, diabetes*, an inadequate blood supply, trauma, compression or stretching of the nerves. Neuropathy is a *degenerative* condition in which the nerves gradually lose their function; symptoms include numbness, weakness – especially in the fingers and toes – and *paraesthesia*, or tingling, depending on the nerve involved.

It is thought that there may also be a *hereditary* predisposition to the condition.

NEUROSIS 128
A *psychiatric* condition that is characterized by a degree of insight into his condition on the part of the sufferer and little disruption of his personality – as opposed to *psychosis*. People who have a neurosis tend to be anxious and vulnerable personalities, while the neuroses may include *obsessions*, *compulsions*, *depression*, and *hysteria* as well as specific *phobias*. Treatment may include tranquilizing drugs as well as *psychotherapy*, sometimes in the form of *behavior therapy*.

NEVUS – *see* NAEVUS

NIGHT BLINDNESS
An inability to see at night which is the result of a disorder of the rods of the retina of the eye. The disorder may be due to a deficiency of *vitamin A*, which is found in carrots – hence the old adage that eating carrots helps one to see in the dark – or to *hereditary* factors.

NIGHT SWEATS 14,138
Profuse sweating at night, which may cause the sufferer to wake up in the middle of the night to find the clothes soaked in sweat. Night sweats are seen in those who have an infection that involves *fever*, such as *pneumonia* – when there is sweating during the day as well – and in *depression*, *tuberculosis* and *Hodgkin's Disease*. Night sweats are generally also an early sign of disease.

NITS
Head lice – see *louse*.

NODE 145
Any small swelling, knot of tissue or small structure may generally be called a node, but the term is normally used to describe the small glands of the *lymph* system and two bundles of specialized fibers in the heart. The lymph nodes, or glands, manufacture certain types of *leucocyte* and act as filters for the lymph system; the sinoatrial and atrioventricular nodes in the heart are natural *pacemakers* of the heart: the impulses that initiate the contraction of the heart muscle arise within them.

NODULE
An aggregation of *fat* tissue as a small lump under the skin.

NOSEBLEEDS – *see* EPISTAXIS

NULLIPARA
A woman who has not had any babies.

NYSTAGMUS 120
A condition in which the eyes oscillate involuntarily, usually from side to side. Nystagmus may be *congenital*, the result of lesions in the cerebellum or brain stem caused by neurological diseases, or follow a disorder of the inner ear. Sometimes nystagmus is caused by poor eyesight; it used to be seen in miners who had to work at the coal face in very poor light. The condition is occasionally seen in people with normal eyesight when they try to look at a number of objects which are moving quickly across their field of vision – it is then called physiological or opticokinetic nystagmus.

O

OBESITY 138,146
An individual is properly said to be obese when his body *weight* is 20% or more higher than would be considered normal, taking into account age, build, height and activity. Obesity is directly caused by an excess of fat, or *adipose tissue*, which in its turn is generally the result of over-eating: the amount of food eaten is more than is needed for the supply of energy to maintain bodily activities and so the products of digestion are stored in the tissue as fat.

Over-eating is normally the result of an underlying *psychological* problem such as *depression* or a lack of confidence rather than greed. Occasionally obesity is caused by a *metabolic* deficiency, but it is now thought that an individual's tendencies to obesity may be explained by a relative lack of brown fat in the body. Brown fat is a 'super-storer' of energy, and dissipates energy in the form of heat – it is found in large quantities in animals that hibernate. In man brown fat is concentrated in the region of the shoulder blades; those who have less brown fat than normal have to store more energy in the form of normal fat, which cannot easily be dissipated as heat.

Unless obesity is caused by a metabolic disorder there is no easy cure for the condition other than a strictly controlled and supervised diet. Slimming pills generally help by speeding up the rate at which the body burns up energy; unfortunately they are amphetamines, and as well as having inherent dangers they may become highly addictive. Unless a diet is undertaken, severe obesity predisposes an individual to *heart disease*, *hypertension*, *diabetes* mellitus and *osteoarthritis*; it may also cause social and *psychological* problems.

OBSESSION
A very strong belief or idea that is firmly held and cannot be shaken or influenced by logical argument; it may force the sufferer to perform specific acts, such as touching all four corners of a table in a set sequence. Many quite normal people have a degree of obsession, but when it begins to dominate the mind a severe *neurosis* may set in – see *compulsion*.

OCCLUSION
The blockage and closure of a hollow organ or tube. A *thrombus*, for example, may occlude one of the *coronary* arteries and cause a *myocardial infarction*.

OCCUPATIONAL DISEASE (also INDUSTRIAL DISEASE) 166
A disease that is caused by the hazards or environment in which an individual works. *Pneumoconiosis*, for example, is an occupational disease of miners, while taxi-cab drivers are particularly prone to *hypertension* and *haemorrhoids*. The best protection against occupational disease is the strict adherence to industrial safety procedures and the use of any protective clothing or equipment that may be provided.

OCCUPATIONAL THERAPY
A form of treatment in which an

occupational therapist assesses the extent of an individual's disability, which may be physical or mental, and then organizes activities and adaptations to the individual's environment so that he or she is better able to come to terms with a disability and live a normal life. The occupational therapist may, for example, help in the *rehabilitation* of someone who has had a serious *stroke* by helping the sufferer to use special equipment such as a wheelchair, or, with the help of a *physiotherapist*, prescribe special exercises that will help to strengthen specific muscles.

OEDEMA (US – Edema)100,144,153
Commonly called dropsy, oedema is an accumulation of tissue fluid – that is fluid that has seeped through the walls of blood and *lymph* vessels into the intercellular spaces of tissues. The condition is often not an indication of serious disease – it may be caused by a relative stagnation of the blood due to poor circulation or gravity, as in oedema in the ankles of those who are constantly on their feet, or *hormonally* induced as in pre-*menstrual* oedema. Occasionally a more general oedema is the result of *heart*, *kidney* or *liver* failure – see *pleural effusion*, *ascites* and *pulmonary oedema*. The condition is often treated with drugs called diuretics that increase the production of *urine* by the kidneys and so reduce the quantity of fluid in the body – see *lymph*, *myxoedema*.

OEDIPUS COMPLEX
A *psychological* condition first described by *Freud* and claimed by him to be a normal part of a child's development, in which there are repressed sexual feelings on the part of a daughter for her father and a son for his mother, associated with feelings of jealousy for the other parent. The situation is normally resolved when the child grows up, if this is not the case it is thought that the unresolved Oedipus Complex causes neurosis and sexual abnormalities.

OESOPHAGUS
(US – Esophagus) 32,50
The gullet – a muscular tube that links the *pharynx* and the *stomach*. The oesophagus may become inflamed, in a condition called oesophagitis. The inflammation is sometimes the result of an infection, normally by candida, or *thrush* in

elderly or very weak individuals. More commonly the inflammation is the result of reflux oesophagitis, when the acid stomach juices rise up into the gullet. The condition is associated with a *hiatus hernia*, and may cause a severe pain behind the breastbone, dysphagia, or difficulty in swallowing, and in severe cases *ulceration* and bleeding. The extent of the problem can be detected by the use of an oesophagoscope – a *fiber-optic* instrument with which the gullet can be examined internally. Treatment is usually by soothing drugs and antacids.

OESTROGEN (US – Estrogen) 98
Female sex *hormones* that are produced by the *ovaries* and in smaller amounts by the *adrenal glands* (and in pregnancy by the placenta), in response to gonadotrophic, or gonad-stimulating, hormones from the *pituitary gland*. Oestrogen controls the female primary and secondary sexual characteristics – the growth and function of the sexual organs, the development of breasts and pubic hair, the distribution of subcutaneous *fat* and the *menstrual cycle*.

The hormone is also produced in small quantities by the male *testes*. An over-production of oestrogen in men may cause *feminization*.

Synthetic oestrogens may be used medically for a number of purposes. They may be given after a *hysterectomy* that also involves the ovaries; to control *menopausal* disorders; in the treatment of some breast *cancers* that are thought to be hormone dependent; and in the treatment of cancer of the *prostate gland* in men. Oestrogen, along with the other female sex hormone *progesterone*, is a major constituent of the *oral contraceptive pill*.

**OOPHORITIS AND
OOPHORECTOMY** – *see* OVARIES

OPHTHALMIA 77,120
An inflammation of the eye. Ophthalmia neonaturum is an inflammation of the eye and conjunctiva of a newborn baby that is contracted as the child passes through the *cervix* of a mother infected with *gonorrhoea*. The condition must be treated immediately with *antibiotics*.

OPHTHALMOSCOPE 120,122
An instrument that can be used to

examine the interior of the eye, especially the *retina*. *Cataracts* may be detected by the use of an ophthalmoscope, but the instrument's main use is in examining the retina, because this is the only place in the body where blood vessels and a nerve may be seen directly.

ORCHITIS 94,155
An inflammation of the *testicles*. Orchitis is a painful condition that may be the result of *trauma* or a *bacterial* infection such as *gonorrhoea* or *mumps* – in which case it is often one-sided. Mumps orchitis can occasionally cause *sterility*, but its incidence is low. Orchitis is treated by support, rest, painkillers and *antibiotics*.

ORGAN
Any part of the body that has a specific function. Organs that have failed can sometimes be replaced, as the result of the development of a fairly new branch of surgery called organ transplantation.

ORGANIC DISEASE
Any disease that has a physical rather than *psychological* cause.

ORGASM
A peak, or climax, of physical and emotional excitement occurring as a result of sexual activity that is accompanied in men by ejaculation. There is some dispute as to the exact nature of the female orgasm, but it is thought to consist of two parts or types – *vaginal* and clitoral – which follow a 'plateau' stage of heightened excitement. Orgasm is commonly followed by a period of physical and mental relaxation; inability to achieve an orgasm in women is known as *frigidity*.

ORNITHOSIS – *see* PSITTACOSIS

OSTEITIS
An inflammation of bone that is normally caused by infection, but is sometimes due to a disorder of the *parathyroid* gland or the formation of a *tumor* – see *Paget's Disease*.

**OSTEOARTHROSIS (also
OSTEOARTHRITIS)** 110
A common *degenerative disease* that affects the larger weight-bearing *joints*, especially in older people. Osteoarthritis is characterized by *atrophy* of the articular *cartilages* of a joint and the form tion of new

outgrowths at the edges of bones. Some degree of degeneration is a natural part of ageing, but osteoarthrosis represents a speeding-up of the process. The condition is associated with *obesity*, and the first symptoms are usually pain in the joints which is worse after exercise but is relieved by rest. Fluid may accumulate inside the joint and eventually the range of movements becomes limited. The condition is differentiated from *rheumatoid arthritis* because there is no *systemic* disease, and usually only one or two joints are affected. Treatment is by painkillers and anti-inflammatory drugs, and a reduction of weight if there is associated obesity. Occasionally arthroplasty, a surgical replacement of the joint affected, may be necessary.

OSTEOMYELITIS
An inflammation of the *bone marrow* that is caused by infection. *Bacteria* may either reach the bone through a deep wound, such as a compound *fracture*, or be carried to the site of infection in the bloodstream. An *abscess* tends to form in the bone which eventually leads to the *necrosis*, or death, of a part of the bone; it may then burst through to the surface of the skin, forming a *sinus* that may discharge *pus* for some time. Acute osteomyelitis is sometimes seen in children, especially on either side of the knee. Symptoms include severe pain at the site of the inflammation, fever and general weakness. Treatment is by drainage of the pus and *antibiotics*; sometimes the affected bone is rested by immobilization in a splint or a plaster.

OSTEOPATHY
A form of treatment that depends on the manipulation of bones and joints and is based on the theory that many pains – especially those of the back – are caused by poor posture or minor anatomical abnormalities which lead to slight derangement of the joints.

OTITIS   116
An infection of the ear, which is called otitis externa when it affects the outer ear and otitis media when the middle ear is involved. Otitis externa is an inflammation of the outer ear in which the canal becomes red, sore and itchy and may discharge. It is treated by special drops that normally contain *antibiotics*, anti-inflammatory agents and anti-fungal agents.

Otitis media is an infection of the middle ear, normally caused by *bacteria* that have reached it through the *Eustachian tubes*. It may result in earache, slight deafness, a raised temperature and a red bulging eardrum; in children the infection sometimes causes *abdominal pain*. Treatment is by antibiotics, but if these do not work the eardrum may have to be incised in a procedure called a myringotomy, in order to allow the accumulation of *pus* to drain away. Occasionally the eardrum may perforate of its own accord to the same effect.

OTOSCOPE   116
An instrument used for an examination of the ear, through which the eardrum can be examined and *otitis* diagnosed.

OVARIES   94,98,155
The female *gonads*, which are positioned in the pelvis at the end of the *Fallopian tubes* and supported by *ligaments*. The ovaries produce the female *hormone oestrogen*, while another female hormone called *progesterone* is produced by the corpus luteum inside the ovary. Each month an *ovum*, or egg, matures inside the ovaries and is released into the Fallopian tubes at *ovulation* – a part of the *menstrual cycle*.

The ovaries may very occasionally be affected by the *mumps virus*, and they become inflamed in a condition known as oophoritis, which may be associated with *salpingitis* and caused by *gonorrhoea, tuberculosis* or other pelvic infections. They may also contain simple *cysts*, called ovarian cysts; these are harmless most of the time, but occasionally need to be removed surgically. Sometimes the ovaries may be the site of *tumors* – which may be either *benign* or *malignant* – which may be responsible for a degree of masculinization.

The surgical removal of an ovary is called an oophorectomy, and may be associated with a *hysterectomy*. If the operation is performed before the *menopause* hormone supplements may be given.

OVERDOSE
A dangerously large dose of a drug that may be accidental but is more usually deliberate, when it is either an attempt to attract attention or a serious suicide bid. The most common overdoses involve sleeping pills and painkillers; they tend to cause drowsiness, a depression of *respiration*, low *blood pressure* and eventually unconsciousness – depending on the amount of the overdose and the type of the drug. The sufferer will be given a stomach *wash-out* and often placed on a *ventilator*. Sometimes, as in the case of a paracetamol overdose, specific drugs may be given to counter any *liver* damage. After recovery from an overdose the patient will normally be given *counselling* or *psychiatric* help.

OVIDUCT – *see* FALLOPIAN TUBES

OVULATION   98
The release of the *ovum*, or egg, from the ovary midway in the *menstrual cycle* – about 14 days before the start of a period. Ovulation is dependent on the level of *progesterone* and *oestrogen* in the body; during pregnancy ovulation does not occur and there are no periods. The oral *contraceptive* pill alters the *hormonal* balance so that ovulation does not take place and conception cannot occur, though there are still periods.

Ovulation may be associated with some slight abdominal cramps, and also causes a slight rise in body temperature – by about 0.5°C. In an investigation of *infertility* a woman will often be asked to keep a daily record of her temperature for a few months to check if she is ovulating, because the days around ovulation are the most fertile of the menstrual cycle. If pregnancy is to be avoided using the rhythm method, intercourse should not take place between at least days 10 and 20, though this method is by no means foolproof – see *contraception*.

OVUM   98
An egg, or female reproductive cell that matures inside a follicle in the *ovary*. One ovum is released from an ovary each month and passes down the *Fallopian tubes* to the *uterus* in a process called *ovulation*. Inside the uterus the ovum may be fertilized by a male reproductive cell, or sperm, and implant in the *endometrium* of the womb to develop as a *foetus*. If the ovum is not

fertilized it is flushed out of the womb along with the endometrium in *menstruation*.

OXYGEN – *see* BLOOD GASES

P

PACEMAKER
A group of cells, or an artificial device, that generates the impulses which initiate the contractions of the heart muscle, or *myocardium*. The natural pacemakers of the heart are the sino-atrial and atrioventricular nodes, at the junction of the superior *vena cava* and the right *atrium* and alongside the intraventricular septum respectively. When these natural pacemakers are defective the heart will beat with an irregular rhythm, called an *arrhythmia*, and may go into *fibrillation*. To restore a natural heartbeat an artificial pacemaker may be surgically implanted, or occasionally placed on the outside of the chest. The device gives off a series of controlled electrical discharges that initiate heart muscle contraction.

PAGET'S DISEASE
Also called osteitis deformans, Paget's Disease causes a chronic inflammation of the bones, making them thick, soft and sometimes bowed.

The disease normally affects the elderly and cannot be cured by any specific treatment.

PAIN   138
A distress or discomfort that can range in degree from the mild to the excruciating. Pain may be a response to a dangerous or *traumatic* outside stimulus – when it is a part of the body's defence mechanisms – or the result of a disease process and the inflammation that normally accompanies a disease. Sometimes pain is *psychosomatic*, or the result of *depression* or *hysteria*, but it is no less real than any other type of pain. *Analgesics*, or painkillers, relieve pain, but do not affect its cause – see *abdominal pain*, *chest pain*, *facial pain*, *groin pain*.

PALLIATIVE
A medicine or drug that relieves the symptoms of a condition without curing it.

PALLOR   162
A lack of skin color that may be the result of constriction of the blood vessels, as in *shock*, or a sign of a disease such as *anaemia*.

PALPATION   132
A technique used in the physical examination of a patient by a doctor in which an abnormal state can be detected by the feel of an organ or part of the body to the touch. An enlarged *liver*, for example, one of the signs of liver damage in conditions such as *alcoholism*, can be palpated below the lower edge of the ribs on the right of the abdomen.

PALPITATION   74
An abnormally strong contraction of the heart muscle, of which an individual is aware; also a strong throb or flutter. A palpitation may be caused by sudden excitement or fear, but sometimes it is a sign of *neurosis*, heart disease – including *arrhythmia*, – circulatory diseases or other disorders.

PALSY – *see* PARALYSIS

PANACEA
A 'cure-all'; a proprietary remedy that purports to cure all diseases but in fact rarely has any beneficial effect on any of them.

PANCREAS   17,32,132,146,155
A gland situated behind the stomach, with its head in a loop of *duodenum* and its tail meeting the *spleen* in the left-hand side of the body. The pancreas secretes pancreatic juice, which flows through a duct to join the common *bile duct* and then enters the duodenum to play an important part in digestion; it also secretes the *hormone insulin*, which controls the level of *glucose* in the blood, and another hormone called glucagon. A malfunction of the pancreas may cause either an over-production or an under-production of insulin, and thus *hypo-* or *hyperglycaemia* respectively, the latter being the cause of *diabetes mellitus*.

The pancreas may become inflamed in a condition called pancreatitis, which may be *acute* or *chronic*. Acute pancreatitis is a severe condition in which the *enzymes* of the pancreatic juice may start to digest the organ itself, causing sudden pain, vomiting and sometimes *jaundice* and collapse.

Chronic pancreatitis may follow *virus* infections such as *mumps* and *influenza*, and is often associated with *alcoholism*.

PANDEMIC
An *epidemic* that occurs in many different parts of the world at the same time, or that affects most of the people within a given country or large area.

PARAESTHESIA
(US – Paresthesia)
Commonly called 'pins and needles', paraesthesia is a sensation of numbness, prickling and tingling that is normally felt in a limb or extremity. It is normally caused by prolonged pressure on the *nerve* that supplies the region in which the sensation is felt – as when the legs are crossed for a long time – but is sometimes the result of damage to nerves.

PARALYSIS   72,132
A temporary or permanent loss of the power of movement and sometimes sensation in any part of the body, that is caused by damage to the *nerve* supply – which may in turn be the result of disease, *trauma*, a *cerebrovascular accident* (C.V.A.) or a *transient ischaemic attack* (T.I.A.). The sudden onset of paralysis following such an event is commonly called a *stroke*.

A stroke involving one side of the brain may cause hemiplegia – that is a paralysis of the same side of the face and the opposite side of the whole body. An injury or lesion of the spinal cord may result in paraplegia, where all the body below the lesion is paralysed. In flaccid paralysis muscle tone and reflexes are lost in the affected area, while in *spastic* paralysis the opposite is the case.

One form of chronic paralysis, called paralysis agitans, or 'shaking palsy', is more commonly known as *Parkinson's Disease*. *Alcoholism* may cause paralysis, as may other forms of poisoning, while changes in the brain stem can cause bulbar paralysis, which affects the muscles of the mouth, tongue and throat. Paralysis of the muscles of the face, caused by interference to the facial nerve is called Bell's Palsy; 'infantile paralysis' is a term, now obsolete, once used to describe a form of *poliomyelitis*. There are many individually named paralyses.

PARAMEDICAL
A trained medical operative who is not qualified as a doctor or a nurse, but is specifically trained to assist or in some cases perform medical procedures. An *occupational therapist* and a *radiotherapist*, for example, are both paramedics. Specially trained paramedics are used much more extensively in America than in Britain.

PARANOIA
A psychotic state in which an individual has systematized and logical delusions of persecution. There is a tendency to brooding, jealousy, suspiciousness and megalomania.

PARANOID   140
Either an individual who suffers from *paranoia* or a condition that is similar to paranoia, in which an individual is convinced that the world is against him, that may accompany disorders of the mind – see *schizophrenia*. Paranoid ideas may also accompany depression.

PARAPARESIS
A partial *paralysis* of the lower limbs.

PARAPLEGIA – *see* PARALYSIS

PARASITE
Any organism that lives on or inside a host organism at the expense of the host, without contributing anything to the host's welfare. Some organisms live inside man but are an important part of the body's systems, such as the bacteria that inhabit the *vagina* and *intestine* – this is not a true parasitic relationship, but a state called *symbiosis*. Common parasites of man include *trichomonas vaginalis*, *worms*, *lice* and *scabies*.

PARASYMPATHETIC NERVOUS SYSTEM – *see* NERVOUS SYSTEM

PARATHYROID GLANDS   144
Two pairs of *endocrine glands* situated just to the side of and behind the *thyroid* gland that secrete a *hormone* called parathormone, which controls the *metabolism* of *calcium* and phosphorus in the body. An increase in activity of the parathyroid gland causes an increase in the level of calcium in the blood – the extra calcium is derived from the bones, which become fragile.

A decrease in activity **lowers** the level of blood calcium and may cause *tetany* as well as lesions in the bones and teeth. In the event of an over-activity of the gland, it may be surgically removed in an operation called a parathyroidectomy.

PARATYPHOID FEVER
One of the *enteric* fevers, paratyphoid fever is an infection that resembles *typhoid* and is caused by a *bacterium* of the same *salmonella* family. Symptoms of the disease vary from a mild *fever* with diarrhoea to those almost as severe as typhoid symptoms, depending on the exact strain of bacterium that is involved.

PARENTERAL
A term applied to a procedure in which nourishment and drugs are supplied directly to the cells and tissues of the body, avoiding the usual digestive processes of the *alimentary tract*. Food substances may be given intravenously, and the procedure is used when a patient is unable to take food by mouth or unable to absorb it once it is inside the digestive system.

PARESIS   94
Either a partial *paralysis* or an alternative term for general paralysis of the insane – see *syphilis*.

PARKINSON'S DISEASE   72
Also known as paralysis agitans, or shaking palsy, Parkinson's Disease is a *chronic* disease of the *nervous system* whose onset is usually gradual. The first sign may be a fine tremor in the extremities, which eventually spreads and becomes continuous. Speech becomes slow and careful and a characteristic walk develops, which is caused by muscular weakness and rigidity – the body leans forward and the steps become faster and faster. The cause of Parkinson's Disease is not yet known, though it normally appears in late middle age; there is no specific cure, but the drug Leva-Dopa often alleviates the condition.

PAROTID GLANDS   145,155
Two of the *salivary glands*, each parotid gland is situated just in front of and below the ear at the point of the jaw. The parotid glands become inflamed in parotitis, which may be the result of *mumps* or an infection of the mouth that has spread to the gland through the parotid duct.

PAROUS
A woman who has had children. When a woman has not had children she is said to be nulliparous.

PARROT DISEASE – *see* PSITTACOSIS

PARTURITION
The act of giving birth.

PASSIVITY FEELINGS – *see* SCHIZOPHRENIA

PATHOGENIC
Producing disease – *bacteria*, for example, are pathogenic organisms.

PATHOLOGICAL
A condition is said to be pathological when it is caused by disease and not by natural circumstances.

PEDICULUS
A *louse*. Pediculosis is the condition in which an individual is infested with lice.

PELLAGRA
A disease caused by a deficiency of *vitamin* B that is common in some parts of the world. Pellagra may cause a deterioration of the *mucous membranes* of the body, a flushing and scaling of the skin, *nausea*, vomiting and diarrhoea, general weakness and symptoms of the *nervous system*. The condition is treated by supplementary vitamin B and a healthy diet.

PELVIS   109
The bony girdle formed by the bones of the hip and the lower spine; also the cavity bounded by this girdle. (The term also denotes the area of the join between the *ureter* and the *kidney*.) The female pelvis is normally larger and wider than the male pelvis, in order to allow the passage of the baby at birth. The size of the female pelvis in relation to the *foetal* head can be determined by pelvimetry. If the pelvis is not large enough to allow normal passage of the foetus a *Caesarean section* may be necessary.

PEMPHIGUS
A condition of unknown origin and many varieties that may be either *acute* or *chronic*, in which areas of skin suddenly become covered with large *vesicles*, which heal to leave pigmented areas. Pemphigus causes

itching and burning sensations and a general feeling of illness.

PENIS

The male genital organ, which is also the organ of *urination*. The penis consists of three columns of spongy tissue – two of which are called the corpora cavernosa and the other the corpus spongiosum – with the *urethra* between them. The penis becomes erect when blood gorges the spongy columns as a result of sexual excitement. If a man is unable to achieve or sustain an erection he is said to be *impotent*.

PEPSIN   33

An *enzyme* produced by the glands of the *stomach* that acts on food to partially break down *proteins*.

PEPTIC ULCER   45

A general term for an ulcer of the *stomach* or *duodenum* – see *duodenal ulcer*, *gastric ulcer*.

PERCUSSION

A method of diagnosis that forms part of a doctor's physical examination of a patient. A part of the body is tapped sharply with the fingers and the resonance and pitch of the resulting sound can give the doctor important information about what lies beneath the skin. The presence of fluid or *pus* can often be detected, as well as any inconsistency in the size and condition of an organ.

PERICARDIUM   86

The outer lining of the heart, that is composed of an outer fibrous layer and an inner membraneous layer. The pericardium becomes inflamed in a condition called pericarditis which may be caused directly by *bacterial* infection, but is more usually associated with diseases such as *rheumatic fever*, *tuberculosis*, *connective tissue diseases* and *myocardial infarction*. The condition may cause pain, mild fever, dry cough, breathing difficulties and irregularities in the pulse; sometimes, in constrictive pericarditis, the pericardium becomes progressively more fibrous until it impedes the normal movements of the heart and surgery is necessary. Another serious complication of the disease is the production of a *serous* exudate which may also impede the heart, requiring surgical drainage of the area. Generally pericarditis is treated by *antibiotics*.

PERINEUM

The area between the genitals and the *anus*, including the internal but superficial muscles of that area.

PERIOSTEUM

A fibrous membrane that covers bone and is divided into two parts. The outer layer contains blood vessels that supply the bone and the inner layer is composed of connective tissue cells that help in the formation of new bone. The periosteum may become inflamed in a condition called periostitis, which may follow *trauma* or infectious diseases and cause pain, *fever*, and inflammation of the overlying skin. The condition is treated with appropriate *antibiotics*.

PERISTALSIS   35

A system of muscular contraction by which substances are moved through the *gastro-intestinal tract*. Peristalsis depends on the presence of longitudinal and circular muscle fibers which contract involuntarily in sequence to give a rippling, wave-like motion along the tube, carrying food along in front of the wave.

PERITONEUM

The membrane that lines the abdominal cavity and the viscera; one particular fold of peritoneum, called mesentery, circles the intestines and attaches them to the posterior abdominal wall. The abdominal cavity within the peritoneal lining is called the peritoneal cavity; it may become filled with fluid, called *ascites*. Sometimes toxic substances or waste products are removed from the body in *peritoneal dialysis*.

PERITONITIS   52

An inflammation of the peritoneum which may have several causes. The organisms that cause the infection may gain access to the *peritoneal cavity* through a perforation of the stomach or the intestines, or through a ruptured *appendix*; as a result of a *trauma* such as a stab wound or an abdominal operation that has caused *sepsis*; or be carried there by the blood. Peritonitis causes severe *abdominal pain*, *fever*, vomiting and a rapid heartbeat. The condition is often extremely serious and demands immediate treatment, including *antibiotic* therapy and commonly surgery.

PERNICIOUS ANAEMIA – *see* ANAEMIA

PERSECUTION COMPLEX   140

A feeling that one is being unjustly treated or is the object of a conspiracy, without any due cause – see *paranoia*, *paranoid*, *schizophrenia*.

PERSEVERATION

The constant repetition of an action, phrase or idea that may be the result of an obsession or compulsion that has become psychotic. but is sometimes caused by brain disease.

PERSPIRATION – *see* SWEAT

PERTUSSIS

Commonly called whooping-cough, pertussis is an *acute* infectious disease of children caused by a *bacillus*, in which acute *catarrh* is followed by characteristic paroxysmal cough that terminates in a noisy 'whooping' inspiration. The *incubation period* is between seven and 10 days and the cough starts at about two weeks. The catarrhal stage is associated with symptoms similar to those of the common cold, while the coughing fits often cause a degree of *cyanosis* and end in vomiting. Pertussis is treated with *antibiotics*; a *vaccination* that is effective is available for the disease, but there may very occasionally be side-effects and there is some controversy about its use.

PESSARY

A medical term that has several different meanings. A pessary may be a *vaginal suppository*, where a drug is introduced to the vagina in the form of a soft pellet that dissolves – often in the treatment of conditions such as *vaginitis*. Another type of pessary may be used to treat a *prolapse* of the *uterus* – a ring of polythene or metal is placed at the top of the vagina to support the uterus. A diaphragm, or 'dutch cap', used as a *contraceptive* device, is also properly called a pessary.

pH

A scale on which the relative alkalinity or acidity of a substance can be rated. The point at which a substance is said to be neither acid nor base but neutral is said to be pH 7; increasing acidity approaches pH 0 on the scale, while increasing alkalinity approaches pH 14 – see *acidosis*, *alkalosis*.

PHARYNX 13

The area at the back of the mouth that is lined with *mucous membrane* and communicate with the nose, with the ears through the *Eustachian tubes* and with the *oesophagus* and *larynx* below. The pharynx becomes inflamed in an upper *respiratory tract* infection called pharyngitis; the condition causes a sore throat and general *malaise*, and is associated with *tonsillitis*.

PHENYLKETONURIA

A hereditary disease of protein *metabolism*, in which one of the many chemical reactions involved is deficient. If undetected phenylketonuria may cause severe mental retardation, but the disease is normally revealed at birth in a routine screening called a *Guthrie test*. The condition is treated by a specially prepared diet.

PHIMOSIS

A narrowing, or *stenosis*, of the opening of the prepuce, or foreskin, of the *penis*. The foreskin cannot be retracted over the glans penis without considerable pain unless the condition is treated by circumcision.

PHLEBITIS 77

An inflammation of a vein. Phlebitis is of unknown origin, but is often associated with *varicose veins*; the condition causes pain and tenderness in the area affected, *erythema* of the overlying skin and sometimes *oedema* in the limb below the site of the problem. There is also a tendency for *thrombi* to develop in the inflamed vein. Treatment is by anti-inflammatory drugs and support.

PHLEGM – *see* SPUTUM

PHOBIA 130

An abnormally strong fear of a situation or object. Agoraphobia, for example, is a fear of wide-open spaces, while claustrophobia is a fear of enclosed spaces. Some people may have a phobia for cats, while those suffering from *rabies* may develop hydrophobia – a fear of water. Phobias can severely limit normal life; they are treated by *behavior therapy* and *psychotherapy*.

PHOTOPHOBIA 130

An abnormally strong discomfort experienced when the eyes are exposed to light – the eyelids shut tightly and the head is turned away from the light source. Photophobia may be associated with diseases such as *measles*, *rubella* and *meningitis*, and conditions such as *migraine*; it may also be caused by drugs that dilate the pupils.

PHYSIOTHERAPY

A form of treatment in which physical and mechanical methods, such as massage, controlled exercise, heat, electricity, and infra-red radiation are used to help restore an individual to health. Physiotherapy is particularly important in the treatment of diseases or *trauma* that have affected the muscles and the joints, and in the *rehabilitation* of an individual afterwards.

PIGMENT

An organic substance that colors material in the body. Bilirubin, for example, is one of the *bile* pigments, while *haemoglobin* is a pigment found in the red blood cells. The term 'pigmentation' normally refers to the distribution of the pigment *melanin* in the skin.

PILES – *see* HAEMORRHOIDS

PILONIDAL SINUS – *see* SINUS

PIMPLES – *see* ACNE

PINK EYE – *see* CONJUNCTIVITIS

PINS AND NEEDLES – *see* PARAESTHESIA

PITUITARY GLAND 144

A small endocrine gland situated at the base of the brain. The pituitary gland secretes a number of *hormones* which regulate growth, reproduction, metabolism and the activity of many other glands in the body, such as the *thyroid gland*, *adrenal glands* or *gonads*, that is *testes* and *ovaries*. The gland also secretes oxytocin, a hormone that stimulates contractions of the muscular wall of the *uterus*, and vasopressin, a hormone that causes the muscular walls of blood vessels to contract and also stimulates the tubules of the *kidney* to reabsorb water.

An over-activity of the pituitary gland may cause *Cushing's Syndrome* and *acromegaly*, while an under-activity of the gland may cause *dwarfism*.

PITYRIASIS

A disease of unknown cause in which the skin becomes scaly. In pityriasis rosea the skin becomes slightly red and scaly, forming ring-shaped patches on the chest and upper arm. The patches may last for several weeks or months before disappearing spontaneously.

PLACEBO

An inactive substance that may either be given as a 'control' in a study of a drug's action, or to a patient in an attempt to satisfy that patient's demand for medicine when the doctor thinks that medication is unnecessary.

PLACENTA

The afterbirth. The placenta develops in the *womb* in about the third month of pregnancy; it consists of a spongy mass of tissue that is pervaded by blood vessels and links the *foetus* and the mother through the umbilical cord. *Antibodies*, nourishment and oxygen are passed from the mother to the foetus up to the moment of birth, when the placenta is expelled from the body and the umbilical cord cut.

Occasionally the placenta is abnormal. A 'battledore' placenta is attached to the umbilical cord at its margin, instead of its center; in placenta praevia the placenta is attached to the lower part of the uterine wall – the condition may lead to bleeding in the last few months of pregnancy, *anaemia*, low *blood pressure* and a rapid *pulse*. The haemorrhage must be controlled and strict asepsis observed if complications are to be avoided; placenta praevia can be diagnosed by the use of ultrasound.

PLAGUE

A term commonly used in the past to describe any disease that was epidemic, infectious and often fatal. Today the word is used specifically to describe a disease caused by the organism yersinia pestis (formerly called pasteurella pestis) and transmitted in the bites of fleas who have themselves been infected by rats. A form of plague known as the 'black death' ravaged Europe in the fourteenth and seventeenth centuries, but is now only of historical interest. Otherwise, plague causes a high fever, mental disturbance, delirium, coma and often death. Bubonic plague is characterized by

PLASMA

the formation of buboes, or inflamed
and swollen *lymph* nodes; in pulmonary plague the lungs are highly
involved and the disease, which is
very virulent, can be spread in drop-
let form. Plague still breaks out in
parts of Asia and Africa, and treatment is by *antibiotics* and specific
drugs.

PLASMA
The liquid component of blood,
made up of *serum* and *blood clotting* factors. Plasma can be produced by spinning blood that has
not been allowed to clot in a centri-
fuge – the *blood corpuscles* and
platelets settle at the bottom, while
plasma can be poured off from the
top. As plasma has no red blood
cells there is no danger of an *anti-
gen-antibody* reaction when it is
given to anybody in a transfusion;
plasma can therefore be used as
emergency substitute for blood
before blood of the correct *blood*
group has been obtained. Plasma is
also given to those who suffer from
haemophilia or blood-clotting problems, as well as to those who are
haemorrhaging severely, because it
contains blood clotting factors. It
can be dried or frozen and kept in
storage for several months; because
plasma is rich in the plasma *proteins* albumen and globulin it is
sometimes given to those who have
a low level of protein in the blood.

PLEURA 15
Two layers of membrane that separate the chest wall and the
lungs. The outer membrane is called
the parietal pleura and in effect
lines the thoracic, or chest, cavity.
The visceral pleura lines the outside
of the lungs. There is a small space
between the two layers called the
pleural cavity and the opposing surfaces of the pleura are lubricated by
fluid, so that they can slide easily
over one another – see *pleural effusion, pleurisy.*

PLEURAL EFFUSION 14,26
An accumulation of fluid in the
pleural cavity that may cause
breathing difficulties. The fluid may
be thin and *serous*, when it is
associated with *heart, liver* and
kidney failure, or thick, containing
protein – when it may be a
result of pulmonary conditions such
as *pneumonia, tuberculosis, carcinoma* of the *bronchus* and *connective tissue diseases*. The effusion is

directly treated by drainage and
then indirectly by an examination of
the cause of the problem.

PLEURISY 14
An inflammation of the *pleura* that
may be caused directly by an infection of the membranes but is sometimes associated with *pneumonia,
tuberculosis* or *viral* infection of the
intercostal . muscles. Pleurisy is
occasionally caused by an invasion
of the membranes by a *tumor* of the
lungs and by an *embolus* that has
reached the periphery of the lung
and led to an *infarct*. In pleurisy the
membranes become swollen and
tend to rub against each other,
especially during breathing or
coughing; the sound made by this
can be heard on examination. There
is also a stabbing pain that is felt
most strongly on inspiration. The
condition is treated by *antibiotics*
and an examination of the underlying cause of the problem.

P.M.T. – *see* PREMENSTRUAL TENSION

PNEUMOCOCCI 14
A family of *bacteria* that often cause
pneumonia and may be a cause of
meningitis.

PNEUMOCONIOSES 19,26
A collection of *occupational* lung
diseases that are caused by the inhalation of mineral dusts – including
silicosis, asbestosis, coal miner's
pneumoconiosis and siderosis – see
silicosis.
Coal miner's pneumoconiosis is
very prevalent in mining communities and is caused by the continual
inhalation of coal dust. The condition is frequently detected on
x-ray examination of miners' lungs,
but in a fairly high proportion of
cases there are no symptoms. In
some cases, however, there is considerable damage, including massive fibrosis of the lungs, which may
lead to death through *emphysema*
and *heart failure*.
Asbestosis is caused by the inhalation of asbestos fibers. The substance was once commonly used in
brake linings, shipbuilding and as
an insulation material in buildings,
but its use has become less prevalent since the identification of the
disease. Asbestosis is associated
with bronchial *cancer*.
Siderosis is caused by the inhalation of iron oxides by people such as

arc welders and silver workers. In
isolation siderosis seldom causes
respiratory problems.
Generally, pneumoconioses may
cause a barrel chest, shortness of
breath – especially on exertion – a
thin and wiry appearance and *cyanosis*. The diseases are treated by
avoiding contact with the causative
agents and by the same techniques
used in chronic obstructive diseases
of the airways such as *emphysema*
and *bronchitis*.

PNEUMONECTOMY 26
The surgical removal of a lung,
usually as a result of bronchial *carcinoma* or severe *trauma*. The
cavity that remains is obliterated by
the formation of fibrous tissue and
the rise of the *diaphragm* on that
side of the chest. The lung that
remains enlarges to some extent and
can usually cope with normal
demands.

PNEUMONIA 14
An infection of the lungs that may
be caused by *bacteria, viruses* or the
aspiration of vomit. Pneumonia
often has a sudden onset, with very
high *fever, rigors*, sweats, headache,
malaise and *anorexia*. At first there
is a dry cough; later the cough may
bring up blood-streaked *sputum*.
The chest is painful and breathing
becomes fast, painful and shallow.
The condition is treated by *antibiotics*, bed-rest and appropriate nursing care.
Pneumonia is common in people
who have been weakened by other
diseases, especially the old. It may
be seen after operations, when the
condition is called hypostatic pneumonia – especially when a patient is
not taught to cough and clear his
upper respiratory tract of
secretions.

PNEUMONITIS 10
An inflammation of the *alveoli* of
the lungs that may be caused by
viral infection or irritant fumes and
occasionally by *roundworm* larvae
which migrate to the area. In this
last case the condition is known as
helminthic pneumonitis.

PNEUMOPERITONEUM 45,52
Air in the peritoneal cavity, which
may be the result of a perforation of
an intestine – as sometimes happens
in *typhoid* – the perforation of the
stomach by an *ulcer*, a ruptured
appendix or a *trauma* such as a stab

214

wound. The air normally gathers underneath the *diaphragm*, where it can be seen on *x-ray*. Pneumoperitoneum in small quantities may also be a consequence of peritoneal *dialysis* or a *laparoscopy*.

PNEUMOTHORAX   10
A condition in which a lung has collapsed because of the presence of air in the *pleural* cavity. This may be traumatic, when the air enters the cavity through a stab wound, or be the result of leakage of air from the lung itself. A pneumothorax may occur spontaneously in young, fit people or may be associated with *emphysema* or other lung diseases. In the latter case the condition is more serious because lung function is already generally poor. Young fit people may only notice a slight shortness of breath.

A tension pneumothorax is a condition in which a valve-like mechanism allows air to enter the pleural cavity but does not let it leave. Consequently pressure builds up in the cavity and eventually the venous return to the heart may be impeded as well as the function of the uncollapsed lung. Pneumothoraces are treated by inserting a tube into the cavity under a water seal and draining the air away.

POLIOMYELITIS (also INFANTILE PARALYSIS)   58
Commonly called 'polio', poliomyelitis is an infectious disease caused by a group of *viruses* that invade the *nervous system* and attack the motor components of the spinal cord and brain stem. The viruses are spread in airborne droplets by healthy carriers or those who are infected and in contaminated food and water. After an *incubation period* of one to two weeks an illness develops that is characterized by *fever*, *malaise*, headache, and sometimes *diarrhoea* and vomiting. Later the temperature rises sharply, the headache becomes worse and there are symptoms similar to those of *meningitis*, with pronounced *alimentary tract* problems and tenderness in the muscles. At this stage the disease may clear up without any further problems, but sometimes *paralysis* appears as the temperature subsides. Any part of the body can be affected by polio, but it is most usually seen in the lower limbs, which become flaccid and eventually *atrophy*.

Poliomyelitis may affect the muscles of *respiration*, impairing breathing to such an extent that the condition can be fatal unless a *ventilator* is used. It also affects the brain stem and the nerves that control swallowing, coughing and the voice in a condition called bulbar polio. The incidence of polio has been much reduced by the general *vaccination* of communities; once the disease has set in, treatment is by bed-rest and nursing care.

POLLEN ASTHMA – *see* HAY FEVER

POLYARTERITIS NODOSA
A *connective tissue disease* of unknown cause that is most often seen in young men, polyarteritis nodosa is thought to be associated with disorders of the *immune* systems. Nodules develop in the walls of arteries, causing inflammation and sometimes eventual *thrombosis* and *necrosis*. The clinical symptoms of the disease include *fever*, pain, *tachycardia* and wasting, but the arterial disruption may give rise to a large number of other symptoms. *Steroid* drugs often help to relieve the condition.

POLYCYSTIC DISEASE OF THE KIDNEY   91
An abnormality of the *kidneys* that tends to run in families, in which the organs are distended and contain large numbers of *cysts* with normal tissue in between them. Initially the problem may cause no symptoms and may only be detected at operation or in an examination; sometimes there is pain in the loins, *haematuria*, *uraemia* and hypertension. Eventually the condition may cause *renal failure*. Symptoms such as *hypertension* may be treated separately, but renal failure is treated by *dialysis* or *transplantation*.

POLYP
A *benign* growth, sometimes with a stalk, or pedicle, that projects from the *mucous membrane*. Polyps may be found in the colon – see *polyposis coli* – in the nose, where they may obstruct breathing and in the *womb*, where they may cause irregular bleeding. Polyps are usually removed by cautery.

POLYPOSIS COLI
A familial disease of the large bowel

in which large numbers of *polyps* form inside the colon. It is important that this disorder should be diagnosed because there is a possibility of *malignant* changes in the polyps. This possibility is sometimes anticipated and a *prophylactic colectomy* performed, in which the affected portion of colon is removed surgically.

PORTAL CIRCULATION   43
The blood vessels that supply the *liver*. The liver itself is supplied by the hepatic artery from the abdominal *aorta*, and blood returns to the heart through the hepatic vein. Blood from the *spleen*, *stomach*, intestines and *pancreas* is carried to the liver by the portal vein, where it is filtered and nutrients are absorbed. This blood then returns to the heart via the hepatic vein.

When pressure builds up in the portal vein, because of liver diseases such as *cirrhosis*, the organs and structures drained by it may swell up, in a condition called portal *hypertension*.

POSTMATURITY
A term that is used to describe a pregnancy in which the baby has been in the uterus for more than 40 weeks. Excessive postmaturity may lead to neonatal problems and it has become common to induce labour at about 40 weeks and 10 days.

POSTPARTUM
The few days immediately after birth, when the *womb* is still recovering and beginning to return to its normal state, are known as the postpartum period.

PREGNANCY   98
The state of pregnancy lasts from conception to *labour*, a duration of about 40 weeks – see embryo, *fertilization*, foetus, labour, ovaries, ovulation, ovum, parous, sperm, uterus.

PREMENSTRUAL TENSION (P.M.T.)   101
A fairly common problem in which women tend to gain weight, have abdominal cramps, breast soreness, general irritability and *depression* and sometimes even suffer *migraines* before a period. These changes may come on at any time in the 10 days preceding a period and are relieved when bleeding starts. Premenstrual tension is thought to be associated with the extra reten-

tion of salt and water that is caused by the powerful *steroid* female *hormones.*

PREPUCE
The foreskin, a flap of skin at the end of the *penis* that covers the glans. In infants the prepuce cannot be retracted, but after the age of five it may be pushed back. The foreskin is often removed surgically at birth for reasons of religion or custom in a circumcision; it may also be removed in later life in the treatment of conditions such as *phimosis.*

PRESBYOPIA
A common condition of the eyes in old age in which sufferers have difficulty in reading at a normal distance and in doing close work such as sewing. Presbyopia is caused by a lack of elasticity in the lens of the eye that makes short focusing difficult.

PRICKLY HEAT
A skin condition seen in hot, humid weather, in which there is an eruption of tiny, itching and tingling red pimples in a *rash* that is normally seen on the face, trunk and thighs.

PRIMAGRAVIDA
A woman who is expecting her first baby. After the birth she is known as primiparous.

PROCTITIS 37,39
An inflammation of the rectum that may be caused by infectious organisms, or certain drugs; it may also be associated with *Crohn's Disease* and ulcerative *colitis* or be a side-effect of *radiotherapy.* Proctitis causes discomfort, *tenesmus, diarrhoea* and occasionally rectal bleeding.

PROCTOSCOPE
An instrument used to examine the *rectum,* in the investigation of problems such as rectal bleeding.

PROGESTERONE 99
A *steroid* hormone that is secreted by the corpus luteum, the endocrine tissue inside a ruptured *ovarian* follicle, in small quantities by the *adrenal glands,* and in pregnancy by the *placenta.* Progesterone is produced as a result of the stimulation of the corpus luteum by luteinizing hormone from the *pituitary gland,* and increases the vascularization of the *endometrium* in preparation for

pregnancy. During pregnancy the hormone is produced by the placenta to maintain the vascular structure. Similar effects to those produced by progesterone may be obtained by synthetic substances known as progestogens.

PROGNOSIS
The likely outcome of a disease and the individual's chances of recovering from it.

PROLAPSE
The descent of a part of the body from its correct position. The umbilical cord is said to have prolapsed when it is the first product of labour; the *rectum* may sometimes prolapse through the anus. In older, post-menopausal women the *womb* may prolapse, collapsing so that sometimes the *cervix* of the *uterus* protrudes from the *vagina.* Such a prolapse may be prevented by a *pessary* and can be repaired surgically, although sometimes a *hysterectomy* may be necessary.

PROPHYLAXIS
The steps taken to guard against or make less likely the occurrence of disease. *Vaccination* and aseptic techniques, for example are prophylactic, while condoms, or male sheaths, are sometimes called prophylactics because their use is a step taken to avoid pregnancy.

PROPRIOCEPTION
The awareness of the position and movement of parts of the body in relation to other parts of the body and the environment. The proprioceptive sense organs, or proprioreceptors, are found in the muscles, joints, *tendons* and inner ear.

PROSTATE GLAND 96
A gland that secretes a thin fluid that is part of *semen,* or the male ejaculate and is positioned around the *urethra* and lower part of the *bladder;* it is only present in men. The prostate can become inflamed in a problem called prostatitis, that may be associated with conditions affecting the urethra such as gonorrhoea. It commonly becomes enlarged in middle age, sometimes obstructing the urethra, making *urination* troublesome and occasionally causing *retention* of urine. The gland is also the site for *tumors* which may be *benign* or *malignant;*

it is either partially or wholly removed in a surgical operation called a prostatectomy.

PROSTHESIS
The replacement of a diseased, damaged or lost part of the body with an artificial substitute. A woman who has lost a breast in a mastectomy will normally be provided with a prosthetic breast.

PROTANOPIA
A form of color blindness in which the color red cannot be distinguished.

PROTEIN
A chemical compound made up of substances called amino acids. Proteins are found in both vegetable and animal foods, though milk, eggs, cheese, meat, fish and soy beans are the best sources; they are broken down during digestion, initially by the *enzyme* pepsin in the *stomach,* into their constituent amino acids.

Protein is man's only source of nitrogen, and is essential for the growth of new tissues and repair of damaged tissues. The enzymes of the body are all proteins, as are *antibodies* and *fibrinogen* – the '*plasma* proteins' – as well as many other substances in the body.

PROTEINURIA
The presence of *proteins* in the *urine,* which may have various causes. The condition generally indicates an increased permeability of the tubules of the *kidney,* which may be caused by inflammation such as *glomerulonephritis.*

PRURITUS 68
Itching – an irritation of the skin which causes a desire to scratch the offending area. Pruritis may be *psychosomatic* or *neurotic* in origin, but can be caused by a large number of diseases and disorders. There are some specific kinds of pruritis, such as pruritis ani, an embarrassing itching around the anus that may be caused by *haemorrhoids, worms,* poor hygiene or *allergies* to washing powder; pruritis vulvae where the female genitals itch, as in vaginitis; and pruritis senilis, in which itching may accompany the degenerative effects of ageing on the skin.

Itching may be caused by a number of skin conditions, such as tinea or ringworm, *eczema* or allergic rashes such as *urticaria*; it may also be the result of *lesions* that affect the skin in diseases such as *herpes* zoster and *chicken pox.*

PSITTACOSIS
Although commonly called parrot disease, psittacosis is a disease that infects budgerigars as well as parrots and can be transmitted to man. The disease is caused by a *virus*-like organism and causes headaches, *nausea, fever,* nosebleeds and lung disorders. Psittacosis can be fatal unless it is recognized and treated with *antibiotics.*

PSORIASIS   112
A common disorder of the skin which has a tendency to run in families, whose cause is unknown. Psoriasis causes pink or reddish patches of itchy, scaling skin, mainly of the limbs and scalp. The condition may be associated with nervousness – it tends to appear at adolescence – and sometimes with *arthritis.* There is no specific cure for psoriasis, but the discomfort it causes can be alleviated by soothing ointments.

PSYCHOANALYSIS
A method in which disorders of the mind, behavior and personality are treated in a way pioneered by Sigmund *Freud*; past emotions and experiences that have hitherto been repressed are brought to the forefront of a patient's consciousness and there dealt with. In particular the repressions that may have developed during the normal sexuality of infancy and childhood are examined; they are brought to light by techniques such as *free association* and *psychotherapy.* Once repressions are recognized as such it is possible for an individual to work out ways of adjusting to them.

PSYCHOGENIC
Of mental rather than physical origin.

PSYCHOLOGY
A science, but not necessarily a medical science, in which behavior and the mental processes that govern behavior are studied.

PSYCHOPATHY
A term that is often used loosely and taken to describe homicidal mania. A psychopath is in fact an individual who thinks himself apart from the rest of society and under no obligation to obey its rules or observe its conventions; he may act antisocially and amorally and be unable to comprehend normal emotions, such as guilt. Psychopaths are often friendly, quiet and obsessive, but they are capable of irresponsible and impulsive action.

PSYCHOSEXUAL PROBLEMS
A sexual problem that has its origins in the mind. In men psychosexual problems are those such as premature ejaculation and *impotence*; in women the problems are generally *frigidity* and *vaginissimus.* Nowadays these problems may be treated in a branch of *psychotherapy* called psychosexual therapy, often with good results.

PSYCHOSIS   140
Mental disorders that are of such severity as to cause disintegration of the personality and loss of touch with reality, delusions and hallucinations. Psychoses may be the result of organic diseases, such as tertiary *syphilis, trauma, senility* or *alcoholism* (Korsakoff's Psychosis). They may, on the other hand, have no known physical cause. They are then called 'functional' – see *mania, manic depression, schizophrenia.*

PSYCHOSOMATIC   142
All illnesses are complicated by the interaction of physical and mental factors, but in psychosomatic illnesses and pains the mental factors predominate. Conditions such as mouth *ulcers, eczema* and *asthma* are thought to be strongly associated with emotional stress, while aches and pains, especially in the back, are often caused by emotional rather than physical problems. Psychosomatic symptoms are seen at their most severe in *hysteria*, and rather less so in *depression.* If after tests symptoms are seen to be psychosomatic in origin *counselling* and psychiatric help may be given.

PSYCHOTHERAPY
A form of treatment for psychological and behavioral problems and the psychosomatic element of physical problems that includes techniques such as *counselling,* suggestion, persuasion, *psychoanalysis* and *behavior* therapy. Psychotherapy depends to a large extent on the strength and nature of the relationship between the therapist and the patient; the aim is to make the patient aware of the significance of his own symptoms in the context of his personality.

PTOSIS
A drooping of the upper eyelid, which may be *congenital* or simply a result of fatigue, but is sometimes a sign of a nervous disorder – when it may be associated with *paralysis* of eye movements – or conditions such as *myasthenia gravis.*

PUBERTY   130,138,160
The stage of development at which secondary sexual chaacteristics become apparent, proper genital reproductive functions become possible and in women the *menarche* is seen. These changes are brought about by an increase in the production of *androgen* and *oestrogen* by the *gonads*, stimulated by the action of the *pituitary glands.* In men the voice 'breaks', muscle mass increases and facial and body hair starts to grow; in women the breasts start to grow and subcutaneous *fat* adopts a characteristic distribution. The *hormonal* changes of puberty may cause skin problems such as *acne,* and also conditions such as *depression,* anxiety and *hysteria*; patterns of behaviour may seem strange and worrying as the adolescent searches for a sexual and personal identity in the adult world.

PUERPERIUM
The 42 days that follow childbirth, during which the reproductive organs in the female return to their normal condition.

PULMONARY   10
Of the lungs. The pulmonary circulation supplies deoxygenated blood to the lungs and returns oxygenated blood to the heart; blood is pumped to the lungs through the pulmonary artery by the right *ventricle* of the heart and returns from the lungs in the pulmonary vein that leads to the left *atrium.* Sometimes the opening of the pulmonary artery from the right ventricle is narrowed in a condition called pulmonary *stenosis,* which may be a part of *Fallot's Tetralogy.* The condition may cause serious problems.

Sometimes one of the blood vessels of the lungs may be obstructed by a pulmonary *embolism.* When the embolus is in a large blood vessel it may cause *heart failure*, otherwise it results in an increase in the blood pressure of the lungs, called pulmonary *hypertension*, and *necrosis* of lung tissue called a pulmonary infarct.

PULSE
An indication of the rate and rhythm of the contraction of the heart muscle that can be felt as a series of pressure waves in the large arteries of the body. The three pulses most commonly taken are the radial pulse at the wrist, the carotid pulse in the neck below the jaw and the femoral pulse in the groin – though pulses can be felt in a number of other places in the body. The pulse rate varies between individuals, but is generally between 60 and 80 beats a minute; the pulse speeds up during physical exertion, illness and stress.

PUPIL   120
The opening at the center of the iris of the eye that contracts in response to an increase in light and dilates when light intensity decreases – the pupillary *reflex*.

PURPURA
A condition in which the subcutaneous blood capillaries bleed into the skin, either because of a defect in the capillaries or because the blood platelets have been destroyed.

PUS
A fluid found in *abscesses* and at the site of infections and inflammations, which may be whitish-yellow or almost green, and is composed of dead *leucocytes*, tissue fluids, *bacteria* – both dead and alive – and dead tissue.

PUSTULE
A blister that is filled with *pus*. Compare *vesicle*.

PYAEMIA (US – Pyemia)
A form of *septicaemia* in which the blood is 'poisoned' by *bacteria* that form *pus*, causing the formation of abscesses in many parts of the body. Pyaemia causes *fever* and may be fatal unless antibiotic treatment is given.

PYELITIS   90
An infection, usually *bacterial*, of the part of the *kidney* in which the *ureter* terminates – the *pelvis* of the kidney. Pyelitis causes urinary difficulties, pain and *fever*; the condition is treated by *antibiotics*, painkillers and fluids.

PYELOGRAPHY (US- Urography)
The *x-ray* examination of the structure of the *kidneys*, using radio-opaque dyes.

PYELONEPHRITIS
A *bacterial* infection of the kidney, which may be *acute*, when the symptoms are chills, pain, urinary difficulties and a high temperature, or *chronic*, where the kidneys become progressively more and more scarred and smaller until *renal failure* results. Acute pyelonephritis is treated by antibiotics and other drugs to relieve pain; when chronic pyelonephritis is severe surgery may be necessary.

PYLORIC STENOSIS – *see* STENOSIS

PYLORUS   32
the lower exit of the *stomach* that opens when the stomach pressure becomes higher than *duodenal* pressure to allow the stomach contents to pass – see *stenosis*.

PYONEPHROSIS
An accumulation of *pus* in the *kidney* that is often the result of a blockage by a kidney stone. The infection often spreads to the nearby tissues.

PYORRHEA
Also called periodontal disease, pyorrhea is an infection of the *periosteum* of the teeth that may be caused by *vitamin* deficiencies, inadequate oral hygiene or other infections of the mouth.

PYREXIA
Fever – an increase in body temperature associated with a hot dry skin, shivering, headache, loss of appetite, nausea, *constipation* or *diarrhoea*, aches and pains all over the body – especially in the joints – and sometimes vomiting. When fever is severe there may be *delirium*, *convulsions* and sometimes *coma*. Fevers may be caused by many conditions, but commonly by *bacterial* and *viral* infections.

The average temperature in man is about 37°C (98.6°F). When a fever is said to be low the temperature is around 37.7°C (100°F); in a moderate fever the temperature is around 38.8°C (102°F); and in a high fever around 40°C (104°F).

PYROSIS – *see* WATERBRASH

PYURIA   90
Pus in the *urine*, which may be seen as a cloudy fluid, and indicates a *bacterial* infection of the *urinary tract* or *kidney*.

Q-FEVER
An infectious disease of cattle, sheep and goats, which may be caught by man if contaminated milk is drunk. The symptoms include *fever*, a headache and lung infections; treatment is by *antibiotics*.

QUADRIPLEGIA
A *paralysis* of all four limbs, that may be the result of injury to the spinal column or of a disease that affects it.

QUICKENING
Intrauterine *foetal* movements that are felt by the mother.

QUINSY
A complication of tonsillitis in which *abscesses*, or quantities of pus, form around the tonsils, causing the neck to swell and difficulties in swallowing and breathing. Treatment is usually by *antibiotics*.

RABIES   58
Otherwise called hydrophobia, rabies is an acute infectious disease that is *endemic* in dogs, cats, foxes, bats and sometimes cattle – though because of strict controls it is not found in Britain. Rabies can be transmitted to man by the bite of an infected animal, but only one in four people bitten by a rabid dog actually contract the disease. (The proportion is higher if the bite is from a cat.) After an *incubation period* that can vary from 10 days to two years the rabies *virus* attacks the *nervous system*, causing initially *malaise*, *fever*, irritability and painful muscle spasms on swallow-

ing. Later there may be *convulsions*, *paralysis*, breathing difficulties and terror at the sight of water – hence the name hydrophobia. Once this stage is reached death normally occurs within a week.

Treatment of rabies is in the first instance the immediate and careful cleaning of the bite wound, then daily injections of rabies *vaccine* and afterwards immune *serum*. The disease can be avoided by eradication of the rabies 'pool' through strict quarantine of animals.

RADIATION SICKNESS 162
An illness caused by exposure to radiation: either in the form of *X-rays*, or as the radioactive radiation that may be the result of a nuclear explosion or leakage from industrial, laboratory or medical radioactive substances. Very high doses are fatal, but lower doses may cause an illness that is characterized by *nausea*, *diarrhoea* and vomiting, *malaise*, bleeding from the *mucous membranes*, *anaemia*, *bone marrow* damage and loss of appetite. There may also be skin burns. Radiation used medically, either as X-rays or in radiotherapy, is extremely carefully controlled.

RADIOTHERAPY 136
The treatment of diseases, which are usually *malignant*, by the administration of radiation. The radiation is focussed onto a precise area, in order to kill the malignant cells. It may, however, also cause distressing side-effects, such as *nausea*, *anorexia* and *diarrhoea* – see *radiation sickness*.

RASH
Spots on the surface of the skin. Rashes may be flat or raised, dark red or pale pink, all over the body or localized, depending on the type of rash and its cause. Sometimes the individual spots of the rash contain fluid; they are then called vesicles and eventually become crusted, as in chicken pox, or *varicella*. Rashes may be *allergic* in origin, as in nettle rash, or *urticaria*, and sometimes are seen after a *vaccination*. They may be caused by specific infections, such as *rubella*, *measles* or *scarlet fever*, or simply due to heat. The term may be used to describe a condition of the skin, such as *eczema* or *nappy rash*, while sometimes rashes are caused by drugs. Then the rash tends to occur in a

particular place, and is known as a fixed drug eruption.

RAYNAUD'S DISEASE 88
A disease of young women that is thought to be caused by spasms of the small arteries that supply the fingers and toes. These spasms, which are often triggered by emotional stress and made worse by cold, cause symptoms that are known as Raynaud's Phenomenon – the fingers turn white then blue, and are cold and numb, then turn red and feel warm and painful. There is no actual change in the arteries involved or the fingers. There is no cure for Raynaud's Disease, but keeping the fingers warm helps and *counselling* and reassurance may keep the problem in check.
Raynaud's Phenomenon may also be seen in all types of people as an early sign of disorders of the connective tissue, or of abnormalities of the blood vessels. In these cases the Phenomenon is unrelated to the Disease.

RECTUM 34,96
The terminal part of the large bowel, that starts at the end of the sigmoid colon and continues for about 5 ins. (13 cms.) to the anus. A rectal examination – called an investigation P.R., or per rectum – may be necessary to help determine the cause of lower *abdominal pain*, to assess the size of the *prostate gland* in men with urinary difficulties and to investigate the causes of rectal bleeding.

Rectal bleeding should always be reported to a doctor. It may be due to piles, or *haemorrhoids*, to small cuts and fissures around the anus, called anal tears, or to severe *dysentery*, when the blood will be mixed with mucus. Other possible causes are *diverticular disease* and *cancer* of the rectum.

Rectal itching may cause discomfort and embarrassment. It can be the result of piles, poor hygiene or *threadworms* – see *pruritis* ani. The rectum may also be a site for the introduction of drugs into the body, in the form of suppositories.

REDUCTION
The process of mending a *fracture* or *dislocation*, in which the two bones are replaced in their correct positions or – in the case of a dislocation – the two articulating surfaces are brought back into contact.

REFERRED PAIN
A pain that originates in one part of the body but is felt in an entirely different place. The phenomenon is made possible by the common pathways that are shared by sensory *nerves* in the spinal cord. Pain from the *gall bladder* may, for example, be referred to the shoulder.

REFLEX
A specific and involuntary response to a stimulus. Reflexes are often tested in a medical examination because they may be affected by any disease that involves the *nerves*. The most well-known reflex is probably the knee jerk, in which the leg automatically extends in response to a sharp tap on the tendon below the knee cap. There are many other reflexes, including the pupillary reflex, in which the *pupil* of the eye contracts in response to light; the corneal reflex, in which pressure on the cornea causes the eyelids to close; the abdominal reflex, in which irritation of the skin causes a contraction of the superficial muscles; and Babinski's Reflex, in which the big toe bends upwards – instead of downwards, which is normal – when the sole of the foot is stroked, to indicate disease or injury to the nerves.

REGIONAL ENTERITIS, REGIONAL ILEITIS – *see* CROHN'S DISEASE

REGRESSION
The return to child-like behavior that may represent an escape from problems or stress in *psychological* conditions.

REGURGITATION
Generally, a flow of fluid or semi-fluids in the opposite way to that which is normal. The term is commonly used to describe the rise of food from the stomach to the mouth; it is also used to indicate the backwards flow, or seepage, of blood in the heart as a result of an incompetent *heart valve*.

REHABILITATION
A process in which people who have been cut off by disease or injury from their normal life are reintroduced to their environment. Rehabilitation may involve long periods of *physiotherapy*, *counselling* and education in new techniques in order that the sufferer can

cope with his disability. It is especially useful for people who have had a serious *stroke* and consequent *hemiplegia* to have a period of rehabilitation before they return home.

Various pieces of equipment may be used to help the sufferer live a normal life, and their use is mainly taught by an *occupational therapist*.

REMISSION
A period in which the symptoms of a disease abate. Remission may be permanent, but the symptoms may on the other hand reappear.

RENAL CALCULUS
A stone in the *kidney*. The stone, or calculus, obstructs either the *pelvis* of the kidney or the *ureter* and is usually composed of *calcium* salts, oxalates and phosphates. Certain factors may predispose to the formation of calculi. These are: *urinary* infections and stagnation of urine; excessive loss of water from the body as a result of working in very hot conditions; conditions that cause an increase in the level of calcium in the blood, such as overactivity of the *parathyroid gland*, *Cushing's Syndrome*, multiple *myeloma*, or *tumors* of the bone. marrow, and *vitamin* D intoxication; certain rare *metabolic* disorders; and an excess of milk or alkaline substances in the diet.

Kidney stones tend to cause pain and *haematuria*, but may cause no symptoms. Depending on their position they may become impacted in the tissues, causing obstruction and *hydronephrosis* and may result in *renal failure* unless treated.

RENAL FAILURE also (KIDNEY FAILURE) 146
An inability of the *kidneys* to fulfil their main function of excreting fluid wastes from the body, which may be caused by *polycystic kidney disease*, hypertension, diabetes mellitus, obstructions such as *kidney stones* or stones in the *ureter*, or infections such as *glomerulonephritis*, renal *tuberculosis* and *chronic pyelonephritis*. Renal failure causes *uraemia* and may be fatal unless there is effective treatment – which may be by removing the cause of the problem, by either *dialysis* or *peritoneal* dialysis, or by *transplantation*. Dietary restrictions will also be necessary.

RESECTION 37,56,96
The surgical removal of a diseased part of the body. Resection is sometimes performed on the gut, in diseases such as *carcinoma* or severe ulcerative *colitis*. Once the diseased area has been removed the two ends are either joined back together, to maintain continuity, or connected to a *stoma* in the abdominal wall, as in a *colostomy* or an *ileostomy*.

Resection of the *prostate* gland is sometimes performed by passing an instrument through the end of the penis and carrying out a 'coring' operation – this procedure is known as a transurethral resection.

RESPIRATION 10,14
The exchange of *oxygen* for the waste product *carbon dioxide*. The term includes the exchange of gases between the air and the blood in the alveoli and the lungs; also the exchange at the cellular level within the tissues.

Though properly the lungs are only one of the sites of respiration – their activity is breathing, not respiration – the act of breathing is often referred to as 'respiration'. The rate and depth of respiration, when the word is used in this sense, may increase in physical exertion, so that more oxygen can be supplied to the tissues, and in psychological disturbances and disease states such as *pneumonia*, blood diseases and heart problems. Respiration may be decreased by *shock*, *coma*, *brain* disorders and poisoning.

RESPIRATORY DISTRESS SYNDROME (also HYALINE MEMBRANE DISEASE) 10
A condition that sometimes affects newborn babies, especially those that are premature, that is caused by insufficient surfactant in the lungs. Because of this deficency high surface tension prevents the *alveoli* from expanding; the result is *dyspnoea*, which is manifested by grunts and inspiratory retraction of the chest wall, and eventually *cyanosis*. The baby is given oxygen and drugs that correct the abnormality; as it matures the problem tends to solve itself.

RESPIRATORY TRACT
The airways of the body, from the nose and mouth through the *larynx*, *pharynx*, *trachea*, *bronchi* and bronchioles to the *alveoli* of the lungs. The tract is imprecisely divided in-

to the upper and lower respiratory tracts, the former comprising the mouth, nose and throat and the latter the lower windpipe and lungs. Upper respiratory tract diseases are generally the common infections of the nose and throat such as *coryza*, the common cold, *influenza* and *laryngitis*; lower respiratory tract diseases are those such as *pneumonia*, *bronchitis* and *emphysema* – though lower respiratory tract diseases may sometimes be complications of upper respiratory tract problems, and vice versa.

RESUSCITATION
The process of reviving a person whose heart or breathing has stopped, as a result of a *heart attack*, drowning, a drug overdose or similar experiences. The first essential is to start the heart pumping once more – if the supply of blood to the brain is halted for more than a few minutes the resulting tissue damage to the brain will be irreversible. This may be achieved by external cardiac massage, or by medical techniques such as *defibrillation* and stimulation of the heart by drugs. At the same time breathing may be started by use of one of the various techniques of artificial respiration – the most common used is 'mouth-to-mouth' – which may later be superseded by the use of a mechanical ventilator, or breathing machine.

RETENTION OF URINE 92,96
An inability to pass water that causes the *bladder* to fill up with urine, and may lead to gross distension of the organ. Retention is commonly seen in older men who have an enlarged *prostate* gland, which acts as a *sphincter* by compressing the *urethra* at the base of the bladder. The condition is also sometimes seen in *cystitis*, when the neck of the bladder becomes inflamed; it may be a complication of spinal injuries or disease when the nerve supply to the bladder is damaged. Retention itself is usually treated directly by *catheterization* of the *urethra*; when the cause of the problem is ascertained it can be treated separately – in the case of prostatism, for example, by a *resection* of the prostate gland.

RETINA 120,146
The innermost, light-sensitive layer of the eye. The retina contains millions of tiny cells called rods and

10,14,17,19,44

cones that detect and differentiate light and convey impressions of seen images to the brain. Sometimes the blood vessels supplying the retina degenerate in a condition called retinopathy that is seen in *hypertension*, *diabetes mellitus* and *toxaemia*. The degenerate vessels leak, and blood and exudates may be seen when the retina is examined through an ophthalmoscope. Retinopathy is relieved by treatment of the condition that has caused it.

Sometimes the fluid in the eye, called vitreous humor, leaks through a hole in the retina and forces it away from the back of the eye. This condition is called a detached retina and is repaired surgically. Treatment of a detached retina is more difficult when, as occasionally happens, the retina is forced away from the back of the eye by a *tumor* or *haemorrhage* located behind it.

RHESUS FACTOR

An *antigen* in the blood that was first identified in the rhesus monkey from which it takes its name. Over 80 per cent of people have this factor in their blood, and are therefore called Rhesus, or Rh positive. Those who do not have the factor are called Rh negative. This is a similar situation to that in the ABO system of *blood groups*, and in the same way a person who is Rh– cannot be given the blood of a person who is Rh+.

The presence or otherwise of a Rh factor has a particular importance in pregnancy. If a Rh– mother has an Rh+ baby some of the *foetal* cells will usually enter the mother's circulation and cause the production of *antibodies*. In a subsequent pregnancy these antibodies will enter the foetal circulation of another Rh+ baby and react with the baby's RH + blood cells to destroy them. If this is severe the baby will be stillborn; if less severe the baby will be *jaundiced* and may develop *kernicterus* in *haemolytic disease of the newborn*. The problem can usually be avoided; following detection by blood tests during or before pregnancy, drugs can be given that suppress the mother's formation of antibodies.

RHEUMATIC FEVER   86

A disease that causes inflammation of *connective tissue*, whose origin is unknown but is related to, and sometimes follows, certain specific *bacterial* infections such as *tonsillitis*. It generally affects children between the ages of 5 and 15, especially those from deprived or overcrowded backgrounds. There is a sudden onset of pain, swelling and stiffness in the joints, with *fever*, sweating and *tachycardia* as well as *malaise*, fatigue and loss of weight; the trunk and shins may also break out in red patches and *chorea* is sometimes seen. Treatment is by bed-rest and *antibiotics*.

Rheumatic fever has serious effects on the *heart*, including a thickening and *stenosis* of the *heart valves*, and sometimes *pericarditis* and *myocarditis*; antibiotics are necessary before any future minor operations, such as tooth extraction, in order to prevent further damage.

RHEUMATISM   112

A general term that covers all soreness, stiffness and pain in the joints of the body, from causes that may include a large number of diseases, such as *arthritis*, *rheumatoid arthritis*, *bursitis*, *trauma*, *rheumatic fever*, and many others.

RHEUMATOID ARTHRITIS   112

A disease of unknown cause that leads to chronic inflammation, first of all of the small peripheral *joints* of the hands and feet and later the larger joints of the wrist, shoulder and elbow. It usually, but not always, comes on at around the age of 40 and women are affected more commonly than men. (A specific form of rheumatoid arthritis, called Still's disease, affects children.) The onset of the disease is gradual; the joint pain is transient and the sufferer may experience *malaise*, fatigue, and weight loss. Eventually the joint damage may cause swelling and characteristic deformity. The condition can be diagnosed by blood tests, a clinical history and *x-rays* and treated by anti-inflammatory drugs, gold, *steroids* and *physiotherapy*.

RHINITIS

An inflammation of the *mucous membrane* of the nose that is normally due to *virus* infections such as *coryza*, the common cold. Rhinitis causes a characteristic runny nose. The condition may also be caused by an *allergy*, when it can be treated by medicinal sprays.

RIBOFLAVIN – *see* VITAMINS

RICKETS

A disease in which *calcium* cannot be absorbed from the intestines in sufficient quantities and is therefore inadequately deposited in the developing bones of children. Rickets is primarily caused by a *vitamin* D deficiency. This vitamin facilitates the intestinal absorption of calcium and is synthesized in the body as a result of the action of ultraviolet light on the skin. The result may be a characteristic bowing of the legs and enlargement of the wrists, associated with a poor *appetite*, *diarrhoea*, vomiting and loss of weight. More rarely rickets is caused by an insufficient amount of calcium in the diet or an excessive loss of calcium from the body. Treatment of rickets is by an improved diet that is rich in vitamin D and calcium, including foods such as cod liver oil, butter fat, milk, dairy products and beans.

Rickets may also be caused by chronic *renal failure* during childhood, when it is known as renal rickets, and may result in *dwarfism* and incomplete growth of the *testes* or *ovaries*.

RIGOR

A severe bout of shivering associated with a high temperature and often followed by sweating, that may occur in any acute *fever*. Rigor mortis is the muscular stiffness and rigidity that is seen in a corpse.

RINGWORM – *see* TINEA

RODENT ULCER – *see* ULCER

RUBELLA (also GERMAN MEASLES)

An infectious *viral* illness, usually of childhood, in which a blotchy red *rash* usually starts on the face and neck and spreads over the body, following a day or two of upper *respiratory tract* symptoms. The rash is seen after an incubation period of 14 to 18 days, and normally only lasts two or three days; the glands at the back of the neck are often enlarged.

Rubella is not normally serious, though it causes discomfort, but the condition can cause serious problems if it is contracted by pregnant women, especially during the first two or three months of pregnancy. At this stage the ears, eyes and heart of the *foetus* are developing, and rubella may cause defects in all these areas. For this reason young women who have not had German measles during childhood are often *vaccinated* against the disease before they start to have their families. Pregnant women who do come into contact with rubella usually have a blood test and then an injection of *serum* that gives artificial *immunity* against the disease.

RUPTURE – *see* HERNIA

S

SADISM
Named after the notorious 18th century French aristocrat the Marquis de Sade, sadism is a sexual perversion in which an individual derives sexual pleasure or mental satisfaction from the physical abuse or mental domination of another person – compare *masochism*.

SAFE PERIOD   98
The time of the *menstrual* cycle when conception cannot occur and intercourse can take place safely: theoretically days one to nine and 21 to 28 of the menstrual cycle. Unfortunately it is difficult to judge the safe period exactly and the method is by no means foolproof, though a device now undergoing exhaustive tests may well provide this information with reliable precision – see *contraception*, *ovulation*.

ST VITUS DANCE – *see* CHOREA

SALIVA   32,155
A secretion produced by the salivary glands in the head. These are the two parotid glands, one at each angle of the jaw, the two submandibular glands, one underneath each jawbone and the sublingual glands beneath the tongue. The saliva is secreted in response to the idea or the actuality of food and contains an *enzyme* called ptyalin that partly dissolves food as the first step in digestion. The saliva also stimulates the taste buds and lubricates food, making swallowing easier. The salivary glands may be involved in infections, such as *mumps*, and their ducts may sometimes become blocked by stony concretions called calculi.

SALMONELLA
A group of *bacteria* that live in the intestines of animals and humans and are *pathogenic* in different degrees and in different ways. Salmonella typhi and paratyphi cause the *enteric* fevers *typhoid* and *paratyphoid* fever respectively. Another form of the salmonella bacterium causes *septicaemia*, while others lead to either a mild *gastro-enteritis* or severe *food poisoning* – see *salmonellosis*.

SALMONELLOSIS
An infestation of the digestive system of man by *bacteria* of the *salmonella* group that causes severe and sometimes fatal *food poisoning*. Salmonellosis can be contracted from food that has been infected by human carriers of the organism and then incorrectly canned.

SALPINGITIS   52,94
An inflammation of the *Fallopian tubes*, or oviducts, that is usually *bacterial* in origin. Salpingitis is often a feature of *gonorrhoea*, but may be associated with other organisms, such as the *T.B.* bacillus; it may also follow other causes of pelvic infection, including acute *appendicitis* and a *septic abortion*. Treatment is by *antibiotics*, but sometimes the tubes remain blocked and lead to subsequent *infertility*.

SARCOIDOSIS
A chronic disease that in many ways resembles *tuberculosis*, in which small granular *lesions* are formed in the tissues. Many organs, including the lungs, *lymph* nodes, eyes and skin may be involved. Sarcoidosis may cause no symptoms whatever, but sometimes there are chest problems with a marked shortness of breath and wheezing. The condition is diagnosed through *x-rays* and skin tests and sometimes requires treatment by *steroids*.

SARCOMA
A malignant tumor of the *connective tissue* – a prefix is usually given to denote the site of the sarcoma. A chondrosarcoma, for example, is in *cartilage*, a liposarcoma is in *fat* and an osteosarcoma is found in *bone*.

SCABIES
Also called 'the itch', scabies is an irritating, itchy skin infection that is caused by the mite sarcoptes scabiei. The mites spread through close personal contact and scabies tends to occur in families. After mites have become established on the body the female mite digs a burrow into the skin and lays about 40 eggs inside it. After a while these eggs hatch out into larvae, which crawl over the body until they become adult, copulate and lay eggs in their turn. Initially the itch caused by the mites is mild, but later it may be severe enough to prevent sleep. Little ridges can be seen on the skin, typically on the web between the fingers, sometimes with a black dot at the end that is the female mite.

Scabies is treated by the application of a benzyl benzoate solution to the whole body, after a bath. The solution is left on for 24 hours and the application repeated within a week. The mites die quickly when out of contact with the body, so any clothes that may be infected are hung up, thoroughly aired and then brushed.

SCARLET FEVER
Otherwise called scarlatina, scarlet fever is an *acute* infectious disease that is caused by *bacteria* and transmitted from person to person, or in the milk of a cow that has *mastitis*. The symptoms include a very sore throat, *fever*, *malaise*, enlarged glands on the neck and a *rash* on the body – typically with a pallid area around the mouth. The tongue is often coated with thick white fur through which the red papillae project, giving it the look of a strawberry – this particular sign is in fact called 'strawberry tongue'. Scarlet fever is treated by isolation, bed-rest and penicillin.

SCHIZOPHRENIA   140
Previously called dementia praecox – a term now obsolete – schizophrenia is popularly thought to be a condition in which there is a split mind or personality. This is not in fact the case. Schizophrenia is a *psychotic* illness that is characterized by a disintegration of the personality. Schizophrenics tend to behave in one of several different ways, though the varying forms of schizophrenia are often interchangeable. 'Simple' schizophrenics are usually apathetic and introverted. They may live and work quite happily in the community, but be thought a little strange. *Catatonic* schizophrenics may alternate between stupor and outbursts

of hysterical excitement, with strange postures and repetitive gestures. Hebephrenic schizophrenics react illogically and inappropriately to situations, often using silly or child-like mannerisms and inventing meaningless words. *Paranoid* schizophrenics suffer from delusions and hallucinations – voices from the sky tell them what to do, and they have a feeling of passivity. They think that they are controlled by outside agencies who can put things into their minds and also read their thoughts.

It is not known how schizophrenia develops, but it is thought that there is some *genetic* predisposition to the disorder. Nowadays the phenothiazine drugs help many schizophrenics to lead almost normal lives.

SCIATICA
A pain that is felt along the course of the sciatic *nerve* – running down the back of the buttock, back and foot. Sciatica may be caused by a prolapsed or slipped intervertebral disc that is pressing on the root of the nerve; it is normally seen in elderly people, especially on lifting weights. The condition is treated by bed-rest and *analgesics*.

SCLEROSIS　　　　　60,80
A hardening of tissues – see *atherosclerosis, arteriosclerosis, multiple sclerosis*.

SCOLIOSIS
An abnormal curve of the spine to one side of the body or the other. A scoliosis may be *congenital*, the result of poor posture during childhood, or caused by a disease of the bones or muscles or a compression *fracture* of a vertebra.

SCURVY　　　　　162
A disease now rarely seen in the western world, that was first noted amongst sailors whose normal diet did not include citrus fruits or fresh vegetables. Scurvy is caused by a deficiency of *vitamin C*; it has a gradual onset, with weakness and exhaustion leading to a sallow color and tender, bleeding gums. Eventually the teeth drop out, the breath becomes very bad and there is much bleeding into the skin, muscles and joints – showing as small red spots or large bruises on the skin. The loss of blood causes *anaemia*, fatigue, and *fainting*. Scurvy can easily be avoided if fresh fruit and vegetables are eaten, or failing that if vitamin C, or ascorbic acid, tablets are taken.

SEBACEOUS CYST　　　145
Also called a wen, a sebaceous *cyst* is a painless, soft raised lump, containing yellowish-white cheesy material, that is mainly seen on the hairy skin of the scalp, face, neck, back and scrotum. Sebaceous glands secrete sebum, which lubricates the skin, and it is thought that a sebaceous cyst is a retention of this secretion within the gland that is caused by a blockage of the gland's duct – though there is some dispute about this theory. The cyst is usually removed surgically, along with all the glandular material, so that it does not form again.

SEBORRHEIC DERMATITIS
A form of *dandruff* in which large amounts of sebum are produced by the sebaceous glands of the scalp; the area becomes covered in yellow-grey oily scales, which itch and sometimes burn. The problem normally clears up after the frequent use of proprietary anti-dandruff shampoos. In babies a similar scaling is quite common and is known as 'milk crust'. The condition is not irritating and clears up if the baby's scalp is washed daily in soap or baby shampoo.

SEMEN
The male ejaculate, composed of *sperm* and secretions from the *prostate gland*, seminal vesicles and Cowper's Glands.

SENILITY
The loss of mental and physical abilities that is sometimes caused by the natural changes of ageing – see *dementia*.

SEPSIS
A *bacterial* infection that causes putrefaction of the tissues. Sepsis is avoided during medical procedures such as operations, wound-dressing and childbirth by the use of strict aseptic techniques. All instruments, towels and dressings are *sterilized*, the operator wears surgical gloves and the 'field', or area of activity, is sluiced down with antiseptic lotion.

Puerperal sepsis, or puerperal infection, is a form of sepsis that sometimes attacks the female reproductive tract after childbirth, causing *malaise, fever, abdominal pain* and *distension*. It is treated by *antibiotics* and painkillers.

SEPTICAEMIA
(US – Septicemia)
A state in which *pathogenic bacteria* circulate and multiply in the blood – also called blood poisoning. The toxins produced by the bacteria cause a high *fever*, general debility, or weakness, sweats, a low *blood pressure* and sometimes *delirium*. Septicaemia is seen much less often these days, as a result of the development of aseptic techniques, and is treated by *antibiotics*.

SERUM
The clear yellowish fluid that is left after blood has clotted, which does not contain any blood cells or *fibrin*. Sometimes serum taken from an animal or human recovering from a disease such as *diphtheria* or *hepatitis* is purified and injected into the bloodstream of a sufferer from that disease to increase the sufferer's *immunity*, because the serum contains valuable *antibodies* and *antitoxins*. In the past such serum was commonly prepared by injecting small quantities of bacteria into a horse; this is less common nowadays because the horse serum may cause a serious reaction in humans.

SHINGLES – *see* HERPES

SHOCK
A general term applied to a state in which a sufferer has a low *blood pressure*, weakness, is cold, sweaty and breathes rapidly, has a weak fast pulse and may lose consciousness. Shock may be caused by a *trauma* and *haemorrhage* that decreases the volume of blood in the body, or by *septicaemia*, where *bacterial toxins* cause *vasodilation*; by *myocardial infarction* or *pulmonary embolism*, where the blood pressure is lowered; by severe *diarrhoea* and vomiting that may lead to dehydration; or by severe and widespread burns, in which serum is lost from the surface of the burned skin. Shock is initially treated by keeping the victim warm and then by attending to the cause of the problem.

SHORTSIGHTEDNESS – *see* MYOPIA

SICKLE CELL ANAEMIA
An inherited disorder of the blood seen in dark skinned races in which

the *haemoglobin* is slightly abnormal. If the *gene* responsible for sickle cell *anaemia* is inherited from one parent only the disease is not severe and there are usually no problems under normal conditions. Under stress, however, such as an operation, *trauma*, or flying in an unpressurized aircraft, the haemoglobin may precipitate into a crescent shape – hence the name of the disease. This causes anaemia, and such episodes of 'sickling' may be associated with *debility*, *fever* and pain. Before an operation black people may have their blood checked for sickle cell disease.

If the gene is inherited from both parents the condition is more severe and children so affected do not normally survive into adult life.

SILICOSIS
One of the *occupational* lung diseases, or *pneumoconioses*, silicosis was first described in the South African gold mines and is caused by the inhalation of dust that contains silica particles. The disease is also seen in rock drillers, foundry workers and metal grinders and involves the formation of fibrous nodules in the lungs. The result is shortness of breath and sometimes *emphysema*.

SINUS   28
A term that is used in several different ways. The most commonly known sinuses are the air filled cavities in the bones of the face and skull which become infected in *sinusitis*. Otherwise a sinus is a normal distension of a blood vessel – usually a vein – or a channel between an infection and either the skin or an organ. The carotid sinus is a specialized pressure-sensitive area of the carotid artery which can sense a rise in blood pressure and set in action, through the brain and the *autonomic nervous system* a slowing of the heart; a pilonidal sinus is an infected tract that is usually found in the hairy skin at the base of the spine, often causing considerable discomfort.

SINUSITIS   28
An infection of the sinuses, especially those at the front of the face, that is usually seen in winter. Sinusitis causes headaches, *facial pain* and a discharge from the nose and may be the result of a number of factors, including *bacteria*, *viruses* and *allergies*. The condition may be

treated by *antibiotics*, but when it is very severe surgical drainage of the sinuses may be necessary.

SKIN GRAFT – *see* GRAFT

SLIPPED DISC – *see* DISC

SMALLPOX
A highly infectious disease that was once extremely serious but is now, following extensive *vaccination* programmes, almost completely extinct. Smallpox is caused by a *virus* called variola that may be spread by direct contact or in air-borne droplets; it causes lesions similar to those seen in *chicken pox*, though they are mainly seen on the limbs and face. The first sign of the disease, after an *incubation period* of between eight and 17 days, is a *fever*, with a sore throat and cough. Three or four days later the characteristic spots are seen – first as small red lesions, the *vesicles*, then pustules which finally form a crust. After a few more days the spots disappear, leaving scars and pock marks. Complications of the disease include *pneumonia*, *heart failure*, and *delirium*; smallpox is treated by isolation, bed-rest, plenty of liquids and specialized drugs. Nowadays vaccination against smallpox is rarely necessary.

SPASM
An involuntary contraction of muscles that is strong and often painful. Muscle spasms may be caused by *metabolic* disturbances, as in *tetany*, or be habitual – see *tics*. Sometimes these may be caused by minor *trauma*, as when the muscles of the back go into spasm after a heavy object is lifted, or by *depression*. Muscle spasms may be treated by muscle relaxant drugs and *physiotherapy*.

SPASTIC
A term that is popularly used to describe an individual suffering from any form of *paralysis*. In fact spastic paralysis is specifically a condition caused by disease or damage of certain *nerves* of the spinal cord, in which there is 'spasticity' in one or more limbs – they are weak and sometimes paralysed, with rigidity, brisk reflexes and a resistance to movement that the individual has not originated himself. The spinal nerves may be damaged by birth injuries, accidents or in-

juries to the spine, and sometimes by nutritional deficiencies.

SPASTIC COLON (also IRRITABLE BOWEL SYNDROME)
A condition in which there is intermittent colicky *abdominal pain*, distension of the bowel, *diarrhoea* and sometimes large quantities of *mucus* in the stools. The cause of the problem is unknown, but it tends to be associated with *stress* and fatigue. Treatment is by specialized drugs and mild tranquilizers.

SPERM
More properly called a spermatozoon, a sperm is the male sex cell that is produced in the *testis* and enters the female *vagina* in the *semen*, or male ejaculate, during sexual intercourse. It contains the 23 *chromosomes* of the male parent that link up with the same number of chromosomes in the female parent's *ovum* at fertilization. In cases where male *infertility*, or sterility, is suspected, the numbers of sperm in a given volume of semen may be counted in a sperm count.

SPHINCTER
A ring of muscles around an orifice. A sphincter is normally in a state of contraction, but may be opened under voluntary or involuntary control to allow the passage of solids or fluids through the orifice.

SPHYGMOMANOMETER
A device used for measuring the *blood pressure*. A cuff is placed around the upper arm and pumped up with air until the flow of blood past the cuff has stopped. As the cuff is deflated the pulse is monitored through a stethoscope and the column of mercury, or dial, connected to the cuff is checked. The *systolic* and *diastolic* blood pressures can both be determined by this method; the technique is not at all painful, but there may be some slight discomfort as the cuff is deflated.

SPINA BIFIDA
A *congenital* deformity of the posterior walls of the vertebrae of the spine. Sometimes the defect is very mild – it may only show up on *x-rays* and cause no problems at all. This condition is called spina bifida occulta. Occasionally the problem is more serious and a part of the cord or the membranes covering it pro-

trudes from the back of the vertebrae, sometimes above the surface of the skin. If only the membranes, or *meninges*, protrude the protrusion is called a meningocele; if both the meninges and spinal cord are involved it is a meningomyelocele.

Spina bifida is usually seen in the lumbar, or lower back, region and when severe may cause *paralysis* of the legs and *incontinence*; there may be associated water on the brain and mental retardation. The condition can sometimes be corrected surgically, depending on the degree of deformity; there are also a number of special centers in which both parents and children can be taught methods of coming to terms with the disability and its consequences and given support and help. Spina bifida can be detected before birth by techniques such as *amniocentesis*.

SPLEEN 158
An organ situated in the upper left-hand corner of the abdomen, weighing approximately half a pound. It consists of a capsule that is filled with a mass of red and white pulpy *lymphoid* tissue and *red blood cells*, within a framework of fibers. The spleen forms red and white blood cells in the foetus, but in adult life only certain types of *leucocyte*; it also filters old, worn out or defective red blood cells from the blood. The organ may be badly injured or ruptured by a jab or kick, and if the problem is not promptly diagnosed and blood *transfusions* given the effects may be very serious. The spleen becomes enlarged, sometimes enormously so, in *leukaemia* and *Hodgkin's Disease*, and to a lesser extent in *malaria*, *typhoid* and *glandular fever*. It becomes infected in a condition called splenitis, which may cause pain and vomiting.

The spleen is removed surgically in an operation known as a splenectomy, which may be necessary in Hodgkin's Disease, or in the treatment of *congenital* spherocytosis, in which the red blood cells are abnormal. A ruptured spleen will normally be removed in an emergency operation.

SMEAR TEST – see CERVICAL SMEAR

SPONDYLITIS 110
An inflammation of the joints of the

spine that is normally caused by osteoarthritis – see *ankylosis*.

SPONDYLOSIS
A degeneration of the intervertebral discs that is usually seen in the region of the neck (cervical spondylosis). Sometimes spondylosis causes no symptoms and can only be seen on x-rays; at other times the condition leads to pain and weakness in the arms. Treatment is by exercises to strengthen the muscles of the neck, or *physiotherapy*, and a supporting collar may be used. In severe cases it may be necessary to resort to surgery.

SPRAIN
An injury to a *ligament* around a joint, which causes considerable swelling and pain but no actual damage to the joint. Sprains are treated by ice-packs, support and rest.

SPUTUM 19
An expectoration from the lower *respiratory tract*, or *saliva* and *mucus* from the upper respiratory tract, that is generally increased in smokers. Sputum becomes green and infected, or purulent, in *bronchitis*; in the treatment of chest infections samples of sputum are sometimes cultured so that the offending *bacteria* can be identified and the correct *antibiotics* prescribed.

SQUINT – see STRABISMUS

STAMMER
A speech impediment in which the sufferer finds it extremely difficult to articulate the initial sounds of a word, and often attempts the first consonants a number of times before there is success. The disorder is often caused by a lack of confidence and emotional problems, becoming worse under stress, but may occasionally be a sign of neurological disease. Treatment is by speech therapy.

STAPHYLOCOCCUS
A common group of *bacteria* that are found on the skin and *mucous membranes* and are often responsible for *boils* and other *abscesses*. Toxins produced by staphylococci may be a cause of *food poisoning*.

STATUS EPILEPTICUS
A continuous succession of fits in

an *epileptic*, with no period of recovery. Status epilepticus is more common in children and may be seen when anti-epileptic treatment has a deleterious effect; the condition is extremely serious and demands immediate treatment.

STENOSIS
The tightening or narrowing of an artery, a heart valve – see *valvular disease* – or any other passage. Pyloric stenosis is a narrowing of the pylorus, or lower end of the *stomach*. Renal artery stenosis is a narrowing of the renal artery supplying blood to the *kidney* which may cause an increase in *blood pressure*.

STERILIZATION 98
A term that in medicine may have several meanings. It may denote the procedure in which medical instruments and dressings are made germfree by washing them in boiling water, or steaming them at high temperature and pressure; otherwise sterilization refers to a surgical technique which makes either a male or a female infertile. Male sterilization is achieved by a *vasectomy*; in female sterilization the *Fallopian tubes*, or oviducts, are either cut, tied off or burned.

STEROID 21,39,112
A general name for a group of drugs or naturally produced substances that have a similar chemical structure. Among the naturally occurring steroids are the sex *hormones* – see *androgen*, *testosterone*, *progesterone*, *oestrogen* – and the hormones secreted by the cortex of the *adrenal glands*, called *corticosteroids*. Synthetic steroid drugs are used in the treatment of problems such as *asthma*, *rheumatoid arthritis*, *temporal arteritis* and *Crohn's Disease*; they may also be used topically, or on the skin, in a number of skin conditions. Some steroids have the effect of suppressing the *immune* responses of the body, and so are often used to prevent rejection of a *transplanted* organ; generally the main function of steroids is to reduce inflammation.

STILL'S DISEASE – see RHEUMATOID ARTHRITIS

STOMA
A mouth or small opening – usually a hole made in the abdominal wall

to form an *ileostomy* or *colostomy* after extensive bowel *resection*.

STOMACH   *32,45*

A muscular bag, lined with *mucous membrane*, at the lower end of the *oesophagus* in the upper left quadrant of the abdomen. The stomach stores, warms and digests food: gastric juices, containing the *enzyme* pepsin, are secreted by glands in the stomach in response to the sight, smell and presence in the stomach of food. After the food is churned up, lubricated and partially digested it is delivered to the *duodenum* in suitable quantities.

The stomach also produces a substance called the 'intrinsic factor' which is necessary for the absorption of *vitamin B_{12}*; in the absence of this factor pernicious *anaemia* develops. The stomach becomes inflamed in a condition called *gastritis*, and the mucous membrane may be affected by a *gastric ulcer*; it may be partially or wholly removed in a *gastrectomy*.

STOMACH CANCER   *56,138*

A fairly common form of *cancer* that affects men over the age of 45 more often than women. Stomach cancer seems to have an association with *blood* group A and in certain cases, to run in families. *Tumors* may develop in any part of the stomach, but most commonly are seen in the lower part, or pylorus, producing an obstruction of the passage and eventual vomiting. Cancer may also affect the body of the stomach and can look like an ulcer in its early stages, though later it is distinctive. Occasionally the wall of the stomach is infiltrated by tumors, making it small and stiff, when it is called a 'leather bottle stomach'. Early on there may be no symptoms except for *dyspepsia*; later stomach cancer shows as *anorexia*, *nausea*, pain and weight loss and vomiting. Stomach cancers are treated by *gastrectomy*, but the outlook after the operation is not good.

STOMATITIS   *162*

An inflammation of a *stoma*. If the stoma is abdominal and caused by an *ileostomy* or *colostomy* the inflammation may be caused by the constant irritation from the disposable bags in which *faeces* are collected. Otherwise stomatitis refers to an inflammation of the mouth or oral cavity. The term is a general description, including angular stomatitis – where the skin at the corners of the mouth becomes cracked and infected, often as a result of a deficiency of iron and *vitamin* B; *gingivitis* – an inflammation of the gums; and *cheilosis*, where the lips become cracked and reddened.

Generally, stomatitis is thought to be caused by nutritional disorders and vitamin deficiencies: these are seen in diseases such as *pellagra*, pernicious *anaemia* and severe iron deficiency anaemia. Stomatitis is also seen as a result of *candidal* infections of the mouth and in the course of general *systemic* diseases, as well as blood diseases such as *leukaemia* and *purpura*. Ulcerative stomatitis, otherwise called 'trench mouth' or Vincent's Angina, is seen in conjunction with poor nutrition and bad dental hygiene.

STOOL

The individual portions of *faeces*, or solid wastes of the body. Stools are often examined and analysed, in order to detect the presence of blood, *mucus*, *bacteria* and *parasites* which may be present in disease states – see *floating stools*.

STRABISMUS

A squint, which may be convergent or divergent – in other words the affected eye may look in towards the nose or out away from it. A squint may be caused by longsightedness, where in order to look at a close object the eyes look towards each other, or by defective vision in one eye. Occasionally the problem is caused by *paralysis*, or interruption of the nerve supply, to one of the six muscles that hold the eye in place – this may only show up when a child is tired, when it is called a 'lazy eye'. If the squint is caused by defective vision spectacles and exercises of the eye may be prescribed; if the squint is severe surgery may be necessary, but it is important that squints should be seen by a doctor and treated early on in life.

STREPTOCOCCUS

A large group of *bacteria*, many of which cause infections. Types of streptococcus cause *tonsillitis*, some forms of *nephritis* and *endocarditis*, and are associated with a number of other conditions. They generally have the ability to destroy red blood cells, and so are called *haemolytic*.

STRICTURE

A narrowing or blockage of a hollow organ or duct, which may be due to a large number of factors, from *tumors* to stones and foreign bodies.

STRIDOR   *10*

A loud, harsh breathing sound that may be heard during certain infections of the *trachea* and *larynx* – a sign that there is some inflammation and obstruction in the passages of the upper *respiratory tract*.

STROKE   *64*

Also called apoplexy, a stroke is the result of a *cerebrovascular accident* (C.V.A.). When the brain, or parts of the brain, are deprived of blood for a short period of time, the resulting damage may vary from temporary weakness on one side of the body to complete *paralysis*, and sometimes death. After a stroke, it may be necessary for the sufferer to undergo a period of *rehabilitation*.

SUBLUXATION

A state in which the two articular surfaces of a joint have slipped slightly out of line, in a partial *dislocation*.

SUFFOCATION – *see* ASPHYXIA

SUN STROKE (also HEATSTROKE)

A state of exhaustion that is caused by the combination of excessive heat or exposure to the sun and a lack of replacement of fluids and salt. There may be *cramps*, vomiting, a high temperature, a low *blood pressure*, a weak pulse and sometimes even *fever* and *delirium*, depending on the amount of heat involved and the reaction of the body's temperature-control mechanisms to it, which can vary from person to person. The problem can be avoided if sensible precautions are taken in hot climates; sunstroke can be very serious, and if fever is present it is normally considered a medical emergency, so it is always best to take medical advice.

SUPPOSITORY

A drug given in the form of a soft pellet that is inserted into the *rectum* or the *vagina*. Sometimes drugs given in this fashion are designed to act locally, as, for instance, in *haemorrhoids* or *thrush*; other drugs that affect different parts of the body may be given as suppositories because side-effects such as *nausea* are often avoided.

SUPPURATION

The formation of *pus*. The suppurative diseases are those such as *septicaemia*, in which pussy *abscesses* are formed in the body as a result of inflammation.

SWAB

A word that has two medical connotations. A swab may be a means of collecting and culturing a *pathogenic* organism so that it can be identified: a piece of cotton on the end of an 'orange stick' is dipped into the discharge or *pus*, or brought into contact with an infected area – for example the throat or the *vagina* – and then sent to the laboratory in a special transport medium so that it can be cultured and examined. The small pieces of gauze that are used to 'mop up' during a surgical operation are also called swabs.

SWEAT

A fluid that is excreted by the sweat glands, sweat is important in the temperature control mechanisms of the body and also as a means of excreting waste nitrogen products. Sweat is secreted in response to stimuli from the sympathetic *nervous system* as a reaction to heat, pain, fear, physical exertion, nausea and certain drugs. In rare cases excessive sweating may be controlled by a sympathectomy, in which fibers of the sympathetic nervous system are cut. Fresh sweat does not smell, but if it is allowed to linger and is not removed by washing, *bacteria* will act on the nitrogenous elements to produce an acrid and offensive odour.

SYMPATHETIC NERVOUS SYSTEM – *see* NERVOUS SYSTEM

SYMPTOM

Any part of a disease or disorder that causes discomfort and is felt by the patient. A symptom that is not noticed by the patient is properly called a sign. When a patient visits a doctor to talk about a symptom he is said to be 'presenting' with that symptom.

SYNCOPE

Otherwise called fainting, syncope is a temporary loss of consciousness caused by a brief interruption of the blood supply to the brain. Syncope may be caused by *metabolic* problems such as *hypoglycaemia* or by circulatory disease, but much more commonly it is a reaction in healthy people to emotional shock, tiredness, prolonged standing or an abrupt change of circumstance – as when one gets out of a very hot bath too quickly. A faint should be treated by putting the sufferer's head between his legs, removing tight clothing and giving access to fresh air; some people may quite normally struggle and have minor convulsions during a faint, which may appear, unwarrantably, to be those of a minor epileptic fit.

SYNDROME

A collection of symptoms, signs and test findings that together constitute a particular disease.

SYNOVIAL FLUID   94,112,155

A fluid produced by the synovial tissues that line a bursa to fill the *joint* cavity and lubricate the joint. Synovitis is an inflammation of the synovial tissues and is the basis of arthritis – it may be caused by *rheumatoid arthritis* or by infections such as *mumps, rubella, tuberculosis* and *gonorrhoea*. Synovitis is treated by special drugs.

SYPHILIS   94

A *venereal disease* that is caused by the spirochaete *bacterium* treponema pallidum, and may be *congenital* or acquired by sexual contact.

Acquired syphilis falls into three stages. Primary syphilis is seen two to four weeks after the disease has been contracted – a chancre, or hard, but painless sore develops, usually on the genitals but sometimes on the fingers or lips. The secondary stage appears about six weeks later – a general infection sets in, with *malaise*, sore throat, headache, *rashes*, wart-like lesions on the genitals, enlarged *lymph* nodes and small *ulcers* on the *mucous membranes* of the mouth, and lasts for several weeks. The third, or tertiary, stage of syphilis may become apparent either within months or within years. Masses of granular tissue called gummae are laid down in a number of organs, including the skin, brain and liver; the heart, blood vessels and the brain also become involved, causing neurological disorders, blindness and general paralysis of the insane (G.P.I.).

The disease is treated by penicillin and *antibiotics* and these days is much more uncommon than was once the case, though it seems that there is an increasing incidence of syphilis among homosexuals.

Congenital syphilis is seen when a mother with the disease gives birth to a child. The baby has a characteristic facial appearance, deformities of the bones and teeth and sometimes involvement of the liver and kidneys. The problem can be detected during pregnancy by blood tests such as the *Wasserman reaction* and if the mother is treated with penicillin the foetus is normally unharmed.

SYSTEMIC DISEASE

A disease that affects the whole of the body rather than one of its parts.

SYSTOLE

A period of contraction of the heart muscles during which blood is pumped out of the ventricles. Systole is the period between the first and second heart sounds – see *blood pressure, diastole*.

TACHYCARDIA

A fast heartbeat. Tachycardia may be caused by drugs such as amphetamines, by *fever*, by the action of the *hormone* adrenaline (US – epinephrine) or by the stimulation of the sympathetic *nervous system*. In the last two cases the heartbeat is speeded up as part of the body's preparation for and response to physical action and stress. For every 1°C rise in temperature there is a rise in pulse rate of 10 beats per minute; a paroxysmal tachycardia may sometimes be brought on by caffeine and smoking. Fast *arrhythmias* such as atrial *fibrillation* are also tachycardias, but are more properly then called tachyarrhythmias.

TACHYPNOEA
(US – Tachypnea)   14,19,21

An increase in the normal rate of breathing – which is about 12 breaths per minute in adults. Tachypnoea may be the result of the increased oxygen demands of the body during physical exertion, or caused by *hysteria*, chest infections such as *pneumonia*, acute *asthmatic* attacks, *chronic bronchitis* and *emphysema*.

TALIPES

Otherwise called a club foot, talipes is a deformity in which the foot is twisted either inwards, outwards, up or down at the ankle. If the deformity is upwards the sufferer walks on his heels; if downwards on his toes.

If the foot is twisted inwards the person affected walks on the outside edge of his foot; if outwards he walks on the inside edge. Talipes may be *congenital* and the result of incorrect positioning of a large baby in the womb – in which case the defect can usually be corrected by exercise and manipulation.

The condition may be acquired, when it is usually caused by a disease that *paralyses* or leads to spasms in the muscles of the lower leg. Otherwise it may be the result of scarring or burning of the tissues of the foot.

TAPEWORM – *see* WORMS

T.B. – *see* TUBERCULOSIS

TEMPERATURE   153

A measure of the heat of the body. Temperature varies between different parts of the body – for example, *rectal* temperature and sublingual (under the tongue) temperatures are usually slightly higher than those obtained from the armpit or the groin. It is also a little higher at night and lower in the early morning. The normal range of body temperatures is between 36.7° and 37.2°C (98° to 99°F).

Temperature is reduced by a cold environment, especially in the elderly and children, and an abnormally low temperature is called *hypothermia*. It may also be reduced in *shock*, a large loss of blood and in *myxoedema*. Body temperature increases in *viral* and *bacterial* infections as well as in *malaria*, *Hodgkin's Disease* and other *fevers*. In fact the word fever, or pyrexia, actually means 'a rise in body temperature'.

Temperature also increases slightly in women at *ovulation*, when it is 0.5°C (0.9°F) higher than normal.

TEMPORAL ARTERITIS (also CRANIAL ARTERITIS, GIANT CELL ARTERITIS)

An inflammation, or *arteritis*, of the temporal branches of the carotid arteries, the main arteries of the head and neck, that is a disease of the *connective tissue*. The condition usually affects people who are over the age of 70 and causes a severe headache, often only on one side of the head. Occasionally the inflammation leads to a *thrombosis* of the arteries that supply the *retina*, causing blindness. Temporal arteritis is associated with a raised *E.S.R.*, which subsequently falls after treatment with corticosteroid drugs.

TENDON

A fibrous cord by which muscles are attached to bones. Some tendons are surrounded by sheaths of tissue that contain *synovial* fluid, to lubricate the tendon and reduce friction. Occasionally these sheaths become infected in a condition known as tendosynovitis; when only the tendon is involved the condition is called tendinitis.

TENESMUS

A painful and involuntary straining to empty the bowels of faeces which has no effect, other than the production of some *mucus* and sometimes a little blood. Tenesmus is sometimes seen in conditions that affect the large bowel, such as *dysentery* and *haemorrhoids*.

TERATOGEN

Any disease, event or substance that causes the development of abnormalities in the *foetus*, or teratogenesis. Teratogens may be diseases such as *rubella*, and overexposure to *x-rays*, or drugs such as thalidomide.

TERATOMA

A *tumor*, usually of the *gonads*, which is made up of cells that are not normally to be found at the site of the tumor. It is thought that such cells may have been misplaced at the time when the developing embryo was differentiating into varying types of tissue and on occasions a teratoma may contain bizarrely misplaced hair and teeth. *Malignant* teratomas of the *testis* are sometimes seen in young men; they are first indicated by a painful swelling of the scrotum, or by the appearance of secondary *cancers*.

Such teratomas normally spread rapidly, and are treated by *radiotherapy*, drugs and the removal of the testis – an orchidectomy. The progress of treatment can be checked by blood tests, because the teratomas secrete identifiable substances into the blood stream. Teratomas are also seen in the *ovaries*, when about 80 per cent are malignant.

TESTIS (also TESTICLE)

A male *gonad*, one of a pair of glands inside the scrotum. The testes consist of numerous seminiferous tubules, in which sperms are produced; the glands also secrete the male sex *hormone testosterone*. They may become infected by the *mumps virus* or *gonorrhoea*, and the inflammation is called *orchitis*. The result may be a hydrocele, or collection of fluid around the gland. Occasionally a testicle is twisted, in a condition called torsion of the testicle. The problem causes extreme pain, and unless an operation is performed as soon as possible the blood supply to the gland may be cut off.

Normally the testes descend into the scrotum from the abdomen in the *foetus*. Sometimes this does not happen and the 'undescended testicle' is moved surgically in order to avoid any risk of *malignant* changes in the gland. Occasionally the testis is the site of a teratoma.

TESTOSTERONE

The principle male sex hormone, or androgen, testosterone is secreted by the *testes* and in small quantities by the *adrenal glands* and the *ovaries* in women. It promotes the growth and development of the male genitals and also the male secondary sexual characteristics, such as muscle mass, a deep voice and facial and body hair.

TEST TUBE BABY

In a technique recently developed to help *infertile* women to bear children an *ovum* is taken from the mother's *ovaries* and placed in a test tube. It is fertilized in the tube by *sperm* from the father and at a very early stage in its development the minute *embryo* is implanted in the mother's womb, where it grows normally.

TETANUS (also LOCKJAW)

An infectious disease caused by the

bacterium clostridium tetani that is found in the soil. When a wound is contaminated, especially with earth that has been heavily manured, spores may enter the body and multiply. They produce a toxin that increases the sensitivity of the motor *nerves* of the spinal cord, and after an *incubation period* of between four and 28 days the first symptoms appear. Initially there may be stiffness in the jaw and neck; later the whole body is affected. Painful spasms and convulsions may be caused by the smallest stimulus and death may follow – either as a result of prolonged convulsions of the respiratory muscles or from complete physical exhaustion.

Tetanus can be avoided by strict cleansing of wounds, the maintenance of *immunity* against the disease by *vaccination* and regular 'booster' injections, by the injection of tetanus antitoxin if there is a possibility that there has been an exposure to the disease and the use of penicillin in high doses.

TETANY
Muscle spasms caused by a decrease in the level of *calcium* in the blood, often affecting the hands and feet. The decrease in calcium levels that leads to tetany may itself be the result of a *Vitamin D* deficiency, of an inadequacy of the *parathyroid* gland (or surgical removal of it) or of hyperventilation, the overbreathing that may be due to *hysteria* or some drug overdoses.

THALASSAEMIA (US – Thalassemia)
An inherited disorder of the blood that is seen in Mediterranean countries and parts of Africa and Asia, and in individuals who originate from those areas. In thalassaemia there is an abnormality of the process in which *haemoglobin* is manufactured in the body; the condition may cause *anaemia* and an enlarged *spleen*. When the *gene* responsible for thalassaemia is inherited from both parents an affected child may be severely ill and even die: in this case the condition is called thalassaemia major. In thalassaemia minor the condition is only inherited from one parent and the problem usually causes no symptoms.

THIAMINE
Vitamin B$_1$ – see *vitamins*.

THIRST
The desire to drink fluid. Thirst is usually the body's response to a need for more fluid; it is experienced after fluids have left the body, as may occur through perspiration on a hot day or through *diarrhoea*. It often accompanies fevers, but may be a sign of untreated *diabetes mellitus*, when thirst is accompanied by polyuria, or copious urine, and polydipsia, or copious drinking. Some drugs can cause thirst, especially atropine and certain antidepressants. Excessive thirst and water-drinking may be part of a *psychiatric* illness that is called compulsive water drinking.

THREADWORM – *see* WORMS

THROMBOSIS
The formation of a *blood clot*, or thrombus, inside a blood vessel. The clot normally consists of *atheromatous* material such as cholesterol and clotted blood. If the thrombus becomes detached from the wall of the blood vessel and is carried to another part of the body in the bloodstream it is known as an *embolus*. The thrombus may eventually block the blood vessel, often leading to serious consequences. When thrombosis occurs in the *coronary arteries* it causes a coronary thrombosis, or heart attack – see *myocardial infarction*. A thrombosis in a leg vein, called a deep venous thrombosis, may cause pain, swelling and heat in the leg; it is worrying because sometimes a part of the clot breaks off and becomes lodged in the lungs – a *pulmonary embolus*. In superficial veins thrombosis may be associated with a degree of inflammation, called thrombophlebitis.

THRUSH
Properly called candidiasis, thrush is an infection of the moist parts of the body by the fungus *candida albicans*. Thrush may affect almost any part of the body, but the term is commonly used to describe an infection of the mouth or *vagina*. Vaginal thrush causes discomfort and a white itchy discharge, while the mouth and throat – especially of young children – may develop white patches. Thrush is treated by anti-fungal agents.

THYMUS GLAND
A collection of *lymph* tissues in the neck that produce special types of *white blood cells* called lymphocytes which play an important part in the body's immune responses. The thymus is large during childhood but starts to shrink at puberty and is gradually replaced by other tissues. Tumors, or thymoma, may develop in the gland, sometimes in association with *myasthenia gravis*.

THYROID GLAND 149,151,153
An *endocrine* gland found in the neck that manufactures the *hormone* thyroxine in response to the stimulus of hormone-releasing factors from the *pituitary gland* and the *hypothalamus*. Thyroxine controls the rate of the body's *metabolism* and an under-production of the hormone during childhood may cause *cretinism*; and under-production in later life causes *myxoedema*. An over-production of thyroxine results in *thyrotoxicosis*. Sometimes the gland becomes enlarged and presses on the windpipe – see *goitre*.

THYROTOXICOSIS (also HYPERTHYROIDISM, EXOPHTHALMIC GOITRE, GRAVES' DISEASE). 149,151
An over-production of the *thyroid hormone* thyroxine that causes a characteristic bird-like appearance, with bulging eyes, *tremor*, brisk reflexes and symptoms involving the eyelids. Thyrotoxicosis may also be associated with a rapid pulse, palpitations, weight-loss, *diarrhoea* and *menstrual* disturbances in women – such as a lack of periods. The condition affects women about eight times more commonly than men.

The condition may arise spontaneously, in which case it is primary toxic *goitre*, or *Grave's Disease*; otherwise it is associated with the formation of hyperactive nodules in the gland which may be *benign* or *malignant*. Treatment of the disorder may be by drug therapy, but if the gland is pressing on the windpipe or is cosmetically unacceptable it may be removed surgical.y in a thyroidectomy. Complications of the operation may include *tetany*, as some of the *parathyroid gland* may be removed; hoarseness, because of interference with the nerve that supplies the larynx; and *myxoedema*, if too much of the gland is removed. An alternative form of treatment for older people is the administration of radioactive iodine – the iodine is taken up by the gland and the radiation kills the thyroid tissue.

THYROXINE – see THYROID GLAND

T.I.A. – see TRANSIENT ISCHAEMIC ATTACK

TIC
A twitch, or habit spasm, usually of the facial muscles that may be caused by structural changes in the tissues, by *psychiatric* disorders or by muscular tension.

TIETZE'S SYNDROME
Also called costochondritis, Tietze's Syndrome is a condition of unknown cause in which the joints between the ribs and breastbone become swollen, causing chest pain. Treatment is by painkillers, but the problem usually clears up on its own.

TINEA
Also called ringworm, tinea is a fungal infection that commonly affects the skin between the toes, when it is called tinea pedis, the skin of the groin (tinea cruris), the scalp (tinea capitis), and the beard (tinea barbis). The condition is contagious and causes severe itching; it is treated by anti-fungal agents.

TINNITUS
A buzzing or ringing in the ears that often affects old people and can be most distressing. Tinnitus is associated with deafness, is a cardinal feature of *Ménière's Disease* and may also be a symptom of an overdose of aspirin or quinine. The condition can be caused by ear wax, high *blood pressure*, or congestion of the middle ear associated with chronic catarrh.

TONSILS
Tonsils are seen in several different places in the body, but those most commonly discussed are the palatine tonsils. These are collections of *lymph* tissue at the back of the tongue, which can be seen in a mirror if the tongue is held down. The tonsils produce *leucocytes* and help to protect the body from infection; they are larger in children and tend to become smaller with age. The tonsils become infected in a common condition called tonsillitis, which may be caused by *bacteria* or *viruses*. The symptoms of

tonsillitis include a very sore throat, *fever*, general *malaise* and sometimes difficulty swallowing and a swollen neck. Small collections of *pus* or *exudates* can often be seen in the tonsils themselves. Sometimes abscesses form around the tonsils and require drainage and surgical removal – see *quinsy*. The condition is treated with gargles of soluble aspirin, and penicillin if the problem has a bacterial cause. If tonsillitis is recurrent and is responsible for a large amount of time lost from school or work the tonsils may be removed in an operation called a tonsillectomy; this operation is not, however, as popular or frequently performed nowadays as was once the case.

TORTICOLLIS
Commonly called wry neck, torticollis is a condition in which spasm of the muscles of the neck causes the head to be held to one side. The problem is sometimes the result of an injury to the muscles during birth, but it may also be due to a severe burn or be *occupational* – people who have to make repeated head movements to follow fine work, such as shoemakers, are particularly prone to torticollis.

TOURNIQUET
A tight cuff that is applied round a limb to constrict the blood vessels and stop the flow of blood to wounds that are below the point of application. If a tourniquet is left on the limb for too long the tissues may start to necrose and become gangrenous – the device should be slackened off every 15 minutes or so and then reapplied if necessary.

TOXAEMIA (US – Toxemia)
Poisoning of the blood by toxins that are the waste products of certain *bacteria*, such as clostridium tetani and *diphtheria* bacilli. Toxaemia results in *fever*, vomiting, *diarrhoea* and *shock*. Toxaemia of pregnancy is another name for *eclampsia*.

TOXIN
Any poisonous substance. Toxins are combated by anti-toxins, while bacterial toxins are the waste products formed by *bacteria*.

TOXOCARA
A roundworm that is primarily a parasite of cats and dogs, but can be

caught through contact with the faeces of these animals and ingestion of the roundworm eggs. In man the worms may cause a number of *systemic* symptoms, such as *fever*, *rash*, vomiting, muscular aches and occasionally convulsions. The small lesion containing the worm may initiate an *allergic* response in the surrounding tissue – if it is near the eye blindness can result. In man the problem can be treated with drugs that kill the worms, but it can be avoided if household pets are 'wormed' at an early age and children, who are particularly prone to infection by the worms, are closely supervised.

TOXOPLASMOSIS
An infection by the protozoan organism Toxoplasmosis Gondii. The organism commonly infests sheep, cattle, dogs and can be acquired by man when undercooked meat is eaten or soil ingested; this form of toxoplasmosis causes very mild symptoms, which may not even be noticed. When an infected woman passes the organism on to her unborn child, however, the problem – *congenital* toxoplasmosis – may be more serious. Sometimes the nervous system of the *foetus* is affected and blindness may be the result. Occasionally the condition is so severe that the foetus dies and there is a miscarriage; at other times the infection may be mild and the child normal, apart from a tendency to eye trouble later in life.

TRACHEA   10
The windpipe – a tube made up of muscle, cartilage and membrane that is the main airway of the body and stretches from the larynx to the chest, where it forks to form the left and right main *bronchus*. The trachea may sometimes become inflamed in a condition called tracheitis that is caused by *bacterial*, *viral* or fungal infections or by the aspiration of vomit.

TRACHEOSTOMY
A procedure in which an incision (called a tracheotomy) is made in the front of the *trachea* to enable a tube to be placed in the windpipe. The tube gives access to the lower *respiratory* tract and is used when the airway is blocked above the tracheotomy by acute inflammation of the epiglottis or *larynx*, by membrane formation as in *diphtheria*, by

laryngeal wounds or *tumors* or by a foreign body; it is also used when the respiratory muscles have been paralysed by conditions such as *polio*, or in prolonged unconsciousness, where it will be necessary to keep a patient on a *ventilator* for a long time.

TRACHOMA   125
A common eye disorder that is *endemic* throughout much of the world, especially the middle east. Trachoma is the result of infection by an organism called chlamydia trachomatis, which causes severe *conjunctivitis*, a clouding of the cornea, dimness of vision and eventual blindness. The disorder, which affects some 400 million people, is treated by *antibiotics*.

TRANSFUSION   162
An intravenous infusion of fluid, usually blood that has been appropriately cross-matched – see *blood groups* – to replace fluid that has been lost, normally as the result of *haemorrhage*. Sometimes iron is transfused, when a severe iron deficiency *anaemia* is resistant to therapy. In an exchange transfusion the complete blood content of the body is replaced – as in *haemolytic disease of the newborn*.

TRANSIENT ISCHAEMIC ATTACK (T.I.A.)
A T.I.A. is usually caused by a small *thrombus* in one of the blood vessels of the brain. The thrombus may briefly cause a blockage in the vessel – giving rise to a 'mini-*stroke*', with loss of vision, difficulty with speech and sometimes loss of consciousness. It then either moves off to another part of the vessel where it does not cause a blockage, or according to some medical opinion disperses altogether. There is no permanent damage, as in a major stroke, and treatment is usually by drugs that prevent the thrombi from forming. It is also important that any *hypertension* or high levels of blood *cholesterol* and fats are controlled.

TRANSPLANTATION
The surgical replacement of a diseased or deficient organ in the body with an organ taken from a donor. Organ transplantation has advanced rapidly over the last decade: the most common transplants are still those of cornea, but kidney transplants are now performed quite frequently. Heart and liver transplants are not yet widely available, though a number of successful operations have been performed. There are two main problems to transplantation. The first is the obvious problem of availability of donors; the other is the body's own defence mechanisms against disease. The organ must be tissue-matched or 'typed', so that the organ that is selected matches as closely as possible the tissues of the recipient. Otherwise, the recipient's defence systems will reject the foreign tissue in an *immune* reaction. If the immune mechanisms are reduced the body will be open to infection, so a careful balance must be drawn.

TRANSSEXUAL
A person who deeply wishes to be of the opposite sex to his or her biological sex. A transsexual usually adopts the behavior, life-style and dress of the desired sex, and after gender identity therapy may undergo surgery to his or her external genital organs and *hormone* therapy.

TRANSVESTITE
A person who derives sexual pleasure from wearing clothes traditionally assigned to the opposite sex.

TRAUMA
A physical trauma is a wound or injury caused by an external force; a *psychological* trauma is an emotional *shock* that causes mental injury or pain.

TREMOR   60,72,132,151
A mild rhythmical shakiness that is usually seen in the hands and sometimes the head. A tremor may be very fine, when it can be shown up by the oscillations of a flat piece of paper that is held on the back of the outstretched hand, and is sometimes caused by *thyrotoxicosis*. Coarser tremors may be found in *multiple sclerosis* and *Parkinson's Disease*, while the condition may also be caused by drugs or *alcoholism*. An essential or familial tremor is a *benign* condition that is seen in families, but is not an indication of physical or mental disease.

TRICHOMONIASIS
A common condition of women caused by a protozoan organism called trichomonas vaginalis that can also be found in the male *urethra* and can be transmitted through sexual intercourse. The infection causes a painful burning and itching of the *vulva* associated with a frothy white *vaginal* discharge and can be embarrassing and distressing. Trichomoniasis is treated by a drug called metronidazole, which may need to be taken by both sexual partners.

TRISOMY 21 (also DOWN'S SYNDROME, MONGOLISM)
An abnormality of the *chromosomes* in which there are three instead of two of the 21st chromosome. The result is mongolism, in which there is *congenital* mental retardation of varying degrees. Physical growth is also retarded and there is a characteristic *facies* – a sloping forehead, slanted eyes, a flat nose and low ears. There may also be congenital defects of the heart.

TROPICAL DISEASE
Any disease that is *endemic* in the tropics and not normally seen in temperate climates, except when carried by travellers – for example *malaria, lassa fever, cholera, yellow fever*. Travellers who intend to visit the tropics should always protect themselves against diseases by *vaccination*, and in the case of malaria by the use of *prophylactic* tablets.

TUBERCULOSIS (T.B.)
An infectious illness caused by mycobacterium tuberculosis, the tubercle *bacillus*. In active pulmonary tuberculosis the bacterium is inhaled and causes cough, *fever*, sweats and general weakness; the condition is very infectious and requires several weeks isolation and prolonged drug therapy. More often, however, the bacterium is inhaled but does not cause clinical illness – a reaction with the *lymph* nodes of the lungs leads to the production of *antibodies* in an immune reaction, which can be detected in a *heaf test*.

Sometimes tuberculosis spreads through the bloodstream to cause widespread disease, in a condition known as miliary tuberculosis. The disease may also affect the *meninges* in tuberculous meningitis – a condition that can be extremely dangerous unless treated swiftly. Bovine tuberculosis is endemic in cattle and at one time was often transmitted to man. Over the last 30 years, however, advances in milk and cattle hygiene have made the condition rare. *Vaccination* has also reduced considerably the incidence of active tuberculosis.

TUMOR
A growth that forms an abnormal lump or swelling in tissue and develops spontaneously. A tumor may be *benign* or *malignant, cystic* or solid – see *cancer.*

TURNER'S SYNDROME
A *chromosomal* disorder in which the sufferer lacks one of the usual female sex chromosomes and is XO instead of the normal XX. Individuals suffering from Turner's Syndrome are of short stature, with a thick webbed neck, poorly developed breasts and pubic hair and have no periods.

TYPHOID
One of the *enteric fevers,* typhoid is an *acute* infectious illness that affects the *alimentary tract* and is caused by the *bacteria* salmonellae typhi and salmonellae paratyphi – usually where the sanitation is poor and the water supply contaminated. Flies may also spread the disease, and certain apparently healthy people may have a chronic reservoir of infection within them and act as carriers.

A few days after catching the disease the temperature rises rapidly, and is normally highest at night; a headache, *malaise* and aching in the limbs follow, associated with drowsiness; after a week a typical rash appears. First of all the sufferer is *constipated,* but then on about the tenth day there is profuse watery *diarrhoea* together with abdominal distension and tenderness. After the end of the second week the victim may become delirious, pass into a *coma* and eventually die. In the temperate climates, however, the illness is rarely so severe, and normally subsides. Typhoid is treated by bed-rest, isolation and *antibiotics.*

TYPHUS
An infectious illness more common in hot climates that is caused by a micro-organism carried by ticks, lice and fleas. Typhus has an *incubation period* of about two weeks, after which there is a *headache,* high *fever,* pain in the limbs and *rigors;* there may also be drowsiness and delirium. The disease is most serious in its *epidemic* form – typhus used to kill whole armies in the past. It can be avoided by good sanitation, the use of insecticides, the control of rats and where necessary the use of protective clothing; it can be treated by *antibiotics.*

U

ULCER   45,77
A breech in the continuity of a surface, which may be either *mucous membrane* or skin. The common, painful ulcers that are found in the mouth, sometimes at times of stress, are called aphthous ulcers – they can be relieved by the use of proprietary remedies. Ulcers may develop around the ankles as a result of poor circulation or *varicose veins,* and are known as venous stasis or varicose ulcers.

Rodent ulcers are a local, malignant form of skin cancer in which an ulcer with a raised, rolled edge forms on the face at the edges of the nostrils, lips or eyelids. They are normally removed surgically and the site repaired by plastic surgery. *Gastric* and *duodenal ulcers,* jointly called *peptic ulcers,* are breeches in the internal linings of the stomach and duodenum respectively, while corneal ulcers affect the cornea, the transparent part of the front of the eyeball.

ULTRASOUND
An investigative technique in which high frequency sound waves are used to show up internal structures, using the same principles as radar. Ultrasound can be used in situations where x-rays would be dangerous, such as the examination of the baby while still in the womb, and to investigate the valves and arteries of the heart.

ULTRAVIOLET LIGHT   160
Light of extremely short wavelength that is present in sunlight and causes sunburn after prolonged exposure. Ultraviolet light also acts on substances in the skin that are precursors to *vitamin* D; medically it is sometimes used in the treatment of *acne* and *psoriasis.*

UNCONSCIOUSNESS
A condition in which a person is insensible, has no knowledge of what is going on around him and cannot be roused to consciousness. Unconsciousness may be caused by a blow on the head, *fainting, haemorrhage,* poisoning or an overdose of drugs, especially hypnotic drugs, or lack of oxygen. It may also be artificially induced as part of general *anaesthesia.*

URAEMIA (US – Uremia)   90
A condition in which large amounts of urea and nitrogenous waste products accumulate in the blood, normally because, through renal failure, the *kidneys* are unable to fulfil their function of filtering them from the blood and excreting them. In such quantities these products are toxic and must therefore be removed artificially by *dialysis.* Symptoms of uraemia include vomiting, *nausea,* drowsiness, and eventual *coma;* if untreated the condition may be fatal.

URETER   90
Parts of the *genito-urinary tract,* the two ureters each connect a *kidney* to the *bladder.* They may be the site of a urinary obstruction if a kidney stone becomes lodged inside them; the stone may cause severe colicky *abdominal pain, haematuria,* or blood in the *urine,* and if untreated *hydronephrosis.*

URETHRA   90,94
The final part of the *urinary tract* which carries *urine* from the *bladder* to the outside of the body. In females the tube is short – only about 2 ins. (5cms.) long. In males it is about 8 ins. (20 cms.) long and also carries secretions from the *prostate gland* and *seminal vesicles,* and *sperm* from the *vas deferens* in its final part.

Sometimes there is a discharge from the urethra, called a urethral discharge, which is a sign of infection and inflammation. It usually occurs in men and may be due to a specific disease such as *gonorrhoea;* more commonly the organism causing the infection cannot be identified and is termed *non-specific urethritis,* or N.S.U.. Treatment is by *antibiotics.*

URINE   90
The liquid wastes of the body that are excreted by the *kidneys,* stored in the *bladder* and expelled from the body through the *urethra* in the act of urination. Specimens of urine

are often tested in the diagnosis of disease – a 'mid-stream' urine specimen can be cultured or examined microscopically to detect *bacteria* that may be causing an infection, while sugar and sometimes *ketones* may be found in the urine of *diabetics*. The urine can be analysed in cases of poisoning or drug overdose in an attempt to identify the toxic substance that has been taken, while a *hormone* found in pregnant women called H.C.G. can be detected in the urine in a pregnancy test – see *haematuria*, *proteinuria*, *dysuria*, *pyuria* .

UROGRAPHY – *see* PYELOGRAPHY

URTICARIA
Commonly called nettle-rash, urticaria is an itchy, raised red *rash* that is normally caused by an *allergy* to a substance such as a drug, fabric or foodstuff. The rash may last for hours or days; it is very troublesome but may be treated by *antihistamines*.

UTERUS 98
The female womb. The uterus is situated in the *pelvis* and connects with the *vagina* below through the *cervix*, or neck of the womb. The organ is normally only about 3 inches long and 2 inches wide at the top, shaped like an inverted pear. Every month the lining of the womb, or *endometrium*, is shed in response to fluctuating *hormone* levels as part of the *menstrual cycle*.

The muscle layer of the womb may be the site of *fibroids* which can cause *menorrhagia*, or heavy periods, as well as gross enlargement of the organ. The uterus may also be the site of *cancer* – either in the body of the womb or in the cervix. Cervical cancer can be detected at an early stage in a cervical smear or 'Pap' test. Occasionally such problems may necessitate a a *hysterectomy*.

In pregnancy the fertilized *ovum* implants in the wall of the uterus and grows there. At 20 weeks the pregnant womb has expanded so much that it reaches the level of the navel and at 36 weeks it is at its largest. After this the baby starts to descend into the pelvis prior to birth.

UVEITIS 37
An inflammation of the uveal tract of the eye, which consists of the *iris* and the choroid layer. Uveitis is a painful condition which can be caused by infection or injury to the eye and may occur in association with diseases such as *ulcerative colitis*, *sarcoidosis* and *ankylosing spondylitis*. The condition may lead to impaired vision or even blindness, but is usually amenable to treatment.

V

VACCINE 166
A substance that when introduced into the body causes the production of specific *antibodies*, so conferring a degree of immunity against a particular disease. Vaccines may contain live *viruses* or *bacteria* whose strength has been reduced or which have been killed by heat or formaldehyde. They are introduced into the body in a process called vaccination, which may involve a subcutaneous injection, as in the case of *diphtheria*, or can be oral, like the Sabin *polio* vaccination which is given on a lump of sugar; sometimes, as in a smallpox vaccination, the vaccine is introduced through a scratch on the surface of the skin.

Different vaccinations may be given at different times during childhood. *Polio*, *tetanus*, *diphtheria* and sometimes *pertussis*, or whooping cough, vaccinations are normally given three times during the first year of life; *measles* vaccine is given at around 13 months, while *rubella* vaccine may be given between the ages of 12 and 13. 'Booster' vaccinations may be given later in life, especially if there has been, or is likely to be, exposure to any particular disease.

VACCINIA
Otherwise called cowpox disease, vaccinia is a disease of cows' udders that is transmitted to man by direct contact or in a *smallpox vaccination*, where the vaccine is based on fluid from the cowpox *vesicles* of cows.

The condition causes lesions that are similar to those of *chicken pox* and smallpox – vesicles followed by crusted *lesions*. An attack of smallpox confers immunity from cowpox – a fact that was first remarked by Sir Edward Jenner in the eighteenth century and led to the first vaccination.

VAGINA 99
A sheath of muscle and membrane that connects the *uterus* to the *vulva*, and is a part of the female reproductive tract. The vagina may become inflamed in a condition called vaginitis, whose most common cause is an infection of the fungus candida albicans, or *thrush*; this condition, as well as problems of the whole female reproductive tract, can be investigated by an examination 'p.v.', or per vagina. Vaginitis causes itching and soreness as well as a whitish discharge. Senile vaginitis is caused by a relative deficiency of *oestrogen* in postmenopausal women, in which the vaginal walls become thinner and drier. The condition is treated by a local application of oestrogen cream.

VAGINISSIMUS
A tightening of the opening of the vagina, either on attempted intercourse or medical examination. It may be caused by physical conditions such as vaginitis, but is more commonly due to psychosexual problems.

VAGOTOMY 45
A resection of the *vagus nerve* – usually the branches that cause production of acid in the stomach, when the operation is performed as a part of the treatment of a *duodenal ulcer*. Following a vagotomy there may be a feeling of faintness after a meal and *diarrhoea*. These side effects can be avoided if a more specific operation called a highly selective vagotomy is performed, in which only the fibers that specifically supply the stomach are cut, rather than the whole nerve trunk.

VALGUS
A term that denotes a deformity away from the midline of the body. In hallux valgus, for example, the big toe bends towards the little toe, often as a result of a *bunion*; in genu valgus, or knock-knees, the feet are wide apart when the knees are placed together.

VALVES – *see* MITRAL VALVE, TRICUSPID VALVE

VALVULAR HEART DISEASE 86,94
Diseases that affect the *valves* of the

heart. There are two forms of valvular disease – stenosis, in which the valves stiffen up and the aperture narrows, and incompetence, where the valve flaps do not meet closely when the valve is closed and blood can flow backwards, or *regurgitate*.

Valve disease is often caused by *rheumatic fever*, but may also be congenital or the result of *syphilis* or *bacterial* or *fungal* infection of the valve. It may also be seen in *ankylosing spondylitis*. The affected valves may eventually cause serious circulatory problems and need surgical repair. This may be by a valvotomy, where a stenosed valve is opened up, or by *valve replacement*. The presence of valve disease can often be indicated by the presence of a heart *murmur*.

VALVE REPLACEMENT

The surgical replacement of a diseased *heart valve* that is causing serious circulatory problems. The replacement may be biological – when it is taken from an animal, such as a pig – or artificial, in which case it is manufactured out of metal or polythene. Valve replacement operations are now performed quite often, and the prospects for survival and recovery are good.

VARICELLA   68

Also called chicken pox, varicella is a highly infectious disease that usually affects children. It has an incubation period of 11 to 18 days, after which there is a short spell of mild *fever*. The next day an itchy red *rash* appears, mainly on the trunk. *Vesicles* develop, which eventually form scabs, and a few more of them appear each day for about four days. After around 10 days the scabs drop off and the person affected is able to return to his normal activities. If the scabs are scratched or picked unsightly pock marks and scars may be left behind.

The *virus* that causes chicken pox is closely related to that of *herpes* zoster – one member of a household sometimes catches varicella when another has shingles, and shingles itself is normally caught by those who have had chicken pox during their youth.

VARICOCELE

Dilated, or 'varicose', veins of the spermatic cord in the scrotum. A varicocele may cause a large swelling of the scrotum and a dull ache.

The condition is sometimes seen in adolescent males, where it does not often require treatment, but when recurrent or persistent it can raise the temperature of the scrotum and so affect the developing sperm, causing *infertility*. In this case surgical removal of the varicocele may be necessary.

VARICOSE ECZEMA – *see* ECZEMA

VARICOSE VEINS   77

Large dilated veins. They may be seen in the *rectum*, where they are known as *haemorrhoids*; in the scrotum, where they are called a *varicocele*; and more commonly on the long saphenous veins of the leg. Varicose veins are thought to be caused by poor venous return. This may in turn be the result of prolonged standing or lack of exercise, since the deep muscles of the leg act as a 'muscle pump' to squeeze blood through the veins and back to the heart. At first the legs tend to ache, especially after a day spent on the feet. Later the ankles may swell and finally large distended veins appear, looking rather like bunches of grapes, which tend to get worse as other veins become involved. The condition may be associated with varicose *eczema* and even *ulcers*.

In the first instance varicose veins can be treated by the use of support stockings; later individual varicosities may be injected with an agent that inflames the walls of the veins, sticking them together and eliminating the space. Eventually the most varicose part of a vein may need to be stripped. One cut is made at the groin and another at the ankle; the ends of the vein are then tied off and the intermediate vein pulled out.

VAS DEFERENS

The duct of the *testis* that carries sperm to the urethra, and is cut in a *vasectomy*.

VASECTOMY

A method of male *contraception* in which the *vas deferens* is tied off with a ligature to deny sperm access to the *urethra*. Ejaculation is unaffected, because the ejaculate is anyway mainly composed of glandular secretions; after vasectomy these secretions no longer contain sperm, although sperms that were already in the vas deferens before

the operation may not be used up for several weeks. Vasectomy has no effect on male potency.

VASOCONSTRICTION

The constriction of blood vessels, which may be caused by drugs called vasoconstrictors or by the stimulation of the sympathetic *nervous system*.

VASODILATION

A dilation of blood vessels, that may be caused by the stimulation of the parasympathetic *nervous system* or by drugs called vasodilators. The blood vessels that dilate are usually peripheral and the increase in their size causes a decrease in *blood pressure*. Vasodilators are therefore often used in the treatment of *hypertension*.

V.D. – *see* VENEREAL DISEASE

VEIN   74

A vessel that drains blood from the *capillary* plexuses at the cellular level of the tissues and returns it to the heart. All venous blood – except for that carried in the pulmonary vein – is deoxygenated, and the passage of blood within the vessels is known as venous return. Blood returns to the heart under the pressure of the circulatory system, but is assisted by the squeezing action of muscles on the veins – especially in the 'muscle pump' of the legs. Valves in the veins prevent a backward flow.

VENA CAVA   74

The largest vein in the body. The superior vena cava collects blood from the head and neck and enters the right *atrium* of the heart; the inferior vena cava drains blood from the abdomen and legs.

VENAPUNCTURE – *see* BLOOD TESTS

VENEREAL DISEASE (V.D.)   94

Also called sexually transmitted diseases, venereal diseases include *syphilis*, *gonorrhoea*, and soft sore, or *chancroid*. N.S.U., or non-specific *urethritis* can be transmitted by sexual activity, but is not necessarily caught in that way; the same is true of *trichomonas vaginalis*. *Warts* around the genitals or anus, called anal or venereal warts, may also be transmitted by sexual contact.

VENTILATOR
A machine that is used to maintain *respiration* artificially when an individual is unconscious or under general *anaesthesia*. Air is pumped into the lungs at a fixed rate and under a specific pressure and then removed.

VENTRICLES   76
The two thick and muscular large chambers of the heart. The right ventricle pumps blood to the lungs through the pulmonary vein, having received it from the right *atrium*; the left ventricle, which is more muscular, receives blood from the left atrium and pumps it through the *aorta* and around the whole body. The left atrium is divided from the left ventricle by the *mitral*, or bicuspid valve; the right atrium and ventricle are separated by the *tricuspid valve*.

The walls of the ventricles may become infarcted after a *coronary thrombosis*, while sometimes the muscular wall becomes very thin and fibrous, to form a ventricular *aneurysm*.

There are also four ventricles, or cavities, in the brain. Two are lateral and the other two medial. These ventricles are continuous with the spinal cord and contain *cerebrospinal* fluid; they may become involved in any infection of the C.S.F.

VERNIX CASEOSA
A layer of greasy material that covers newborn babies and is made up of *sebaceous* secretions from the skin.

VERRUCA – *see* WARTS

VERTIGO
A sensation in which the outside world seems to be spinning around, or an individual feels that he is spinning around in a static world. The condition may be caused by labyrinthitis, an infection of the organs of balance inside the ear, or by lesions of the brain stem. Vertigo is sometimes experienced as part of *Ménière's Disease* and can often be extremely disabling; it can be treated by specific drugs. The term is often used inexactly as a synonym for dizziness or giddiness.

VESICLE   68
A small, superficial blister-like lesion that is filled with clear fluid – unlike pustules, which contain *pus*.

Diseases such as *varicella* and *herpes* zoster cause the formation of vesicles, and are said to be vesicular.

VIRILISM
Masculinization of a female, where she increases muscle mass, acquires a deeper voice and may grow hair on the chest and face. Virilism may be caused by a *hormonal* disorder or sometimes by an *ovarian tumor* that secretes male hormones.

VIRULENCE
The 'strength' in terms of infectivity of a *pathogenic* organism such as a *virus* or *bacteria*.

VIRUS
A minute organism that may be responsible for a wide variety of diseases and infections, from *coryza*, the common cold, to *smallpox*.

Viruses are smaller than *bacteria* and cannot be seen with an ordinary microscope. They consist of a central core of D.N.A., or deoxyribonucleic acid, surrounded by a shell of *protein*, and have the ability to replicate inside a living cell. Viruses, and therefore virus diseases, cannot be affected by *antibiotics*, but these drugs may sometimes be given to combat any complications that may be caused by bacterial infection.

VISCERA
The abdominal contents.

VISION   70,124,126
Eyesight. Vision may be affected by *cataracts*, *glaucoma*, a detached *retina*, retinopathy, *papilloedema*, *migraine*, *hysteria* and many diseases that affect the eye; double vision is known as *diplopia*. Specific diseases of the eye are treated by an ophthalmic surgeon.

Poor vision can be the result of a defect of the eye rather than a disease. Sometimes the defect is *congenital*, but it may develop as part of the ageing process. The result may be shortsightedness, or *myopia*, longsightedness, or *hypermetropia*, or *astigmatism*. These, as well as many other forms of poor vision, may be diagnosed by the use of special charts that measure visual acuity, or sharpness. The various conditions can usually be treated by specific optical lenses, either in glasses or in contact lenses.

VITAMINS
Substances which are essential for health and cannot, with certain exceptions, be manufactured in the body. They therefore need to be ingested in the diet. Vitamins A, D, E and K are known as the fat-soluble vitamins, while B and C vitamins are water soluble.

Vitamin A is necessary for growth, healthy *mucous membranes*, the development of bone and night vision. It is found in egg yolk, milk, liver, cod liver oil, carrots and tomatoes, but is also manufactured in the body from a precursor called carotene. A deficiency of vitamin A leads to a general lack of resistance to infection, and when severe to blindness.

Vitamin B is actually a complex of a number of vitamins. Vitamin B_1 is otherwise called thiamine and plays an important part in *carbohydrate metabolism*. A deficiency leads to beriberi, but the vitamin is found in cereals, beans, meat and nuts. Vitamin B_2, or riboflavine, is important in *respiration* at the cellular level. It is found in liver, milk and eggs, though an isolated B_2 deficiency is not usually important. Vitamin B_6, or pyridoxine, is found in most foods and a deficiency is very rare. Vitamin B_{12}, or cyanocobalamin, can only be absorbed in the presence of an intrinsic factor that is secreted by the stomach. This factor tends to be lacking in people who have had a *gastrectomy*, and the resulting deficiency may cause pernicious *anaemia* and if severe, degeneration of the spinal cord. The vitamin is found in liver, kidneys and dairy products but also synthesized in the gut by intestinal *bacteria*.

Vitamin C, or ascorbic acid, is essential for the maintenance of healthy cells and tissues. It is found in oranges and other citrus fruits; a deficiency causes *scurvy*. Some people think that huge doses of vitamin C increase the body's resistance to infections of the upper *respiratory tract*; there is some argument about this claim, which is not generally regarded as proven.

Vitamin D plays an important part in the metabolism of *calcium*, and therefore in the growth and maintenance of bone. It is manufactured in the body by the action of sunlight on a precursor in the skin, but is also found in dairy products and cod liver oil. A deficiency of Vitamin D causes diseases of the bones, such as *rickets*.

Vitamin K is found in fishmeal, spinach, and cereals. It plays an important part in the *blood-clotting* process and a deficiency of the vitamin, though rare, may cause bleeding disorders.

Vitamin E is present in so many foods that a deficiency is unlikely. It is an essential nutrient, though its functions are unknown.

VITILIGO
Also called leukoderma, vitiligo is a skin condition that is more common in the black races in which patches of skin lose their pigmentation and become milky-white. The condition is sometimes called piebaldism; its cause is unknown and there is no cure.

VOCAL CORDS   24
Folds of fibrous tissue in the *larynx*. Sounds are made by the flow of air from the lungs over the vocal cords, which vibrate variably under the control of a branch of the *vagus nerve*. The voice may be affected by an inflammation of the cords, as in *laryngitis*, or by a thickening and coarsening of the cords, as in *myxoedema*. Occasionally the vocal cords may have nodules. These may be innocent, but they are sometimes *cancerous* growths. In this case a laryngectomy may be necessary, but speech is still possible if the sufferer learns the technique of producing sounds by swallowing air and belching it up.

VULVA   94
The female external genitals, consisting of the labia majora and minora, the clitoris and the entrance, or vestibule, of the *vagina*. The vulva may become inflamed in a condition called vulvitis, which is often caused by a *candidal* infection, or *gonorrhoea*.

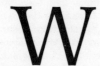

WARTS   94
A small commonly seen skin lesion that is caused by a *virus*, tends to appear on the face, fingers or elbows and may be soft or hard. Warts on the soles of the feet are called plantar warts, or verrucae – any type of wart is properly called a verruca,

but the Latin term is normally only used to describe plantar warts. Warts may be seen on the genitals and around the anus, when they are known as condylomae, or venereal warts – see *venereal disease*.

There are many folk remedies for warts, and some of them may appear to work. In fact it is more likely that the wart has disappeared spontaneously, as most warts do. Medically, they are treated with a paste that dissolves the hard outer layer of the wart and cauterizes the remainder, which can then easily be scraped off.

WASH-OUT
Otherwise called a gastric lavage, a wash-out is a process in which the contents of the stomach are removed. A tube is introduced into the stomach through the mouth and *oesophagus*, water is poured into it and – using the tube as a siphon – the gastric contents are removed, usually for analysis. The procedure is common after an overdose of drugs or poisoning, but if the subject is deeply drowsy or unconscious he will need to be *intubated* so that the airway is protected.

WASSERMAN REACTION
One of the first blood tests for *syphilis*, the Wasserman Reaction has now generally been superseded by more modern tests. The term is still sometimes used loosely to describe any blood test for the disease.

WASTING
A decrease in muscle size and tone, or muscle *atrophy*. Wasting may be caused by a prolonged period of immobilization in a plaster cast or splint that has been applied for orthopaedic reasons or by a degeneration of the nerve supply to a limb or a muscle. It can be a result of a number of neurological diseases including *syringomyelia* and *poliomyelitis*, and occurs in diseases that directly affect the muscles, such as *muscular dystrophy*. Wasting is treated by removal of its cause; otherwise the condition may be improved by *physiotherapy*.

WATERBRASH   45
The belching, or eructation, of acidic fluids from the stomach that is part of heartburn and is a symptom of *dyspepsia* and also sometimes of a *duodenal* ulcer – see *pyrosis*.

WEIGHT   136,138,146,151
Body weight depends very much on the height and build of an individual, so that it is almost impossible to give a 'normal' weight. Generally a woman over 25, 5ft 5in tall, fully clothed and of a medium frame will weigh on average 9¼ stone (130 lbs), while a man over 25, fully clothed, 5ft 10in tall, with a medium build will weigh, on average, 11½ stone (160 lbs.). Normal weights, however, when fully clothed, may range from 6½ stone to 12½ stone in women, and from 8 stone to 14½ stone in men, depending on height and build.

Weight may increase as a result of glandular or *metabolic* malfunctions of the body or of *depression*, when overeating is a common symptom – see *obesity*. Weight is also gained in pregnancy.

Body weight decreases in nearly all illnesses and diseases, mainly because people who feel ill usually lose their appetite. It may decrease more significantly, however, in conditions such as *chronic diarrhoea*, *malabsorption*, *thyrotoxicosis*, *anorexia* nervosa, starvation, *fevers*, *tuberculosis*, untreated *diabetes* mellitus and *carcinoma*. A severe loss in weight is always a cause for concern and a doctor should be consulted. It is also sensible to ask a doctor for his advice before embarking on a crash diet, because a rapid loss of weight may sometimes be dangerous.

WEIL'S DISEASE   14
Also called leptospirosis, Weil's Disease is a *zoonose*, or disease that can be transmitted to man from animals. The disease starts with a headache, aching limbs, *nausea* and *vomiting* and sometimes skin *rashes*. Later more serious symptoms may occur, including *jaundice*, *meningitis*, *myocarditis* and *pneumonia*. The majority of sufferers recover after the first phase of the illness and avoid the more serious complications. As Weil's Disease can be caught by contact with contaminated *urine* and *faeces* from rats, field mice and hedgehogs, farmworkers and sewage and abattoir workers are particularly at risk.

WEN – *see* SEBACEOUS CYST

WHEEZING   19,21
A musical or sonorous sound made

by the passage of air through obstructed airways – the pitch of the sound depends on the aperture of the tube involved. Wheezing may be heard on inspiration or exhalation, and is common in *asthmatics* and in those suffering from an *acute* attack of *bronchitis*. In asthma the tubes are narrowed as part of an *allergic* response; in bronchitis the lining of the bronchioles becomes inflamed and clogged up with mucus and *pus*.

WHITLOW
A small *abscess* caused by infection that may be seen at the tips of the fingers or toes, often beside the nail. Whitlows can be very painful, and are usually treated with poultices that draw out the *pus*; sometimes the area has to be lanced, or opened up with a scalpel and then drained.

WHOOPING COUGH – *see* PERTUSSIS

WILSON'S DISEASE   72
An inherited disorder of copper *metabolism* in which a high level of copper accumulates in the body and is deposited in the brain and the liver. Wilson's Disease causes similar symptoms to *Parkinson's Disease*, as well as mental retardation, *jaundice* and *cirrhosis*. The condition is treated with drugs that remove the excess copper from the body.

WISDOM TOOTH
The third and last molar tooth at the end of the jaw. The four wisdom teeth normally appear in early adult life, but may not be seen until the late twenties; occasionally they remain impacted throughout life and are never seen. If the wisdom teeth cannot break through the gum cleanly and take their place – because of an arrangement of the other teeth that does not allow them sufficient space – they may have to be removed surgically under local or general *anaesthetic*.

WOMB – *see* UTERUS

WORD BLINDNESS – *see* DYSLEXIA

WORMS
A term used loosely to describe a *parasitic* infestation of man, which may in fact be by one of three separate types of worm, or a combination of them – threadworms, tapeworms and roundworms.

Threadworms are the commonest of all parasites of children. The male threadworm is smaller than the female – which is still only half an inch long. Threadworms are found in the *faeces* and may be passed on by contamination of food and water as a result of poor hygiene; they live in the colon and *rectum* and cause rectal itching. Roundworms may be caught in the same way but are much larger – 10 ins. (25 cms.) long. Two or three may live in the small intestine of an infected person. They cause few symptoms other than an increase in appetite and sometimes *diarrhoea* and colicky *abdominal pain*; occasionally a round worm may be vomited up.

Tapeworms are common parasites that infest humans after passing through an intermediate stage inside pigs, cows and even dogs and sheep. If inadequately cooked meat is eaten the intermediate stage of the parasite may be ingested. Once in man the tapeworm grows, hooking itself onto the wall of the intestine – usually in the large bowel.

Worms are treated by special drugs that paralyse the parasites – they can then easily be passed out of the body in the stools.

WOUNDS
Any cut or abrasion may be termed a wound, but more generally the word is used to describe bodily trauma that are the result of violence or accident. The treatment of wounds depends on adequate debridement, or cleansing and removal of dead tissue, as well as blood replacement, *antibiotics*, surgical repair and often stitching. A *tetanus vaccination* is also often given after a wound.

WRY NECK – *see* TORTICOLLIS

X-RAYS
Short wave-length electro-magnetic radiation that can be used in medicine either diagnostically or therapeutically. X-rays can be used diagnostically because they show up bones and dense substances clearly but soft tissues are poorly defined.

X-rays and other forms of radiation can also be used therapeuti-cally in the treatment of cancer – see *radiotherapy*.

XANTHOMA
(also XANTHALESMA)   146,153
Fatty deposits that are sometimes found in the upper eyelids of elderly people. They are harmless themselves, but are sometimes found in association with *diabetes* or *myxoedema* and may be a sign of a high level of *cholesterol* in the blood – see *eyelid nodules*.

XANTHOPSIA
A condition in which all objects appear to have a yellowish tinge. Xanthopsia is sometimes caused by an excess of the drug digitalis, especially in the elderly who tend to accumulate the drug in their bodies.

YAWS   94
A tropical disease caused by a micro-organism called a spirochaete which is similar to the organism that causes *syphilis*. Yaws is transmitted by direct, but not necessarily sexual, contact with a sufferer through small cuts and abrasions in the skin, often in the feet. Initially yaws causes fever, pain and itching and later small lesions appear on the face, hands legs and feet which may turn into deep ulcers.

Without treatment, normally by *antibiotics*, the condition may lead to serious deformities of the bones and skin.

YELLOW FEVER
A severe tropical disease that is transmitted by mosquitoes and affects mainly the *liver* and *kidneys*. Symptoms include *fever*, headache, *vomiting*, joint pains and *jaundice*, but the disease can be prevented by *vaccination*.

ZOONOSES
Infections that are primarily diseases of animals but which can be caught by man – for example *Q-fever*.

ZOSTER – *see* HERPES

Index

Page numbers in bold print indicate the main references in the text; those in italic print indicate references to illustrations.